Reasoning in Medicine

Reasoning in Medicine

An Introduction
To Clinical Inference

Daniel A. Albert, MD
Ronald Munson, Ph.D.
Michael D. Resnik, Ph.D.

Part of the Johns Hopkins Series in Contemporary Medicine and Public Health

Originally published by The Johns Hopkins University Press

Reprinted 2014 by Labrador Books

ISBN: 978-1500573867
ISBN-10: 1500573868

The name Labrador Books and its symbol are trademarks of Labrador Books

A Labrador Book

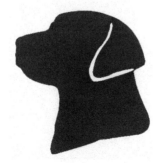

The authors' discussion of . . . concepts . . . is particularly rewarding. In the chapter on inductive inference the meaning of probability is teased out of four separate concepts . . . The chapter hypotheses, laws, and theories includes a particularly good discussion of the ways in which we conceptualize what we do in medicine. . . . The chapter on disease provides a similarly insightful frame of reference for a concept too often taken for granted. One of the true delights of this book is that it is unabashedly interdisciplinary. –Kevin Patrick, M.D., M.S. *JAMA*

I believe his book successfully accomplishes the aim of providing an introduction to medical reasoning. It is . . . suitable not only for physicians and surgeons, but also for other interested members of the health-care team. –Carl F. Anderson, M.D., *Mayo Clinic Proceedings*

The authors have arrayed the understanding and issues involved in the basic concepts and rules of thought in science and medicine. They have indicated the complexity of the world, the pitfalls of medical thinking, and the shortfall of philosophic accounts of thinking. They have also identified some strong methods for medical decision making. Their ten-year effort is a solid contribution to the literature. –Edmund L. Erde, Ph. D. *Journal of Medical Humanities*

Daniel A. Albert, M.D. is Professor Medicine and Pediatrics and Chief of Rheumatology at the Dartmouth Institute of Dartmouth-Hitchcock Medical Center. He has published numerous papers on rheumatologic disorders in adults and children, as well as articles on various conceptual issues in medicine and on the use of decision analysis in making diagnostic and management decisions.

Ronald Munson, Ph.D. is Emeritus Professor of the Philosophy of Science and Medicine at the University of Missouri—St. Louis. In addition to articles on the philosophy of biology and medicine, his publications include *Raising the Dead: Organ Transplants, Ethics, and Society, The Woman Who Decided to Die: Challenges and Choices at the Edges of Medicine,* and *Intervention and Reflection: Basic Issues in Bioethics.* His is also the author of the novels *Nothing Human, Fan Mail, Night Vision,* and *The Harvard Game.*

Michael D. Resnik, Ph. D. is Emeritus University Distinguished Professor at the University of North Carolina, Chapel Hill. He has published numerous articles on logic and the philosophy of mathematics, as well as the books *Frege and the Philosophy of Mathematics, Choices: An Introduction to Decision Theory, Mathematical Objects and Mathematical Knowledge,* and *Mathematics as a Science of Patterns.*

To all our children: Alexis
Justin

Rebecca

David

CONTENTS

Acknowledgments

This book is the outcome of a decade-long enterprise by the three authors. We each have different backgrounds (clinician, philosopher of science, logician) but share a common interest in the character of clinical medicine. Although the differences in our perspectives may account for the length of time we took to complete this project, we believe that those differences also contributed greatly to the understanding of clinical medicine that we present here.

The late Ernest Nagel is one of those responsible for inspiring this project, and a great number of other people have provided us with substantial advice and help. The following individuals were kind enough to read the manuscript, in whole or in part, and to comment on it: Abigail Albert, Roy E. Albert, Arthur S. Elstein, Richard Grandy, Miriam Munson, Mark Silverstein, and Douglas Stalker. We are also grateful for the comments of the anonymous reviewers solicited by the original publisher. Of course the responsibility for all errors and omissions remains ours alone.

Part of the work on this book has been supported by grants and awards to the individual authors from the University of Chicago, University of North Carolina Research Council, and University of Missouri—St. Louis Office of Research Administration. A Kenan Leave allowed one of the authors (Resnik) time to work on this book.

CHAPTER 1   *Orientation*

Over the centuries, the theoretical and practical aspects of medicine have changed dramatically. What has not changed are the two fundamental intellectual tasks of the physician: making a diagnosis and deciding on the best form of treatment for a patient's problem.

The scarcity of information about these basic cognitive activities stands in sharp contrast to the enormous wealth of information that we have accumulated about the mechanisms of diseases and the most effective modes of treatment. This book attempts to redress the balance to at least a slight degree. It is an introduction to the cognitive aspects of clinical medicine. More specifically, it is concerned with clinical inference—with the legitimate conclusions that can be drawn from information about a patient, obtained directly by physical examination and history taking or indirectly by laboratory studies.

"Clinical medicine is an art as well as a science." This is the response almost any practicing physician is likely to give if asked to explain how he or she arrived at a diagnosis after considering a large body of complex and diverse information about a patient. It is also the response almost every physician regards as appropriate when asked to account for the choice of one mode of treatment out of a wide range of possibilities.

Whether or not the response expresses some deep truth about the nature of clinical medicine, it surely captures a widely shared perception. In the view of most physicians, the reasoning processes in clinical medicine contain a somewhat mysterious and inexplicable component. Clinical reasoning is seen as something that goes beyond rules and rubrics, protocols and algorithms. It is taken to involve elements of intuition and creativity that cannot be replaced by explicit or "mechanistic" procedures.

Since the time of William Osler, this notion has permeated clinical medicine and helped shape its general intellectual tone and attitudes. The great diagnostician who draws upon years of experience and vast resources of knowledge to make correct pronouncements on puzzling cases has become virtually a cult figure within clinical medicine. He or she serves as an emblem of possibility and represents for other clinicians the combination of traits that all must admire. Such a clinician is the virtuoso performer of the art of medicine.

The notion that medicine is an art as well as a science underlies the traditional endorsement of the need to teach clinical medicine by example, rather than from abstract principles alone. According to traditional thinking, only when clinicians in training are directly involved with an accomplished clinician in caring for sick people can they gain the experience necessary to perform reliably on their own. They must acquire the sort of habitual responses, gut feelings, and implicit knowledge needed by any competent clinician. They must acquire the right kind of perceptions so that when they look at a patient, they are looking through the eyes of a clinician. Whether with the help of such experience they too can become virtuoso performers, and not just members of the orchestra, only time can tell.

REASONING AND THE MATRIX OF CLINICAL MEDICINE

In recent years, a variety of efforts have been made to chip away at the "art" component of clinical medicine and replace it with something more like science. It is important to realize that endorsing such efforts does not mean accepting the view that clinical medicine is "nothing but" science. No matter how successful such efforts are, there will always be a place for intuition, creativity, implicit knowledge, and guided experience in the practice of clinical medicine—as indeed there is in the practice of the traditional empirical sciences. At most, the basic issue concerns the relative size of the "art" and "science" components. By the 1930s, the science component was much larger than it was in the 1830s, and during the last half century, it has continued to increase in size. The art component has by no means ceased to exist, for more and more we have come to realize that no amount of information can take the place of judgment.

However, even the most ardent defender of the notion that clinical medicine involves art has no wish to deny that it also involves rational processes. These processes form the focus of this book. Our aim is to dig deep into the clinical mind and to lay bare the processes of reasoning and inference that are (or can be) involved in arriving at and in justifying clinical decisions. Ours is not a psychological or sociological study. Rather, it is an exercise in analysis and explication. We are not concerned with how clinicians most often reason so much as with how they reason when they reason well or successfully. In this sense, our aims are more prescriptive than they are descriptive.(Of course, in instances of "good medicine" the two are the same.)

We present an analysis of clinical reasoning that is anchored in a fictional but realistic case of a young woman who gets sick and becomes a patient in a teaching hospital. Her case history is detailed from the point of view of the medical resident involved in her care. The reasoning of this resident, the attending physician who supervises the resident, and the others in the clinical team caring for the patient serve as the reference point for our analysis.

Clinical reasoning and decision making take place within a dense and complicated conceptual matrix. For one thing, contemporary medicine, whatever else it might be, is scientific medicine. It is dependent upon the laws and theories of the empirical sciences of physics, biochemistry, and biology to provide an understanding of the mechanisms involved in both normal functioning and disease processes. Clinical medicine relies upon scientific data in doing its job and uses many of the methods typical of the sciences in arriving at defensible judgments.

Furthermore, clinical medicine employs patterns of reasoning and statistical techniques that are not unique to it but that have been developed and deployed in other disciplines. Then, too, clinical medicine makes use of concepts-such as the general notion of disease-that play a largely unacknowledged but nevertheless crucial role in the enterprise.

To restrict our view of clinical reasoning in a way that fails to consider the elements that make up the conceptual matrix within which it occurs is like attempting to tell the story of King Lear without mentioning his daughters—the result is no more than a parody or caricature. To avoid this outcome, we cast our nets wide and pull in for examination some of the more significant of the topics that form both the background and the substance of clinical reasoning. The process of evaluating a patient involves gathering data; verifying the data; invoking rules, laws, and theories; formulating and testing hypotheses; deriving conclusions; and arriving at warranted decisions. We address each of these topics in the context of our case and bring in other cases or examples when needed. The case is at the center of the web, but we trace out many of the interwoven strands that form the entire structure.

What emerges from our analysis, we believe, is a deepened appreciation of the subtlety and conceptual complexity of clinical reasoning. The ways in which the good clinician acquires, evaluates, and employs information to reach conclusions about diagnoses and treatments seem almost inexplicable, but in fact the processes involve intellectual methods that can be explicitly stated. Recognizing the nature and function of these methods removes some of the mystery from clinical reasoning, but it does not deprive it of its wonder. Instead, the recognition makes it clear that the source of the wonder is in the processes, not in the product. The ability to arrive at correct conclusions about amazingly complex systems on the basis of clinical examination will always be an impressive accomplishment.

THE SEQUENCE OF TOPICS IN THIS BOOK

The next chapter presents the case that serves as our reference mark for subsequent discussion. In an attempt to capture some of the complexities and uncertainties that are characteristic of actual cases encountered in clinical practice, the case is presented in the form of a series of dramatized scenarios. Interviews with the patient and conferences between the resident responsible for the patient's care and the attending physician raise virtually all the issues we will be concerned with in the remainder of the book. (A clinicopathological case report, a postmortem conference, and an autopsy report follow the case presentation.)

For the most part, the sequence of chapters after the case presentation follows the stages in the process of actual clinical reasoning. We begin with the evaluation of the patient, move to establishing a diagnosis, and end with decisions about managing the patient's illness. Thus chapter 3 discusses ways of acquiring and evaluating clinically relevant data from patient interviews, physical examination, and laboratory testing. Chapters 4 and 5 discuss the use of clinical data and other information in, respectively, inductive (probabilistic) and deductive arguments to arrive at defensible clinical conclusions.

The entire process of acquiring data and reasoning about them takes place within the broader framework of the scientific enterprise, and chapter 6 discusses causal laws, hypothesis testing, and theories and their connection with clinical medicine. In chapter 7 the central theoretical concept of medicine—disease—is examined in detail, and an analysis of the concept in terms of biologically programmed processes is developed and defended.

The specific inferential task of establishing a diagnosis for the illness of a particular patient is addressed in chapter 8. Several models of diagnostic reasoning are discussed, and a cyclical model is presented as an accurate and correct account of the process. Because physicians must eventually translate some of their inferences into action, they must arrive at management plans for their patients. Chapter 9, which is devoted to decision analysis, addresses the issues that are involved in reaching such decisions.

The final chapter serves as a summary of the previous chapters by interpreting the initial case history from their perspective. The illumination of those chapters is brought to a focus here, and the sorts of theoretical and conceptual presuppositions that physicians rely on in acquiring and evaluating data, arriving at diagnoses, and deciding on courses of therapy emerge with considerable clarity.

The chapters can be read independently, so it is not necessary to be familiar with earlier discussions to follow accounts in a later chapter. To make this possible, we have introduced some redundancies, such as the statements of Bayes' theorem in both chapters 4 and 9.

Merely listing the sequence of topics does little to indicate the richness of the content of clinical medicine. Each phase of the process of clinical reasoning involves aspects that are peculiar to medicine, but each phase also involves more general principles. As we mentioned earlier, these principles are often ones shared with other disciplines, disciplines that superficially seem distant from clinical medicine. Thus, we find ourselves encountering topics in statistics, formal logic, the philosophy of science, and decision analysis.

A thorough understanding of the character of clinical medicine requires that we explore the matrix within which it operates. In the end, the distance between clinical medicine and a variety of other intellectual disciplines is more apparent than real. Just as Moliere's Monsieur Jourdain was surprised to learn that he had been speaking prose all his life, some clinicians might be startled to learn that they have been implicitly employing modes of reasoning they were not aware of.

We should also mention something that this book does not attempt. According to a naive, though appealing, notion, a work that successfully elucidates the process of clinical reasoning ought to be a logically formal account-one that employs axioms, theorems, definitions, proofs, and so on. From this perspective, some observers have bemoaned the vagueness of medical vocabulary, the redundancy of medical information, and the generally intractable character of the clinical process.

However, such shortcomings are only apparent. The actual process of reasoning by clinicians permits successful inferences even in cases in which formal and rigid automated systems have been disappointingly inaccurate. (We have more to say on this topic when we discuss computer diagnosis.) Given the phenomenal complexity of the human body and the myriad ways in which it can become dysfunctional, it seems almost miraculous that an experienced clinician can arrive at detailed physiologic explanations and perform successful interventions based primarily upon what a patient says she or he feels. With our dependence on natural language for information about symptoms and with our limited understanding of many illnesses, the obstacles to a purely formal account of the clinical process seem insurmountable. Thus, it is not our aim to present anything like a "formalized" account of clinical medicine or even to offer a concise set of guidelines for clinical reasoning.

Nevertheless, the analysis of clinical reasoning is not an all-or-nothing process. The alternatives are not logical formalism on one side and pure intuition on the other. We follow a middle road. We show that there are guiding principles of inference that can anchor clinical reasoning and that observing these principles will help to improve the care of patients.

PRACTICAL AIMS OF THIS BOOK

To care for patients properly, clinicians must employ a variety of intellectual skills that go beyond the mere possession of medical knowledge. They must gather data, assess its reliability and relevance, decide whether other data are worth acquiring, weigh diagnostic and therapeutic alternatives, and in general, exercise judgment about the best interest of their patients.

Typically, medical students and house officers have been assumed to possess the foundations of these skills. Consequently, they have been instructed in the body of medical information, and then, by observing experienced physicians applying this information, they have learned the rudiments of the clinical process. However, recent studies suggest that medical students and beginning physicians may not possess an adequate foundation of the general principles needed to acquire relevant skills effectively. This is particularly the case in the area of statistical inference, and it seems reasonable to believe that it is true in other areas as well.

This work is not a handbook of any sort, and it is not intended to remedy deficiencies in statistical inference or in any of the other areas addressed. To perform such a task would require a much more detailed treatment than is appropriate for our aims. However, we hope to show that there are a number of general principles directly relevant to patient care that constitutes important subjects for medical education. Our assumption is that it is better for the individual to learn these principles independently before being called upon to apply them in the clinical arena. We hope that the formal teaching of these principles will relieve part of the burden of conveying them that typically falls during the apprenticeship period of medical education. If this is so, then the result should be to ease the transition from preclinical to clinical training.

This book is primarily aimed at physicians and physicians in training. Yet we hope its audience will extend beyond this group to include many others with a professional interest in medicine. We believe that nursing professionals, medical sociologists and psychologists, and philosophers of medicine and science will all find much of interest and value to them in a close consideration of the elements of clinical reasoning.

In order to accommodate a broad audience, we have made an effort to avoid both jargon and unnecessary technical language. We have tried to write in clear, straightforward prose, and when special medical, statistical, or logical concepts were needed, we provided explanations in the text itself. As a consequence, terminologies of different conceptual schemes are employed in our analyses. We have made no effort to unify these terminologies. It is not clear that this could be done without losing the advantages of the different approaches, and furthermore, the result might well be more confusing than helpful. We have tried to be both comprehensible and useful to all who have a serious interest in medical reasoning. Clinical medicine is only one of many disciplines that must translate abstract principles into reality, and we believe that even those who are not clinicians will find it worthwhile to consider how the process takes place in clinical medicine.

Quite apart from the practical usefulness this book may have for medical students and physicians, we hope that it will also have an intellectual usefulness for all readers. The therapeutic demands placed on medicine make it easy to overlook or undervalue the fact that contemporary medicine is a scientific and intellectual discipline. Physicians are not and ought not be mere technicians who follow set procedures. To return to our earlier image, clinical activities are embedded in a matrix of laws and theories, empirical rules, patterns of reasoning, modes of analysis, and specific and general concepts. An appreciation of the components of the matrix and their relations to clinical practice is a goal worth achieving for more than practical reasons.

Scientific medicine is no longer in its infancy, even though it is not yet in its maturity. It is a complex and sophisticated discipline that is amazingly effective in pursuing its goal of promoting the welfare of those who are ill. Yet at present we have nothing like an adequate understanding of the character of the discipline itself. Medicine in general, and clinical medicine in particular, is only just now undergoing the sort of self-scrutiny and analysis of its own methods, concepts, and aims that characterize established disciplines such as physics and biology.

We will be glad if this book can contribute in even a small way to promoting medicine's self-scrutiny. In our view, it will be impossible to read the discussions of the topics in the following chapters and not come away with a deeper appreciation of the intellectual character of clinical medicine. This appreciation, we hope, will encourage further inquiry and analysis and so help promote the development of an anatomy of medicine itself.

RECOMMENDED READING

Elstein, A. Medical Problem Solving and Analysis of Clinical Reasoning. Cambridge, Mass.: Harvard University Press, 1978. A study by a cognitive psychologist.

Feinstein, A. R. Clinical Judgment. 1967. Reprint. Melbourne, Fla.: Krieger, 1974. Analysis using Boolean algebra.

Morgan, W. L., and G. L. Engle. Clinical Approach to the Patient. Philadelphia: W. B. Saunders, 1969. Commonsense clinical recommendations.

Murphy, E. A. The logic of Medicine. Baltimore: Johns Hopkins University Press, 1976. An eclectic approach.

Wright, H. J., and D. B. Macadam. Clinical Thinking in Practice. London: Churchill Livingston, 1979. A British approach.

Wulff, H. Rational Diagnosis and Treatment. Oxford: Blackwell, 1976. Elegant, concise, but somewhat difficult treatise.

CHAPTER 2

The Case Report:
Mrs. Halprin

The case presented in this chapter is a wholly fictional but realistic portrayal of an illness and of the diagnostic and therapeutic measures taken to deal with it. We have cast the presentation in the form of a dramatized scenario, in the hope of capturing some of the doubts, uncertainties, and richness of detail that are characteristic of the actual clinical situation.

The case report unfolds in historical order. We follow the changes in the fictional Mrs. Halprin's illness and give an account of the decisions and actions of her physicians as they cope with it. The narrative presentation of the events is interrupted by interludes in which we comment on the lines of reasoning taken by her physicians. At the end, a clinicopathological case presentation rehearses in a concise form the circumstances and events of the illness and the efforts to treat it.

The case of Mrs. Halprin serves as a reference point in the discussions of the following seven chapters. In the final chapter, we reexamine the case in the light of those discussions. This provides us with the opportunity to comment on the ways in which the diagnostic inquiry was conducted and how diagnostic and management decisions were reached.

NARRATIVE CASE PRESENTATION

August 15: Admission and First Examination

Dr. Julie Barton was twenty-seven years old and a second-year medical resident at Boston Central Hospital. Two things about practicing medicine constantly surprised her. First, she was amazed that she liked it so much, something she had had her doubts about during the hard years of medical school. Second, she was repeatedly impressed by the fact that it was actually possible to make sense out of the incredible variety of signs, symptoms, and findings associated with illnesses. To be able to arrive at a diagnosis after reviewing the patient's history, performing a physical examination, and interpreting laboratory results never failed to amaze her. Of course, the magic didn't work in every case, and it was that fact that provided both the continuing frustration and the fascination of clinical medicine.

Late in the afternoon on a Wednesday in August, Julie walked into room B-1203 and introduced herself to Mrs. Clara Halprin. The room was semiprivate, but at the moment Mrs. Halprin was its only occupant. She was propped up in bed reading a mystery novel, and although she was in no apparent distress, she looked moderately ill. Her face was pale and the lines around her mouth were pulled downward in an expression of unhappiness.

"I'm Dr. Barton, "Julie said. She shook hands with Mrs. Halprin, and they exchanged smiles. "I want to ask you some questions about how you're feeling and get some information that might help us figure out why you're sick."

"All right," Mrs. Halprin said. "But didn't Dr. Kline tell you all about me?" Dr. Kline was Mrs. Halprin's private physician.

"We have some information from him, but we like to be thorough and get it for ourselves. It won't take long. After I ask you some questions, I'm going to examine you."

Julie began by asking about Mrs. Halprin's daily life and habits. Julie guided the conversation with her questions. She didn't want Mrs. Halprin to ramble, but at the same time she wanted her to talk freely. In Julie's view, it was better to have patients tell you too much than too little.

As Mrs. Halprin talked, Julie was able to form a picture of her daily life and the history of her present illness. Mrs. Halprin was thirty-one years old and married. Her husband, Mark, was a thirty-three-year-old computer programmer. They had been married for nine years and had two children-Jennifer was six and Kevin eight.

"I'm really surprised to be in a hospital," Mrs. Halprin said. "I've always made it a point to take care of my health. I don't smoke or drink, and I don't take any medicines regularly. I try to make sure that we get well-balanced meals." Her efforts had seemed to pay off, for she and the rest of her family were in generally good health.

For the month before her admission to Boston Central, Mrs. Halprin had not been entirely well. "It never occurred to me that I might get sick," she told Julie. "Before it happened, I was a lot more worried about how Jennifer would adjust to moving from kindergarten to first grade in September. Now I'm worried about myself."

The summer had started pleasantly. Mark had accumulated some extra vacation time, and that made it possible for the family to drive down to Falmouth and spend a couple of days on the beach. Mark took scuba-diving lessons at nearby Woods Hole, and Clara had been content to sun herself on the beach.

The days at Falmouth were the last good times the Halprin family had had together. "About three weeks after we got back, I started feeling ill. At first, I thought it must be just a summer cold. I had a sore throat, a runny nose, and a cough. I never coughed up anything, but I seemed to cough all the time. It kept me from sleeping well, and during the day I always felt tired." Previously, when the children took their naps, she had used the time to read or do work around the house. But now she found herself taking a nap with them.

After about a week, Mark had asked her, "Why don't you go see Dr. Kline?"

"I thought he was just tired of seeing me drag around all the time," Mrs. Halprin told Julie. "I told him I thought it was just a virus. But he said maybe it wasn't and Dr. Kline could at least give me something to make me sleep better."

Two days after her husband's suggestion, Mrs. Halprin left Jennifer and Kevin at the house of a neighbor and consulted their family physician, Dr. Gerald Kline. Dr. Kline did a brief physical examination and took a throat culture.

"I think you probably have an upper respiratory tract infection," Dr. Kline told her. "I'm going to give you a prescription for an antihistamine and Septra. That's an antibiotic that contains sulfa, and it ought to knock out any infection. If you're not feeling better in three or four days, give me a call."

Almost immediately, Mrs. Halprin felt much better. "I was glad I let Mark talk me into seeing Dr. Kline, and I was sorry I hadn't gone to him earlier." For about three days, Mrs. Halprin seemed entirely well.

"For the first time since we got back from Falmouth, Mark and I spent an evening alone. We went to dinner at an Indian restaurant, saw an early movie, then stopped for ice cream at a place in Somerville. We had to wait in line for a long time, and by the time we got back home that night, I was feeling more tired than I had since seeing Dr. Kline."

She expected to feel better after a night's sleep, but the next morning she felt just as tired. She was so lacking in energy that it was all she could do to take care of the children that day until Mark could come home from work and relieve her of the responsibility.

"Sometime during that day, I began to feel slightly feverish. I didn't feel chilled or shivery, just flushed." Along with the fever, her joints began to feel stiff and achy. Even walking or lifting dishes caused her discomfort.

"Mark and I both decided that I had simply overexerted myself and had a slight relapse." She continued to take the antihistamine and the antibiotic that Dr. Kline had prescribed and expected that she would get better in another few days.

Four days after her reversal, Mrs. Halprin called Dr. Kline again. She described how she was feeling, and he told her to discontinue the medications he had prescribed.

"It sounds like you may be having a drug reaction," Dr. Kline told her. "Take aspirin three or four times a day if you need it for the pain in your joints.

If you don't start feeling better soon, I'll want to see you at the office again." Mrs. Halprin followed Dr. Kline's instructions, but she failed to improve.

"Had you ever taken any sulfa drugs before?" Julie asked. "If you did, did you have any reaction to them?"

Mrs. Halprin shook her head. "That was the first time."

"Are you sure about that?" Julie looked somewhat skeptical. "You've never had a urinary tract infection?"

"Never," Mrs. Halprin said. "I've been lucky in that respect."

"Please go on with what you were telling me. You didn't get any better after you discontinued the drug?"

"In some ways, I got worse," Mrs. Halprin said. During the next two weeks, she developed a mild, unproductive cough, much like the cough she had had when she first felt ill. But now the cough would sometimes be accompanied by a sharp pain in the chest.

"I also began to have stomach pains and cramps," she said. The pains weren't severe, but they were sufficiently frequent that they added to her general misery. She was glad, at least, that she wasn't bothered by diarrhea or constipation, which at first she believed might be the cause of the pains and cramps.

"What really scared me was when I woke up one morning and found that my arms and thighs were covered with a rash. It was very red and itchy."

The itching wasn't intolerable, but the rash was so dramatic that Mrs. Halprin couldn't ignore it. She immediately made arrangements to consult Dr. Kline once more.

Dr. Kline again examined Mrs. Halprin and listened to her account of her symptoms. In the end, however, he remained uncertain about the nature of her illness.

"He was honest with me," Mrs. Halprin told Julie. "He said he didn't know what was wrong and that he wanted to make arrangements for me to be admitted here. He said the hospital is set up to run some sophisticated diagnostic tests and that I would get the best care possible from experts."

Mrs. Halprin was reluctant to go into the hospital at first, because of the difficulties it would cause for her family. Her husband assured her that things could be worked out. "I can take the kids over to my sister's house, then pick them up after work."

"I let myself be persuaded," Mrs. Halprin said. "Quite frankly, I don't feel well enough to do everything I have to do at home. I figured it would be better to come to the hospital and get well so I could then get on with things."

"I think you made the right decision," Julie said. "We'll do everything we can to get you well. Now, if you don't mind, I'd like to examine you."

Proceeding in the manner that had become more and more familiar to her with experience, Julie began her physical examination of Mrs. Halprin. She paused from time to time to make notes to herself, and as she worked, she asked Mrs. Halprin specific questions. She asked about Mrs. Halprin's parents and grandparents and about her close relatives. She asked if Mrs. Halprin had frequent headaches. Whether she had any allergies or ever experienced difficulty in breathing. She finished her questions by asking if Mrs. Halprin had ever had any other rashes or shown sensitivity to the sun or had hair loss, sores in her mouth or nose, weight gain, or swelling or pain in her joints.

As Julie completed her examination, Charles Covici came into the room. Charles was a third-year student at nearby Eastern medical school, and he too would play a role in caring for Mrs. Halprin. Julie introduced him.

"We're going to need some blood and urine from you," Julie told Mrs. Halprin. "We're also going to take some smears from your throat, cervix, and rectum and send them to the lab to be cultured. None of this will hurt, so don't be worried."

"When will you be able to tell me anything?" Mrs. Halprin asked.

"We won't know anything until tomorrow at the earliest," Julie said. "We'll have to get back the lab results first."

Mrs. Halprin nodded. "It's all right if my husband comes to see me this evening, isn't it?"

"Of course," Julie said. "Just try to relax as much as you can, and don't hesitate to let us know if you start to feel worse." She shook hands with Mrs. Halprin and tried to make her smile reassuring.

August 16: Clinical Conference and Second Examination

At ten o'clock the following morning, Julie Barton went to the small staff conference room down the hall from Mrs. Halprin's room. She poured herself a cup of coffee and waited for Dr. Harold Williams and Charles Covici to arrive. Harold Williams was a senior member of the Boston Central Hospital staff and associate professor in the Department of Medicine at Eastern University School of Medicine. Mrs. Halprin's records would list Dr. Williams as her attending physician. Although Julie Barton's training was at the stage in which she was expected to play a major role in the decision-making process, the primary responsibility for seeing to Mrs. Halprin's welfare fell to Dr. Williams. Julie felt glad to be working with Dr. Williams. He was a thin, slightly stooped man in his early forties with a gentle manner and a ready smile. Despite his unprepossessing appearance and manner, he had an established reputation as a clinician and teacher. He was patient, thorough, and willing to explain why some lines of inquiry might be more rewarding than others.

Charles Covici came in at the same time as Dr. Williams. Both poured themselves coffee and joined Julie at the conference table. After a minute or so of small talk, Dr. Williams got down to business.

"All right, Julie," he said. "Suppose we start with Mrs. Halprin."

Julie spread out her notes so she could refer to them. She described Mrs. Halprin as appearing moderately ill but not in any apparent distress. Her temperature was 100.4° F. Her heart rate was 100 beats per minute, and her respiratory rate was 18per minute—neither quite normal. At 100/70, her blood pressure was normal.

Julie mentioned the red, itchy rash that had appeared on Mrs. Halprin's legs and described it in precise terms. "Skin examination revealed an erythematous, slightly raised papular rash," she said. "It is confined to the extremities, lower greater than upper, and is slightly pruritic."

Julie reported that, except for a slight redness at the back of Mrs. Halprin's pharynx, the rest of her head, eyes, ears, nose, and throat were normal. However, the lymph nodes in the hollow above her clavicle (the superclavicular fossa) were slightly swollen. Yet they were not, Julie said, "tender, rubbery, or matted."

Julie mentioned that she had found Mrs. Halprin's chest to be dull to percussion. The dullness could be heard primarily on the lower left side. However, there was no sound of a "rub," the sound made by the pleural covering of the lungs when it becomes inflamed. On the left side of Mrs. Halprin's sternum, Julie reported hearing a systolic flow murmur.

"Mrs. Halprin has no swellings or masses in her abdomen, although there is a suggestion of fullness in the left upper quadrant," Julie said. "Her arms and legs are normal, and the neurologic examination was unremarkable. She says that the joints of her wrists, knees, and ankles ache and are painful to bend, but the joints are not appreciably swollen."

Julie glanced at Dr. Williams to indicate that she had completed her summary. Dr. Williams nodded and gave her a reassuring smile. "Thank you very much," he said. "Before we hear the initial lab results, let's stop for a moment and think about what we might be up against. Mrs. Halprin has a four-week history of a systemic disorder of an uncertain etiology. Are there any leads we might want to think about following up?"

"We know she's been to the seashore recently," Charles said. "On the basis of that, plus her history and physical examination, I would say she may have viral hepatitis. I'd order liver function tests to check that possibility."

Dr. Williams nodded. "The possibility is surely there," he said. "I'm glad that occurred to you, but we must consider others as well."

Charles nodded in agreement. The truth was that he was glad he had been able to come up with a single genuine possibility. He was keenly aware of how little of a practical nature he knew about clinical medicine.

"There are at least three reasons we need to explore other avenues," Dr. Williams continued. "First, there are other disorders besides viral hepatitis that fit this sort of clinical presentation. Second, liver function tests will neither exclude nor confirm the diagnosis, especially if we're seeing that disease in its beginning stages. And finally, there are other features in this patient's presentation that lead away from viral hepatitis and toward other possibilities."

"You mean features such as her unproductive cough?" Charles asked. "Exactly," Dr. Williams said.

"Let me say something here," Julie began. "I agree that we should consider viral hepatitis prodrome. But I think two other possibilities are worth our attention. First, she may be having a drug reaction to the sulfa she's been taking. And second, she may have subacute bacterial endocarditis -SBE." "Those are fine suggestions," Dr. Williams said. He glanced at Charles. "Notice that the second one could account for the pulmonary symptoms which would be unusual if there were hepatitis prodrome." Dr. Williams paused for a moment to make some notes for himself. He clipped his pen to the pocket of his shirt, then glanced at Julie and Charles to see if either had anything to add. "All right," Dr. Williams said. "Let's go talk to Mrs. Halprin and see if we can learn anything else that might help us."

Mrs. Halprin was propped up in bed when the three of them entered the room. She put down the book she had been reading and glanced nervously from one person to another.

"Hello, Mrs. Halprin," Julie said. "This is Dr. Williams, the head of our clinical team. And you remember Charles Covici."

"How have you been feeling?" Julie asked. She automatically put her hand on Mrs. Halprin's wrist, not so much to check her pulse as to provide some general reassurance. "Did you sleep all right?"

"Fairly well," Mrs. Halprin said. "My rash kept me awake some, and it still hurts when I move my arms and legs. But I'm in pretty good spirits. My husband called this morning to tell me the children were doing fine, and he's going to visit me later this afternoon."

"That's very nice," Julie said. She stepped back so that Dr. Williams could be nearer Mrs. Halprin.

"I've heard about your problem." Dr. Williams said. "I'm sure you're tired of questions, but I'd like to ask you a few more, if you don't mind. Now, as I understand it, you've been ill for about four weeks, and most recently you've developed a rash on your legs."

"That's right."

"Before all of this began, you were at the seashore?"

"I did go to the beach," Mrs. Halprin said. "But I was there only for a couple of days."

"Did you have any seafood while you were there?"

"Yes, I did. I like shellfish a lot, and I had clams on the half-shell for dinner."

"What about other members of your family?" Dr. Williams asked.

"None of them had clams, that's for sure. Mark thinks raw clams are gross, and the children would never touch them. I think they all had hamburgers." "I see," Dr. Williams said. "That sounds like my children when they were younger. Now, do you know if you're allergic to any medications? "

"None that I know of."

"Do you know if you've ever taken a sulfa antibiotic?"

"I believe I did. After I talked with Dr. Barton I remembered that about eight or ten years ago I had a bladder infection, and I think Dr. Kline told me I was getting sulfa. I didn't have any reaction to it."

"Did you visit a dentist recently? Have a tooth filled or anything like that?" asked Dr. Williams.

"I got my teeth cleaned about two months ago, but I didn't have any fillings."

"That's good," Dr. Williams said. "Have you had any trouble with your hair or mouth?"

"I got canker sores when I got my cold, but that always happens to me. And now that you mention it, I do think my hair is falling out more than usual. I noticed that my brush seems filled with it."

"All right, Mrs. Halprin," Dr. Williams said. "Let me stop the questions for a minute and check a few things about your physical exam. This will be very brief."

Starting from Mrs. Halprin's head, Dr. Williams quickly ran through some of the same steps that Julie Barton had performed more slowly. When he was finished, he folded his stethoscope and slipped it into the side pocket of the long starched coat.

"Mrs. Halprin, have you noticed any weakness in your muscles-say, when you're climbing stairs or getting out of your chair?"

"Not really. I get winded when I go up stairs, but I don't feel particularly weak."

"All right," Dr. Williams said. "You've been very cooperative and helpful. Now we're going to try to figure all of this out."

"You still don't know what's wrong with me?" The disappointment was clear in her voice.

"There are a number of possible causes of your illness," Dr. Williams said. "We're going to be investigating them over the next several days. Right now, it's too early to tell you what's wrong. We should have a much better idea in two or three days."

"I guess that means you can't tell me when I'll get better."

"Not right now," Dr. Williams said. He squeezed Mrs. Halprin's hand. "Not until we have a better idea of what's wrong with you."

After leaving Mrs. Halprin, Dr. Williams and his team reassembled in the small conference room. Julie and Charles sat opposite each other and left the chair at the head of the table for Dr. Williams.

"We've learned something new," Dr. Williams said. "Because of the dental procedure recently performed on Mrs. Halprin, we now know she has a source for subacute bacterial endocarditis." Dr. Williams glanced at Charles. "And what else should we consider?"

"I don't want to sound like a broken record," Charles said. "But there's some evidence of a potential exposure to viral hepatitis. That will depend on whether there has been a public health hazard involving shellfish in the Woods Hole area."

"Very good," Dr. Williams said. He smiled encouragingly at Charles. Julie knew it was her turn to become the target of Dr. Williams's questions. She wasn't surprised when he said, "Julie, can you tell us about the lab data we've got now?"

Julie turned back the top page on her clipboard and began her terse summary. "Mrs. Halprin's hematocrit is 27 percent. She has normal red blood cell indexes and marked anisocytosis. Her white blood cell count is 4,200, with a normal differential count, except for 8 eosinophils."

Julie realized that only a few years before she would have had no understanding of the data she was now so confidently reporting. The hematocrit is a measure of the volume of packed red blood cells in a sample of blood. At 27 percent, Mrs. Halprin's hematocrit is low, indicating that she is anemic. The white blood cell count is the number of white cells in a cubic milliliter of blood. A count of 4,200 put Mrs. Halprin in the "low normal" range. Eosinophils are special cells found in the blood that are associated with allergic reactions. Eight is a high number.

"Platelets were 143,000, and the erythrocyte sedimentation rate is 68," Julie continued. "Urine analysis showed 5 to 10 white cells, 2 to 5 granular casts, and 5 red cells per microscopic field." Platelets are small cells that participate in the clotting of blood, and Mrs. Halprin shows a "low normal" platelet count.

The sedimentation rate is a measure of how fast red blood cells in a sample settle out and form a sediment, a general indication of inflammation.

"There was a 2+ out of 4 proteinuria," Julie said. "Electrolytes and glucose were normal, but her blood-urea-nitrogen was 35, and serum creatinine was 1.4. The cardiogram showed nonspecific changes, and the chest x-ray showed blunting of the left costophrenic angle."

Julie recognized that Mrs. Halprin's urine contained protein (proteinuria) in an amount that usually reflects kidney disease. Similarly, the figure of 35 for the BUN (blood-urea-nitrogen) was high and is a typical indicator of kidney disease. The blunting of the angle formed by the junction of the ribs and the diaphragm (the costophrenic angle) might indicate either scar tissue or the accumulation of fluids in the chest.

Julie looked away from her notes and at Dr. Williams to indicate that she was finished with her review. "That's all useful information," he said. "But, like the physical exam results, it's still quite nonspecific. We would be interested in hearing about what you thought and what you did."

It was the sort of question Julie had come to expect during her training. Just saying that a test or procedure was "standard" or "usual" was never an adequate justification. There always had to be a good reason for doing anything. To try to fish for answers to a diagnostic problem merely by ordering a variety of lab tests was considered almost as bad as missing an obvious diagnostic possibility in favor of one less likely.

"All right," Julie said. "First of all, as we mentioned earlier, viral hepatitis prodrome is possible and worth exploring. Consequently, I ordered liver function tests, hepatitis antigen, prothrombin time, and an assay for immune complexes."

"That all sounds reasonable," Dr. Williams said. "Did you stop there?" "No, I didn't. I also considered the possibility of a drug reaction. I didn't think it was likely because of the length of time between Mrs. Halprin's stopping her medicine and the appearance of the rash. But I went ahead and asked the dermatologists to consult on this." "That sounds good," Dr. Williams said.

"I think lupus is also a possibility. She has diffuse alopecia, a vasculitic rash, mucosal ulcers in her mouth, and a recent history of sun exposure. Therefore, I ordered antinuclear antibody and complement studies. Also, I obtained blood cultures to check for bacterial endocarditis. Finally, I thought DOI-disseminated gonococcal infection-ought to be considered, so I cultured her cervix, rectum, and pharynx."

"Excellent," Dr. Williams said. "You've brought up some possibilities that we definitely need to consider. At this early stage, we want to be careful to keep the door open. Now tell me, did you initiate any therapy?"

"No, I didn't," Julie said.

"I think that was a good decision," Dr. Williams said. "Mrs. Halprin is in no immediate distress or danger, and we don't want to muddy the waters with some nonspecific therapy. Whatever we're faced with, we've got a good chance to see it bare. Now at this point, I would like to discuss the pros and cons of the diagnostic possibilities you've mentioned. Then I'd like to add a few more of my own."

Dr. Williams looked at Charles, who nodded to show that he was following the discussion. Julie felt sympathy for him. It was impossible for anyone in his position not to feel lost or disoriented a large part of the time. There was just so much to know and think about that only experience in actual clinical inquiry and decision making could provide a guide.

"Let's take viral hepatitis prodrome first," Dr. Williams said. "It's got a number of factors in its favor. It is a common disease, the temporal sequence of events is acceptable, and the clinical features are compatible for the most part." Julie watched Charles make some notes on an index card. She knew that Charles would later do some reading on the diseases mentioned.

"Now, what is there against the diagnosis?" Dr. Williams asked. "For one thing, although she ate shellfish, viral hepatitis has not been a problem in the Woods Hole area recently. What's more, there's the possible presence of pulmonary disease and, perhaps, renal disease."

Dr. Williams paused to see if the others were following him. Satisfied that They were, he went on. "Another disorder related to viral hepatitis, polyarteritis nodosa, is less likely, because the patient is female, is not hypertensive, and shows no evidence of neuropathy. Of course, that disease could explain the abdominal pain, since it can involve bowel ischemia, cholecystitis, or pancreatititis. I know the textbooks say otherwise, but the eosinophilia is an unusual manifestation of polyarteritis nodosa, except as an overlap with hypersensitivity vasculitis. It makes sense for us to obtain an amylase from Mrs. Halprin, but I don't think we had better count too much on its solving our diagnostic problem."

Julie made a note to herself. If an additional test was to be performed, it was her responsibility to see that it was carried out. The presence of the enzyme amylase would indicate the likelihood of pancreatic or small intestine disease, for in diseases of both sorts an excess amount of amylase is liberated.

"Another rare complication of viral hepatitis is the syndrome of mixed cryoglobulinemia. It ordinarily has a different rash associated with it, but since cryoglobulins are immune complexes and it causes renal disease, we should try to measure them."

Julie nodded and wrote another note for herself. The initial tests of materials obtained from Mrs. Halprin were ones suggested by her account of her symptoms and Julie's physical examination. Now that more data were available about the functioning of her organ systems, it was reasonable to perform more laboratory tests in order to explore the most promising avenues opened up by the first round of testing.

"We've mentioned a drug reaction," Dr. Williams went on to say. "I doubt that it could account for all this patient's problems or for the temporal sequence of events. Still, the eosinophilia is suggestive, and we're not ready to rule out anything reasonable yet."

Dr. Williams stopped long enough to pour himself a cup of coffee. Julie used the time to write numbers beside the diagnostic possibilities discussed so far. Charles seemed to be having a hard time staying awake. His eyes were closed and his head nodded, but as soon as Dr. Williams sat back down, Charles shook himself and looked alert.

"Julie recommended that we consider the possibility of lupus," Dr. Williams said. "It was a good suggestion, Systemic lupus erythematosus is a relatively common disease. As many as one out of every thousand women in some populations are afflicted. And the disease could account for most of Mrs. Halprin's findings—constitutional, pleural, abdominal, articular, dermal, lymphatic, and hematologic. Either the sun or the sulfa or her respiratory tract infection could have caused the disease to flare. That's the way it often is with lupus.

"However, there are things to be said on the other side," Dr. Williams continued. "Her eosinophilia is uncharacteristic, and she lacks the more specific signs of lupus. We would expect to see a malar rash." Dr. Williams touched his cheek to indicate the location of such a rash. "We might expect to see mucosal ulcers or perhaps cytoid bodies in the retina. As it is, we have *some* evidence for three or four of the eleven criteria for lupus, and the presence of four of the eleven is said to be 96 percent sensitive and specific for the diagnosis. Yet we still haven't evaluated all eleven. We don't have a good history of photosensitivity, oral ulcers, a false positive test for syphilis, hemolysis, or an antinuclear antibody. We should do all of these tests."

Julie wrote down the names of the additional tests she would have to make arrangements for.

"Whenever you think of SLE, you should also consider SBE," Dr. Williams said. "In both of them, the manifestations are primarily due to the inflammation caused by the vascular deposition of immune complexes—an immune complex diathesis, as we say. However, the SBE, as well as in DGI, there might be features resulting from microembolic phenomena—for example, Roth spot, Osler's nodes, and the pustular skin lesions of DGI. These featuers different from SLE and from this patient's findings.

"Let me mention another dark-horse diagnosis: Henoch-Shonlein purpura. This would account for Mrs. Halprin's urticarial rash as evidence for glomerulonephritis and for abdominal pain after viral syndrome. However, we should notice that she is older than most patients with that disease and, what's more, her rash is not confined to her lower extremities."

Julie watched Charles write down the name of the disease. It was surely one that he would have to do some reading about.

"While I'm going with other possibilities, let me mention hypersensitivity angiitis. This is a syndrome that follows viral infection or exposure to a drug or allergen. It is associated with prominent pulmonary, skin, and renal manifestations and with eosinophilia. Yet Mrs. Halprin's other hematologic abnormalities are less common in this disorder."

Dr. Williams finished his coffee and looked into the bottom of the Styrofoam cup. "I think we can also exclude Goodpasture's syndrome," he said. "The clear chest x-ray and the lack of hemoptysis and skin rash, especially in a woman, rather much preclude it."

He put the cup aside and pushed the hair back from his forehead. Julie was impressed with the way in which Dr. Williams could continue to come up with possibilities. She was familiar with all the diseases he had named, but somehow most of them simply hadn't occurred to her in considering the findings in this case.

"Another rare eosinophilic disorder is Churg-Strauss disease," Dr. Williams said. "It's a granulomatous vasculitis seen in patients with long-standing asthma. But this is not a condition our patient reports." He nodded to himself, as though he had made up his mind about something. "Finally, I have no reason to believe that we are seeing a fungal or neoplastic disease. Though if I had to choose one, it would be angioimunoblastic lymphadenopathy. But it just occurred to me to mention Lyme disease. We have to consider this in any patient who has spent any time on Cape Cod, especially the islands. The more we learn about this disease the more protean its manifestations become, although it's true that she didn't have the characteristic rash. The lymphadenopathy raises the question of AIDS, although she is not in a high-risk group."

Dr. Williams glanced a Julie and Charles. "Do either of you want to add anything?" They both shook their heads. "All right, then. I guess we can end for now. I think we'll know a lot more about this patient in the next few days."

Comments on the Events of August 15 and 16

Mrs. Halprin was admitted as a patient at Boston Central Hospital on

Wednesday, August 15. She was given a physical examination and materials were collected for laboratory study. On Thursday, she was seen on morning rounds by the attending physician and members of the admitting team. Her case was presented by the resident, various diagnostic possibilities were discussed, then Mrs. Halprin was visited by the admitting team. They asked her more questions, she was examined again, then the team adjourned for a conference.

This is a relatively standard sequence of events. To get a better understanding of what is involved in the presentation, examination, and consideration of diagnostic possibilities, it is useful to consider in more detail just what went on in Mrs. Halprin's case.

The Case Presentation

During the morning report at a teaching hospital like Boston Central, a member of the admitting team (a resident, intern, or medical student) presents the case to the attending physician. (Other physicians on the ward or others with a special interest in the case may also be present.) The presentation and discussion of the case are part of the normal operating procedure in internal medicine, surgery, pediatrics, and other specialties directly connected with patient care. Specialties that are more test oriented, such as pathology, clinical chemistry, and radiology, do not always employ the case presentation method.

The case presentation itself is highly stylized and generally conforms to a format developed during the course of this century. It ordinarily consists of five sections: the chief complaint, a history of the present illness, the past medical history, a review of systems, and the social and family history. A few comments on each of these are enough to indicate their general character.

The Chief Complaint

The chief complaint is a one-sentence statement of why the patient sought medical attention. By convention, the complaint is stated, as nearly as possible, in the patient's own words.

For Mrs. Halprin, the chief complaint might be stated in this way: "This thirty-one-year-old white female was admitted to the hospital because of fever, rash, and joint pains."

The History of the Present Illness

The aim of presenting the history of the present illness is to give a complete picture of the patient's problem viewed within the context of the patient's life over a period of time. Just what happened within recent time to bring the patient to this point?

The patient is assumed to be the source of the history. If he or she is not, then this fact is mentioned. Furthermore, the patient is assumed to be a reliable and competent observer.

Giving a concise and complete history of the present illness requires a skill that takes years of experience to develop. The physician must gather materials by means of an interview with the patient that is often rambling and incomplete. He or she must then select the relevant information from what has been said and present a rationally reconstructed history that follows chronological order. Although irrelevant details must be omitted, data that are relevant but apparently inconsistent must be kept. Furthermore, the history must include data the physician obtained by asking the patient specific questions about important details the patient may not have noticed or may simply have neglected to mention.

A history of the present illness can go wrong in many ways. It may contain too much detail or too little detail. It may include irrelevant information or fail to include relevant information. Habit, theoretical bias, or even social prejudice may lead to errors of omission or commission in the presentation of the information. Finally, the chronological organization may be faulty, so an incorrect and misleading sequence of events is presented.

The Past Medical History

The next item in the case presentation format, the past medical history, consists of a short recitation of important aspects of the patient's general medical history. It is this longer-range history that helps supply a context that might be relevant for understanding the present illness. Allergies, operations, medications, and pregnancies fall into this category.

A Review of Systems

The review of systems (ROS) is the portion of the presentation in which the physician reports the results of a series of questions asked the patient about various symptoms. The symptoms asked about are all ones that are connected with organ systems.

The Social and Family History

The last item in the case presentation is the social and family history. The physician summarizes for the listener information about the patient's home environment, occupation, place in the community, medically relevant habits, and diseases of close family members.

Taken together, these five items constitute what is usually referred to as he patient's history. In general, the oral account of the case presentation is an abbreviated form of a more detailed written statement that is a part of the patient's chart. (A medical chart is the entire written record of information about the patient. In addition to the patient's history, it also contains such items as records of laboratory tests and results, medications prescribed, and progress notes.)

The Physical Examination

Like the case presentation, the physical examination is also a stylized reconstruction of data. In this case, the data are obtained from the maneuvers and observations performed by the physician on the patient at the bedside. A fairly uniform series of observations make up a general physical examination. However, variability in the standard sequence is not unusual. When some parts of the examination are not likely to be productive, they may be curtailed. Other parts that hold the promise of providing more useful information may be pursued in greater detail.

The report of the results of the physical examination usually starts with a brief statement of the general appearance of the patient. The aspect of the patient's overall condition that is most striking to the examiner is the one that is mentioned. For example, a patient may be described as obese, wasted, anxious, comatose, and so on. This key expression is then followed by a phrase that indicates the severity of the patient's condition. For example, a patient may be described as appearing healthy, chronically ill, in acute distress, and so on. This initial description is then typically followed by a statement of the patient's vital signs. Mrs. Halprin, for example, was said to have a temperature of 100.4° F, a heart rate that at 100 beats per minute was above normal (tachycardia), an elevated respiration rate of 18 breaths per minute, and a normal blood pressure.

Next, anything out of the ordinary about the skin is mentioned. (Mrs. Halprin was described as having an itchy, raised, bumpy rash on her legs and arms.) Then findings regarding the head, eyes, ears, nose, and throat are reported. (Mrs. Halprin had a redness at the back of her throat.)

Lymph nodes are then felt for in a variety of areas: neck, underarms, groin. If they can be felt, this is mentioned.

Neck and chest examinations are next. In Mrs. Halprin's case, the examiner noted a dull sound when he tapped on the lower portion of the left side of her chest. This indicated that there was a solid or liquid, not just air, in the chest cavity. But, as Dr. Barton reported, there were no sounds to indicate that the linings of the lungs and chest cavity were inflamed.

During the chest examination, the examiner listened through a stethoscope to Mrs. Halprin's heart (auscultation) at the left side of her sternum. This revealed an unnatural sound (a murmur) during the contraction (systolic) phase of the heart's cycle.

At this point, joints, muscles, and neurological responses may be considered. The examination showed that although Mrs. Halprin complained of joint pains, she had no objective signs of an inflammation in the tissues lining the joints of her wrists, knees, and ankles (synovitis). Otherwise, the rest of her examination was normal.

Possible Diagnoses

A knowledgeable person may use the data presented in the history and physical examination to generate a series of possible diagnoses. These possibilities may account for some or all of the data. Furthermore, questions may be raised about the data themselves. Are certain observations reliable? Are certain features not mentioned present or absent?

With the data from the history and physical examination available, the admitting team may stop to recapitulate the data and discuss the situation. Or they may wait until the laboratory data are presented. In Mrs. Halprin's case, Dr. Williams chose to pause to reflect on what they knew so far. Doing so provided an opportunity to teach, something frequently performed by a Socratic dialogue between the attending physician and other members of the group.

Charles Covici, the medical student, believed that he could account for the findings in Mrs. Halprin's case by a diagnosis of viral hepatitis. Dr. Williams gently chided him for limiting the set of diagnostic entities he was willing to consider. Furthermore, Dr. Williams pointed out that Covici suggested attempting to confirm the diagnosis by relying on a nonspecific test.

Dr. Barton, the resident, mentioned two possibilities as candidates for a diagnosis: a drug reaction, and a disease with variable manifestations-subacute bacterial endocarditis (SBE).

Rather than hear the laboratory data at once, Dr. Williams chose to visit with the patient. He did so because of the need to clarify some of the details mentioned in the case presentation. He confirmed that the patient had eaten raw seafood, which is a potential source of viral hepatitis. He found that in the past Mrs. Halprin had taken a sulfa-containing drug without incident. He learned that she recently underwent a dental procedure. This is a worthwhile finding, for dental work can liberate bacteria into the bloodstream and thus may be responsible for an infection of the heart valves (SBE).

Dr. Williams also got positive responses to two questions relevant to a diagnosis of SLE: Mrs. Halprin had had sores in her mouth and had had some hair loss. When he performed an examination, he noted pallor and an enlarged spleen, but did not think her lymph nodes were enlarged. He thought the inflammation in Mrs. Halprin's joints involved the tissue covering the tendons, as well as the tissue of the joints—tenosynovitis. While none of these observations led Dr. Williams to a specific diagnostic conclusion, they influenced what he thought were more or less likely diagnostic possibilities.

During their conference, the members of the clinical team, under the leadership of Dr. Williams, reviewed the additional findings obtained from examining and interviewing Mrs. Halprin. Dr. Williams pointed out that they had learned about possible sources for hepatitis (the shellfish) and endocarditis (the dental procedure). He also called attention to physical findings that suggested SLE (hair loss, rash, etc.).

The laboratory data available to the team were those secured as a part of a standard evaluation of newly admitted patients. A complete blood count showed that Mrs. Halprin was anemic (too few red blood cells). There was a suggestion that her cells were variably shaped (anisocytosis), although a sign that they were being fragmented (schistocytosis) was not mentioned. Mrs. Halprin's white blood cell count was slightly low (leukopenia), but her blood also showed an unusually high proportion of cells that mediate allergic responses (eosinophils). Her platelets (blood cells that help clotting) were below normal, and the rate at which the red blood cells fell when her blood was left standing (sedimentation rate) was an abnormally fast 68mm/hour. This is a nonspecific finding that is typical of systemically ill patients; it sometimes varies with the severity of the illness.

Mrs. Halprin's urine showed the presence of white and red blood cells, as well as fragments of clumped cells called casts. Urine is normally free of cells, and Mrs. Halprin's condition is sometimes known as active inflammatory sediment. The kidneys normally act as an efficient filter of the blood, but Mrs. Halprin's kidneys seemed to be leaking protein. This is a common finding when the kidneys are inflamed (nephritis). The measures of Mrs. Halprin's salts (electrolytes) and sugar (glucose) were normal, but blood products that are ordinarily eliminated by the kidneys were accumulating. This is an indication of decreased kidney function.

The electrical activity of Mrs. Halprin's heart, as recorded on the electrocardiogram, was not normal, but the changes were not ones associated with any particular disease process. Her chest x-ray showed a rounded or blunted area where her diaphragm meets the chest wall. This is probably due either to the accumulation of fluid or to an old scar on the surface (pleura) of the lungs.

After reviewing the laboratory data, Dr. Barton chose several diagnostic possibilities. She then suggested acquiring evidence that would make one or more of them either more or less likely. She also chose less likely possibilities. These were all ones that either are reversible by therapy or have very serious consequences. (SBE is an example that fits both categories. Its consequences may be fatal, but it is also treatable.)

To help determine the likelihood of hepatitis as a diagnostic possibility, Dr. Barton ordered blood studies that tell something about the function of the liver (liver function tests). Liver damage reveals itself both in diminished liver function and in the presence of specific chemical changes. This led Dr. Barton to order tests for the presence of liver-produced clotting factors (prothrombin time) and for the presence of viral hepatitis in the blood (a protein known as hepatitis antigen). The clotting factor test was chosen because it is a reversible cause of serious bleeding. Consequently, if there was an indication that Mrs. Halprin was suffering from liver damage, there would be a need to provide her with therapy.

Dr. Barton also ordered a test for immune complexes. These complexes are ones that are formed by protein molecules produced by the immune system (antibodies). They bind to foreign substances (antigens) such as invading viruses. When the antibodies form complexes with the antigens, their removal from the body ordinarily results. The complexes are ones that should be found in a generalized viral infection, and they have been found in the earliest stages of viral hepatitis. These complexes have also been implicated as the cause of many manifestations of disorders in a large number of "experimental models" of disease, for if the complexes become deposited in tissues, they produce inflammation.

Dr. Barton considered it unlikely that Mrs. Halprin was having a drug reaction. Nevertheless, Dr. Barton asked the dermatologists to examine Mrs. Halprin's skin to determine whether the rash on the lower part of her body was consistent with a drug reaction.

Systemic lupus erythematosus occurred to Dr. Barton as a diagnostic possibility. Accordingly, she ordered two tests that are often positive when that disorder is present: the ANA (antinuclear antibody) test, which determines the presence of antibodies against the nuclear material of cells, and a measure of complement components (these are parts of the biochemical system involved in the inflammatory response).

Finally, Dr. Barton attempted to locate a source for an infectious agent that might be affecting Mrs. Halprin's heart valves. Thus, Dr. Barton had Mrs. Halprin's blood cultured for bacteria, and smears taken from her cervix, rectum, and throat were cultured for gonorrhea.

Dr. Barton ordered no therapy for Mrs. Halprin simply because she did not know what to treat. Mrs. Halprin was not in a life-threatening situation, and had Dr. Barton initiated any therapy at all, she would be contributing more confusion to an already confusing situation. Symptoms would be suppressed, changes due to drugs or drug reactions might appear, and Mrs. Halprin's condition would be obscured by an overlay of therapy. A less-compelling argument could have been made to start antibiotics.

As attending physician, Dr. Williams must function in the dual role of diagnostic inquirer and teacher. In keeping with both of these responsibilities, he reviewed the pros and cons of each diagnostic entity Dr. Barton proposed. He noted the relevant clinical features displayed by Mrs. Halprin, the temporal sequence of events of her illness, the prevalence of disease in her geographic area, and the epidemiologic aspects of diseases in connection with Mrs. Halprin's age, gender, and race.

Dr. Williams also tried to fit together various pieces of information. He mentioned diseases thought to be due, in some instances, to chronic viral hepatitis infection-polyarteritis nodosa and mixed cryoglobulinemia. Because of the lack of several clinical features, he believed these were unlikely diagnostic possibilities, but he suggested tests that would provide more relevant information about them.

Dr. Williams's discussion of SLE was more positive, but he was worried by the presence of the allergic blood cells (eosinophils), which are not characteristically associated with the disease, and by the lack of other clinical signs. Dr. Williams expressed similar doubts about subacute bacterial endocarditis (SBE) and disseminated gonococcal infection (DGI). Dr. Williams mentioned some clinical features displayed by Mrs. Halprin that are both suggestive of Henoch-Shonlein purpura and hypersensitivity angiitis and also inconsistent with them. Finally, he dismissed both Goodpasture's syndrome (a rare disorder in which antibodies attack the lung and kidney) and Churg-Strauss disease (a multisystem disorder of inflamed blood vessels-vasculitis-associated with long-standing asthma) on clinical grounds. We can assume he mentioned them for teaching purposes. As an afterthought, he mentioned Lyme disease (an infection transmitted by tick bite) and AIDS.

August 17: The Report to Dr. Williams

The day after the clinical conference, Julie Barton met briefly with Dr. Williams to bring him up to date on Mrs. Halprin's condition.

"Have there been any significant changes with Mrs. Halprin?" Dr. Williams asked.

"Not really," Julie said. "But we do have some additional information. First, her rash did seem at least temporally correlated with sun exposure. Second, her liver function tests and prothrombin time are normal, and her hepatitis antigen is negative."

"Is that it?"

"No, there's some more," Julie said. "Her creatine phosphokinase, amylase, and total eosinophil count in her blood were normal. VDRL was positive, but only at a one-to-one dilution. Finally, the Coomb's test and all her cultures were negative." Julie realized that the normal level of creatine phosphokinase meant that Mrs. Halprin did not show the characteristic evidence for injury to muscle or brain tissue. Furthermore, as the level of amylase indicated, she didn't show evidence of disease of the pancreas or small intestine. Both substances are enzymes associated with those particular organ systems, so damage to the organs typically results in liberating abnormal amounts of the enzymes.

The VDRL test for syphilis may be positive when syphilis is not present but lupus is. Consequently, a positive test result might be informative, even though it might not indicate syphilis. The Coomb's test suggested that Mrs. Halprin's red blood cells were not being destroyed by antibodies.

"I think we know enough now to say that we can safely rule out viral hepatitis prodrome," Dr. Williams said. "And the lower-titer VORL does suggest lupus, if the fluorescent treponemal antigen test, which is more specific for syphilis, is negative."

"The dermatologists saw her," Julie said. "They thought that the rash looked vasculitic, but their biopsies won't be back for several days."

"All right," said Dr. Williams. "Other remote possibilities we should keep in mind are mycoplasma and Epstein-Barr virus syndromes. Both involve systemic illnesses of a variety of sorts." Julie wrote down the names on an index card and slipped the card back into the top pocket of her coat.

"Did you discuss the laboratory data with the patient?" Dr. Williams asked. "We told her that an infection was unlikely but that we were still unsure of the diagnosis. She reports that she still feels weak and has joint pain, but seems reasonably comfortable."

"Fine," Dr. Williams said. "Let's keep her and Dr. Kline informed."

"Dr. Kline thought we ought to handle it from now on," Julie said.

August 18: The Report to Dr. Williams

Early the next morning, on the fourth day after Mrs. Halprin's admission to Boston Central, Julie met with Dr. Williams and Charles Covici. Her role as resident made it her job to present to the others the most recent clinical information about their patient.

"Mrs. Halprin has a low-grade fever to 100.2° F and mild pleuritic chest pain," she said. "We are still not giving her any medications."

Julie glanced at Dr. Williams .He nodded his approval, and she went on with her report. "We have some interesting lab data," she said. "Her antinuclear antibody is positive at 1:320, with a homogeneous pattern. Both the complement components C3 and C4 levels are depressed. FTA, cold agglutinins, and monospot tests were negative."

Charles turned to Dr. Williams and asked, "Doesn't the ANA confirm the diagnosis of lupus?"

"Not really, but it makes it very likely," Dr. Williams said. "Subacute bacterial endocarditis is unlikely, unless we have a positive culture." He glanced at Julie.

"All final culture reports are negative," she said.

Dr. Williams nodded. "That suggests that systemic lupus erythematosus is more probable than endocarditis. We can say that much. But I don't think we've totally excluded a drug reaction or Henoch-Shonlein purpura." Dr. Williams turned to Julie. "Now what do you plan to do about Mrs. Halprin's chest pain?"

Julie had anticipated the question. She knew that such pain might result from an inflammation of the lining of the heart or from a clot in the lungs.

"We plan to evaluate her for both pericarditis and pulmonary embolus," she told Dr. Williams.

"That's very proper," he said, "I also think assays for antibodies to native double-stranded DNA, cryoglobulins, and immune complexes would be helpful to diagnose SLE."

"They've been ordered," Julie said. "Mrs. Halprin's renal function is not normal. She had two grams of protein in a twenty-four-hour collection, and her creatinine clearance is 75 ml per minute. We didn't find any evidence of hemolysis by haptoglobin."

"All right," Dr. Williams said. "We're doing all the right things. We'll just keep after this problem."

Comments on the Events of August 17 And 18

The data reported on August 17 virtually eliminate the possibility that Mrs. Halprin is ill because of viral hepatitis or a bacterial infection. In several respects, the data point toward lupus. Dr. Williams was still reluctant to arrive at lupus as a diagnostic conclusion while other possibilities still seemed worth considering. He pointed out that in their previous clinical conference he failed to mention two other types of infection (mycoplasma and Epstein-Barr virus) that should be checked out, and were subsequently discussed in terms of the negative cold agglutinins (mycoplasma) and monospot (Epstein-Barr) tests.

The following day's data favored SLE even more strongly. The antinuclear antibody test, which assays for antibodies against one's own cells (autoantibodies), is very sensitive for SLE but not specific. Thus, as Dr. Williams observed, Charles Covici was mistaken to believe that SLE was "confirmed." In spite of the high likelihood of SLE, which can inflame the heart (pericarditis), Dr. Williams believed it wise to evaluate Mrs. Halprin for another common cause of pleuritic chest pain that has vastly different therapeutic implications, namely, a clot in the lungs (pulmonary embolus). The additional kidney tests permitted the degree of inflammation and the degree of dysfunction to be quantified. Furthermore, the haptoglobin test showed that there is no evidence of premature destruction of red blood cells (hemolysis).

August 19: Consultation

Julie made it a point to see Dr. Williams as early as she could on Sunday morning, August 17. She went directly to his office and interrupted him in the process of writing a grant proposal.

"I wanted to let you know about Mrs. Halprin," Julie said.

"All right," Dr. Williams said. He put aside his papers with no apparent reluctance and gave Julie his full attention. "Did she have a bad night?"

"Yes, she did. She spiked a fever to 102°. She complains of more joint pain, and her rash is more pronounced. We think she has pericardial Rub, but there's no evidence of tamponade." Julie knew that tamponade resulted when there was so much fluid collected in the pericardial sac around the heart that heart function was inhibited.

"Did you start any medication?" Dr. Williams asked.

"We debated starting her on prednisone, but finally we decided to give her indomethacin." The choice had been between a steroid hormone and an aspirin-like drug. Julie had opted for the drug least likely to produce major systemic changes.

"Let's go see her." Dr. Williams said.

Mrs. Halprin was lying quietly in bed, neither sitting up nor reading. Dr. Williams put his hand around her wrist and smiled.

"Good morning," he said. "I guess you didn't have a good night."

"I felt terrible, especially when my temperature went up. But I'm much better now. The medicine must have helped."

"Let me listen to your heart for a moment," Dr. Williams said. When he had completed his examination, he turned to Julie and said, "The rub is still there."

"What does that mean?" Mrs. Halprin asked.

"It means you have some inflammation around your heart," Dr. Williams said. "It should decrease with the medication, but we would like to do some tests to verify that and to see if any fluid has collected in the sac that holds your heart. The test uses sonar. It doesn't hurt and it isn't dangerous. We also need to make sure you don't have clots in your lungs. Dr. Barton will tell you more about it later today."

Mrs. Halprin nodded. "All right. I'm ready to do most anything to avoid spending another night like last night."

"I'm sure you are," Julie said. "But these tests are no big deal."

Julie and Dr. Williams walked back to his office. Dr. Williams sat behind his desk, and Julie took the visitor's chair. Dr. Williams seemed somewhat abstracted. Julie sat quietly, waiting until she had his attention. "I wanted to tell you we've got the results from those additional tests," she said. "The anti-DNA antibodies and immune complexes were positive, but cryoglobulins were negative."

"As we initially suspected, she has SLE," Dr. Williams said. "When a young woman presents with a subacute systemic disorder characterized by constitutional symptoms, rash, arthritis, polyserositis, and nephritis, there are many possibilities. But there is only one probability—SLE." He glanced at Julie. "Of course, one must exclude infectious diseases and other immune complex disorders, but the problem is not as confusing as it seems to be."

"But there aren't any pathognomic features of SLE, are there?"

"No," Dr. Williams said. "And because of that, the American Rheumatism Association has developed a list of eleven criteria, the ones I referred to during one of our conferences on this patient. When four out of the eleven criteria are satisfied, the result is 96 percent sensitive and specific for SLE."

"Should we just limit ourselves to the criteria?" Julie asked.

"No, because there are many features of SLE that aren't mentioned by the criteria, yet they can be quite helpful in establishing the diagnosis. I have in mind such factors as hypocomplementemia." Julie recognized the condition mentioned. Hypocomplementemia was present when a patient showed low levels of complement, a group of blood-serum proteins that play a role in the inflammatory process.

"I'll schedule Mrs. Halprin for an echo," Julie said.

"All right," Dr. Williams said. "And continue the medication. Keep me informed about any changes, and we'll reassess the situation on a day-to-day basis."

Comments on the Events of August 19

Mrs. Halprin's condition worsened overnight. Because of this, Dr. Barton was pushed toward initiating therapy. Because Dr. Barton had good reason to believe that SLE is the cause of Mrs. Halprin's problem, she ordered treatment with an aspirin-like drug-indomethacin. She also considered the perhaps more dangerous drug prednisone, an anti-inflammatory corticosteroid, but opted for the more conservative therapy. Mrs. Halprin was informed that other tests on her heart and lungs would be necessary.

A test for antibodies to DNA was positive, showing that Mrs. Halprin has a feature that rarely occurs in diseases other than SLE. Tests for immune complexes were also positive. These lab data are characteristically taken to "confirm" a diagnosis of SLE. With this information in hand, Dr. Williams then reconstructed the argument in favor of SLE as a diagnostic explanation for a multisystem disorder with inflammation of the skin (rash), joints (arthritis), lining tissue (polyserositis), and kidney (nephritis).

August 21, 8:30A.M.: Consultation

In the two days since her last discussion with Dr. Williams, Julie had grown more concerned about Mrs. Halprin. Some changes had taken place that made Julie feel she should talk to Dr. Williams again.

She went directly to his office with Charles Covici before the start of morning rounds. She always seemed to be interrupting him, but Dr. Williams put aside the papers he was working on and gave them his full attention. If he was annoyed by the interruption, he didn't show it.

"It's about Mrs. Halprin," Julie said. "Her chest pain and fever improved, her lung scan was negative, and her echocardiogram showed only a small pericardial effusion. We were thinking of sending her home, but some other things have occurred that make me think that's not such a good idea."

"Specifically?" Dr. Williams asked.

"She's gained five pounds, developed ankle edema, and decreased her urine output. According to the latest numbers, her sediment remains active and her BUN has jumped to 65. Creatinine is up to 2.2."

"That's unfortunate," Dr. Williams said.

Julie nodded. She had expected Dr. Williams to confirm her own doubts. "Diagnostically, the major possibility seems to me to be worsening renal insufficiency secondary to active lupus nephritis."

"That seems right. It's either nephritis alone or in conjunction with the Indocin® (indomethacin). What does this suggest to you?"

Julie and Charles sat down in the visitor's chairs. "I think the basic decision is whether we're going to do a renal biopsy," Julie said.

"Yes," Dr. Williams said. "But don't forget that we have a host of therapeutic choices that may or may not relate to the biopsy decision. There's no specific study that's going to answer our problem for us. To take a logical approach, we're going to have to incorporate the notions of benefit, risk, and efficacy in our process of decision making."

Dr. Williams got up from his desk and erased the blackboard behind him. "First, let's stop the Indocin (indomethacin)," he said. "I think there's little to lose and potentially much to gain by doing that. Assuming that's true, let's outline some strategies."

Dr. Williams picked up a piece of chalk and sketched out the range of possibilities. (See fig. 2.1.) When he was done, he brushed the chalk off his fingers and sat back down at his desk. "There are many other logical possibilities," Dr. Williams said. "But the ones here are the most reasonable strategies I can think of."

"Those are all pretty standard, aren't they?" Julie asked.

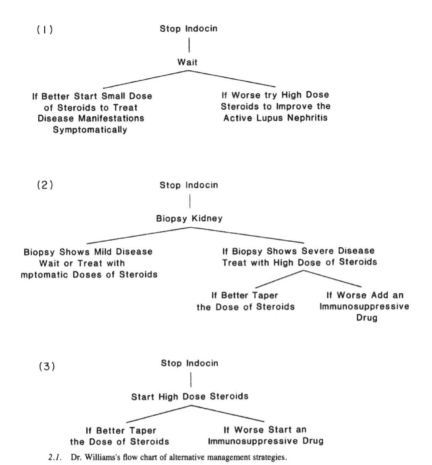

2.1. Dr. Williams's flow chart of alternative management strategies.

"For the most part. There are several more experimental treatments I haven't mentioned. If these fail, we still have them in reserve. I'm thinking, in particular, about massive pulse doses of corticosteroids and plasmapheresis."

"So how can we decide how to proceed?" Charles asked. All the possibilities listed seemed quite reasonable to him.

"Here's one general rule," said Dr. Williams. "It's not a good idea to initiate more than one therapeutic modality at a time, unless the treatments are a sensible physiologic combination or unless the patient is in the rapid evolution of an irreversible process."

"So that should dictate that we stop the Indocin (indomethacin)?" Julie asked.

"Well, it suggests it. For future management, we would like to know whether Mrs. Halprin's current decline is due to the indomethacin. As a separate issue, we can then determine whether her nephritis responds to steroids." Dr. Williams glanced at Julie and Charles to see if they were following his reasoning. Julie nodded to show she was.

"That's why I would be against strategy two," Dr. Williams continued. "If she was rapidly losing all kidney function and needing dialysis, it would be a different story. But that's not the case."

"What about biopsy?" Julie asked.

"Strategy three is appealing if, and only if, you believe that the histologic appearance of the biopsy is a good guide for future therapy. You might think that it could provide prognostic information or indicate what therapies might be most useful."

Dr. Williams swiveled his chair around to face Charles and Julie. "There is a third reason to perform a diagnostic test that is often an unconscious motive of either the physician or the patient."

"Curiosity," Charles suggested.

"Something like it. Everybody seems to feel a 'need to know' as much about the problem as possible, on the grounds that any knowledge is potentially useful. This is a motivation that is hard to deal with in an analytic framework."

"But biopsy is sometimes useful," Julie said.

"Sometimes," Dr. Williams said. "The usefulness of a biopsy in helping achieve the best patient outcome is something that can be evaluated by decision analysis. Basically, what we want to know is whether the results will redirect our strategy to a more effective therapy."

"And doesn't that happen?" Charles asked.

"Not always. For that to happen, it is necessary for there to be different and effective treatments for different biopsy results. What's more, we have to be unable to predict the biopsy results beforehand by using other data. Finally, the test cannot have an excessive rate of mortality or morbidity."

"And those criteria aren't met here?" Julie was guessing.

"The last one is. Renal biopsy is a reasonably safe procedure. But renal biopsy in systemic lupus erythematosus doesn't always satisfy the first two."

"But they're relatively common," Charles said. "Biopsy seems to be about the first thing that comes to mind when there's evidence of kidney dysfunction.

At least the nephrologists are anxious to biopsy Mrs. Halprin."

"I know," Dr. Williams said. "I think biopsy and other pathologic tests have a great appeal. Partly, it's because of the long tradition of correlating clinical findings with the underlying pathology. And partly, people like biopsies and other such tests for purely visceral reasons. Somehow it seems more satisfying to see actual results, rather than to have to interpret them from a number. Even though I might not need the information biopsies provide, I can appreciate why physicians are inclined to do them."

Dr. Williams stood up. Julie realized that the pedagogical part of the session was done. It was now time to take some action.

"I think we have little to lose by pursuing strategy one," Dr. Williams said.

"However, we need to discuss these issues with Mrs. Halprin. I would like for you to do that, then come back to see me this afternoon."

August 21, 2:00P.M.: The Report to Dr. Williams

Julie caught Dr. Williams just as he was leaving his office. He seemed to be in a hurry, so she kept the conversation as brief as she could.

"I talked with Mrs. Halprin about the biopsy," Julie said. "Quite frankly, I was a little surprised by her response. Most patients are reluctant to agree to any invasive procedure, even when we think it's necessary. Mrs. Halprin was just the opposite."

"I would guess she's read something about lupus, talked with other patients, and reached the conclusion that it's important to know how bad her kidneys are," Dr. Williams said. "On the basis of what we know, I'm going to guess that biopsy will show that she has mild histologic disease. I expect her to improve when Indocin (indomethacin) is stopped."

"I'll keep that in mind," Julie said. She hesitated. She didn't want to delay Dr. Williams, but she couldn't avoid mentioning something that had been bothering her. "There seem to be so many ways to present options to patients, and every way seems biased in one direction or the other. How do you achieve informed consent?"

Dr. Williams shook his head. "I don't really know. You have to be fair, you have to explain a lot, and you have to treat the patient like an intelligent adult. But beyond that, I don't know much else to say."

Hearing Dr. Williams say that made Julie feel better.

August 24: The Report to Dr. Williams

Three days later, at the beginning of the morning report, Julie brought Dr. Williams up to date on Mrs. Halprin's condition.

"Your guess was right," Julie told him. "The biopsy showed mild disease and we stopped the Indocin (indomethacin). She is now clearly improving."

"Have you been giving any other medication?" Dr. Williams asked.

"We put her on low doses of steroids, and now I plan to send her home. I'll follow her as an outpatient, of course."

"That's a good decision."

With her basic report out of the way, Julie went on to ask for the guidance she felt she needed. "I'm not clear on what features of her disease I should follow to monitor its activity or severity."

"A very reasonable concern," Dr. Williams said. "The features that correlate with disease activity are different in different patients, even when they have the same disease. But certain parameters may indicate a need to change therapy."

Julie nodded. "Are there any general rules? Or is it all just guesswork?"

"There are some general indications. Constitutional and serositic manifestations are ameliorated by nonsteroidal agents or low-dose steroids."

Dr. Williams paused to let Julie make notes. "Serious visceral involvement, such as gastrointestinal, renal, pulmonary, or nervous system manifestations require higher doses of corticosteroids. If they are resistant, then immunosuppressive agents have to be used. Articular and dermatologic manifestations of SLE commonly respond to hydroxychloroquine, a drug used to treat malaria."

"And we should rely on lab data, as well as clinical findings?"

"Lab results can be a useful guide," Dr. Williams said. "Sedimentation rate, white cell count, hematocrit, complement levels, and DNA binding often reflect general disease activity or specific renal activity. In the case of Mrs. Halprin, you'll just have to follow her carefully and find out what happens to her over the course of the next several weeks or months. But she should do well."

Julie had never had the experience of following a patient with lupus for a long period of time. From a professional standpoint, she was looking forward to it. It would be an experience from which she could learn a great deal. She was also looking forward to telling Mrs. Halprin that she could go home.

August 24 and 25: Discharge

Mrs. Halprin felt well enough to smile when Julie, Charles, and Dr. Williams came into the room. She still had a decidedly ill look, but her bed was raised and she was watching TV. She turned off the sound.

"How are you feeling?" Dr. Williams asked.

"I'm doing all right, I guess," Mrs. Halprin said. "I still feel quite weak. I don't seem to have much energy at all, although I slept pretty well."

"Do you think you feel well enough to go home?" Julie asked.

Mrs. Halprin's face brightened noticeably. "I think I'd like to," she said. "I miss the kids a great deal, and although my husband comes to see me every day, it's not the same as being at home."

"I know it's not," Julie said. "I need to setup a schedule with you to visit the outpatient clinic, but we think you could get along quite well at home."

"When can I leave?"

"I thought tomorrow morning, if you find that acceptable." "I'll call Mark at work and let him know," Mrs. Halprin said.

The next morning, Julie met with Clara and Mark Halprin to discuss some of the aspects of Mrs. Halprin's illness and to answer their questions about it. Julie reminded Mrs. Halprin that lupus is a disease that can vary greatly in severity, but is often mild in its effects. Mrs. Halprin would have to stay out of the sun as much as possible, take her medication as prescribed, and report any symptoms. Otherwise, she should try to live as normal a life as possible.

In response to questions from the Halprins, Julie reassured them that lupus is not a disease that is inherited. However, she pointed out, people in families in which there are rheumatic diseases are at increased risk for those diseases, for reasons not wholly understood. To provide additional information, Julie gave Mrs. Halprin specially prepared pamphlets from the American Rheumatism Association and the Lupus Foundation about her disease.

"I'll be seeing you next week," Julie said to Mrs. Halprin. "But that doesn't mean you shouldn't call us if you start feeling ill before then. We think you'll do just fine at home, but we're here in case you need us."

"You've all been very nice," Mrs. Halprin said.

December 2: The Conference with Dr. Williams

Over the course of the next three months, Julie followed Mrs. Halprin's condition during her regular visits to the outpatient clinic. At first, Julie found it pleasant to see Mrs. Halprin improve and resume many of her usual activities. She clearly enjoyed being with her family and living a more or less normal life.

But Mrs. Halprin's improvement was not enduring. She got through a few serious episodes as an outpatient, but eventually she was readmitted to Boston Central. Her husband brought her late one evening, and Julie was called at once.

The next morning, Julie went to see Dr. Williams. As usual, he was surrounded by a mass of papers, but also as usual he put them aside.

"I want to bring you up to date on Mrs. Halprin," Julie said. "We've been seeing her as an outpatient, but we readmitted her last night. When she left, we started her on low-dose steroids and hydroxychloroquine as you suggested, and initially she improved. But then she had several small flares, and some of them were associated with mild infections."

"What did you learn from the lab data during that time?"

"Her disease activity correlated with the sedimentation rate and inversely correlated with complement levels." "What about renal function?"

"It's been compromised, in spite of increasing her steroids to high doses," Julie said. "You may remember that when the function stabilized at 20 percent of normal, we gave her the option of immunosuppressives or intravenous high-dose pulse corticosteroids."

"What did she choose?"

"She went for the corticosteroids, because of her fears about the increased risks of cancer and birth defects with immunosuppressives. So we gave them to her in the monthly one gram of Solumedrol protocol that's currently under investigation in a multicenter trial."

Dr. Williams nodded to show that he was familiar with the protocol. "What sort of results has that produced?" he asked.

"She's only received one dose. Unfortunately, it didn't work at all, and Mrs. Halprin has become uremic."

"Is she on dialysis?"

"That's the problem," Julie said. "Despite intensive counseling by the nephrologists and the dialysis team, she remained adamantly opposed to dialysis. Now she is semicomatose, and we aren't sure if it's due to the uremia alone or whether there is now central nervous system involvement with lupus." "What does her family have to say about dialysis?" Dr. Williams asked. "I've talked to her husband and to her parents; her children are too young to consult. The family is in favor of dialysis, at least temporarily."

Dr. Williams sat quietly for a moment. Julie began to wonder if he hadn't forgotten she was there. At last Dr. Williams said, "In my view, Mrs. Halprin's fears of dialysis are exaggerated and you should disobey her wishes in favor of the family's. She is still young and has a potentially useful life ahead of her. The alternative would surely lead to her death. If she were elderly or had undergone dialysis for a trial period and didn't wish to continue, then that would be a different matter."

Julie had already reached that conclusion herself. She had come prepared to argue that Mrs. Halprin should be put on dialysis, and she was relieved to find Dr. Williams in agreement with her.

"I'll start the ball rolling," Julie said.

December 28: The Conference with Dr. Williams

Julie was able to catch Dr. Williams as he was leaving for Logan Airport. He would be gone for three days, and she wanted to be sure he was aware of the most recent information on how matters stood with Mrs. Halprin. In truth, Julie hoped Dr. Williams would be able to suggest something that might be done to improve Mrs. Halprin's situation.

"We dialyzed Mrs. Halprin to a stable metabolic status, but she has remained comatose," Julie said. "We tried both high-dose steroids and immunosuppressives for presumed CNS lupus, but we got no results."

"I see," Dr. Williams said. "I think you've done about everything that's reasonable to do. But let's think about all this a little more. What did the spinal fluid show?"

"It had an elevated protein of 100 mg percent and a normal glucose of 40 percent. The white blood cell count was 30, 90 percent lymphocytes. Cultures are negative so far."

"Did Mrs. Halprin become hypoxic or hypotensive at any time?"

Julie shook her head to indicate that at no time had Mrs. Halprin experienced a dangerously low level of oxygen or blood pressure.

"Were any imaging studies done?" Dr. Williams asked.

"Yes," Julie said. "She had a CAT scan with dye infusion. It showed no specific abnormalities."

"I suppose she's never been hypoglycemic."

"That's correct."

"And the EEG is normal?" "Nonspecific changes," Julie said.

Dr. Williams nodded. "You'll have to assume it is central nervous system lupus," he said.

"Since you've eliminated most other possibilities, you could try to increase the probability of this diagnosis by doing a brain scan to look for increased uptake or by checking for depressed complement levels in her spinal fluid. But such tests haven't proved to be very useful. Too bad we don't have our magnetic resonance imaging equipment."

"Is there anything else?" Julie asked.

"Not really. You'll just have to wait and see what happens. It often takes weeks to wake up from coma secondary to lupus, but keep your eyes open for other causes of coma. CNS lupus in the face of renal failure is uncommon, and we may be missing something."

Julie felt herself growing angry and disappointed. "I suppose we may have to face the question of just how long we should maintain her in the hope of recovery."

"I don't think we have much choice in the matter."

"I guess not," Julie said. "But it's difficult to stand by and see her hopes grow dimmer while her family is progressively ruined emotionally and financially."

"It is hard," Dr. Williams agreed.

January 20: The Report to Dr. Williams

Harold Williams was already in the small conference room when Julie entered. He was sitting at the table and sipping black coffee from a styrofoam cup.

"Mrs. Halprin just died," Julie said. "She never regained consciousness.

She developed pneumonia four days ago, then became septic." Julie paused, then said, "I've made arrangements for an autopsy to be performed this afternoon."

"That's very sad," Dr. Williams said. "I hope we will at least learn something."

Julie sat down opposite Dr. Williams and flipped through the pages of her clipboard. She had a case to present, and she wanted to be sure she remembered the details. But it was going to be hard to concentrate.

January 20, 4:00P.M.: The Autopsy

By arrangement, Dr. Barton and Dr. Williams met at the morgue to watch the autopsy performed by Dr. Hope, the pathologist. The autopsy proceeded with an examination of the gross-organ pathology. Dr. Hope demonstrated findings consistent with pneumonia, and the examination of the abdomen revealed nothing unexpected .However, when the skull was opened, they found the brain covered by a layer of gray tissue.

"I wonder what that is." Dr. Barton asked.

THE CLINICOPATHOLOGICAL CASE PRESENTATION

A thirty-one-year-old white female was admitted to Boston Central Hospital because of fever, rash, and joint pain.

She was well until one month prior to admission, when she developed an upper respiratory tract infection .Her physician prescribed an antihistamine and Septra® (trimethoprim-sulfa) and she improved for three days. She gradually developed low-grade fevers without chills, malaise, and joint pain, and all medications except aspirin were discontinued. Over the next two weeks, she developed a nonproductive cough, pleuritic chest pain, and abdominal cramping without diarrhea, constipation, hematochezia, melena, or dark urine. Three days prior to admission, she developed a pruritic rash and was referred here. There was no history of drug abuse, extramarital intercourse, known exposure to hepatitis, or allergies. The patient did admit to recent aphthous stomatitis, mild diffuse alopecia, and recent travel to Cape Cod.

The patient appeared moderately ill but in no distress. Her temperature was 100.4° F, pulse 100/minute, respirations 18, and blood pressure 100170. She had an erythematous pruritic papular, confluent rash confined to the proximal anterior portion of each extremity, lower greater than upper. There was mild pharyngeal erythema but no mucosal ulcers were observed. There was mild diffuse adenopathy without discretely enlarged nodes. The neck was unremarkable. Chest exam revealed left basilar dullness to percussion without a rub, and a systolic flow murmur was heard at the left sternal border. Pelvic and rectal exams were unremarkable. Articular exam was within normal limits, in spite of pain at the wrists, ankles, and knees. She was alert, oriented, and cooperative, but anxious. No focal neurologic findings were demonstrated.

Hematocrit was 27 with anisocytosis but normal red cell indexes. White blood cell count was 4,200 and 66 neutrophils, 26 lymphocytes, and 8 eosinophils. Platelets were 143,000 and the erythrocyte sedimentation rate was 68. Urine analysis was notable for a specific gravity of 1.027, 5 to 10 white blood cells, 2 to 5 granular casts, and 5 red blood cells per microscopic field. There was 2+ proteinuria. Sodium was 143 mg/dl, potassium 4.3 mg/dl, chloride 103 mg/dl, bicarbonate 24 mg/dl, glucose 105 mg/dl, urea nitrogen 35 mg/dl, and creatinine 1.4 mg/dl. An electrocardiogram showed nonspecific ST-T wave changes, and a chest x-ray showed blunting of the left costophrenic angle. Liver function tests, creatine phosphokinase, amylase, absolute eosinophil count, Coomb's test, cultures of blood, pharynx, cervix, and cold agglutinins were normal or negative. VORL was positive at 1:1 dilution but not greater, and the fluorescent treponemal antigen was negative. The antinuclear antibody was positive at a 1:320 dilution with homogeneous pattern; DNA binding was elevated at 56 percent; and both C3 and C4 were depressed at 70 and 9, respectively. Her urine contained 2 grams of protein in a 24-hour collection, and the initial creatinine clearance was 75 ml/min. An echocardiogram revealed only a small pericardial effusion, and her course in the hospital was complicated by transiently worsened renal insufficiency secondary to indomethacin. A renal biopsy revealed mild focal proliferative glomerulonephritis, and she was discharged on 10 mg prednisone a day, and hydroxychloroquine.

She had several flares in the next three months, resulting in increasing renal insufficiency. However, the patient refused immunosuppressive agents and did not respond to either high-dose prednisone or intravenous pulse methylprednisolone.

Her final admission was prompted by uremia. She lapsed into coma and did not regain consciousness in spite of intensive dialysis. Terminally, copious thick, green secretions were aspirated from the lung and the patient expired. An autopsy was performed.

Case Discussion

Case discussant (Dr. Harding): Today we will alter the usual CPC format by substituting short discussions both before and after the pathological proceedings instead of a longer discussion prior to the autopsy findings. The patient clearly had systemic lupus erythematosus, as was demonstrated by an elaborate diagnostic evaluation on her first hospital admission. While one can quibble with the details of her management over the next several months, our current state of knowledge suggests that she received appropriate therapy, including low-dose steroids followed by higher doses when she failed to respond, chloroquine, pulse doses of corticosteroids, and eventually dialysis. While she refused immunosuppressive drugs, it was unclear whether these were considered during her final illness. It is equally unclear that they would have been effective terminally. At least part of our task today is to determine the cause of her final illness and to suggest any possible therapy for it. For this, we will need more information about laboratory data during her final admission.

Dr. Barton: Her renal status on admission was as follows. Her BUN was 150, creatinine 14.4, urine output less than 100 cc/day, with a specific gravity of 1.010, 4+ protein, 2 to 5 hyaline casts, and 10 to 20 RBC per high-powered microscopic field. She was acidotic with pH 7.25, serum bicarbonate of 12, sodium of 131, potassium of 5.9, and chloride of 112. Hemodialysis and sodium citrate corrected her metabolic abnormalities until the day she expired, when she again became acidotic. Her depressed mental status was evaluated with a lumbar puncture which showed normal opening pressure, 30 WBC, 90 percent mononuclear, protein of 100 mg%, and glucose of 40, with a peripheral blood glucose of 131. EEG was abnormal with diffuse slowing but no focal abnormalities. Brain scan and subsequent computerized axial tomography (CAT), with and without contrast material, showed no abnormalities. We concluded that the patient had renal failure secondary to SLE glomerulonephritis, CNS disease secondary to SLE, and terminally purulent bronchopneumonia.

Dr. Harding: My thinking would have been much the same as yours. I would have considered either lupus or uremia as the cause of the depressed mental status and would have tried, as you did, to reverse both processes. Would you tell us what steps were taken to exclude infection in this final illness?

Dr. Barton: The patient had multiple blood and urine cultures, which were negative. Culture of her CSF also showed no growth and the gram stain was negative.

Dr. Harding: Thank you. Let us hear the pathological findings now.

Pathologist (Dr. Hope): 1 will review the pathological findings by organ system. First, in the skin of the extremities, there was a vasculitic skin rash with involvement of venules. There was nuclear debris in the living cells of the blood vessels that is commonly called leucocytoclasia. In addition, there was immunoglobulin G and M and complement component deposition at the dermal-epidermal border on immunofluorescent staining. These findings are all consistent with the diagnosis of systemic lupus erythematosus. In the visceral organs, first the kidney showed typical light microscopic changes consistent with diffuse proliferative glomerulonephritis, and on immunofluorescent and electron microscopy there was evidence of immunoglobulin and complement and fibrin deposition in the glomeruli. The spleen showed typical onion-ring lesions of splenic vessels, consistent with SLE. The lungs showed a necrotizing purulent bronchopneumonia bilaterally with numerous gram positive and gram negative organisms on stain. Cultures postmortem demonstrated mixed flora of staph aurous and *Pseudomonas aeruginosa.* On opening the calvaria, we were surprised by the finding of a purulent exudate covering the entire leptomeninges. The brain was edematous but no focal abscesses were noted. On microscopic evaluation, there were numerous large, spherical bodies seen best on India ink preparations, both free in the spinal fluid and embedded in the fibrinoid exudate. Our cultures are still negative after one week of incubation; however, the original CSF from the lumbar puncture grew *Cryptococcus neoformans* after two weeks of incubation several days after expiration. Serological testing of the CSF for Cryptococcus antigen sent to the Centers for Disease Control, in Atlanta, was reported to be positive, again postmortem. We conclude that the patient had severe, active systemic lupus erythematosus and cryptococcal meningitis, and died from respiratory insufficiency secondary to diffuse bilateral bronchopneumonia.

Dr. Harding: Without belaboring the obvious, I will state that this patient's tragic course serves to remind us of a number of principles. In patients with lupus, especially those treated with corticosteroids or immunosuppressive drugs, the chance of opportunistic infections such as cryptococcal meningitis is always real. Second, although lupus can cause virtually any clinical finding in a given patient, not all findings in patients with lupus are due to their underlying disease. Third, the failure to consider a diagnostic entity such as treatable occult infection is often the worst error of omission in a patient's management. Last, in most circumstances, it is wiser to be aggressive diagnostically and conservative therapeutically than vice versa.

RECOMMENDED READING

Texts on Lupus for a Lay Audience

Carr, R. I.Lupus Erythematosus. Washington, D.C.: Lupus Foundation of America, Inc., 1986.
Phillips, R. H. Coping with Lupus. Wayne, N .J.: Avery Publishing Group, Inc., 1984.

Texts on Lupus for Physicians

Lahita, R. G., ed. Svstemic Lupus Erythematosus. New York: Wiley, 1987.
Ropes, M. W. Systemic Lupus Erythematosus. Cambridge, Mass.: Harvard University Press, 1976.
Schur, P. H., ed. The Clinical Management of Systemic Lupus Erythematosus. New York: Grune and Stratton, 1983.
Wallace, D. J. and E. L. Dubois. Lupus Erythematosus. 3d ed. Philadelphia: Lea and Febiger, 1987.

Interviewing

(See also references to chap. 11.)

Bates, B.A Guide to Physical Examination. Philadelphia: Lippincott, 1983.
Coulehan, J. L., and M. R. Block. The Medical Interview: A Primer for Students of the Art. Philadelphia: F. A. Davis, 1987.
Enelaw, A. J. and S. N. Swisher. Interviewing and Patient Care. 3d ed. New York: Oxford University Press, 1986.
Engel, G., and W. L. Morgan. Interviewing the Patient. Philadelphia: W. B. Saunders, 1973.
Koran, L. "The Reliability of Clinical Methods." New England Journal of Medicine 293 (1975): 642-46, 695-701.
Platt, F. W., and J. C. McMath. "Clinical Hypocompetence: The Interview." Annals of Internal Medicine 91 (1979): 898.

CHAPTER 3   *Data*

Physicians often seem obsessed with data. They argue incessantly about the historical, physical, and laboratory details of patients' illnesses. They collect, collate, search out, investigate, accumulate, discard, and finally synthesize a morass of information. Then they worry about its accuracy, precision, and relevance to their patients. Literally hundreds and even thousands of observations are made, even in relatively routine clinical circumstances. In fact, it has been estimated that more than five hundred separate pieces of data are collected in a brief clinical encounter.

To take one example, sweating is an important clinical detail. Beads of sweat often appear on the forehead of someone in intense pain .Generalized sweating is a normal accompaniment of a febrile illness. Sweaty palms often result from anxiety. The absence of sweat can indicate dehydration, some forms of shock, and even some rare diseases such as familial dysautonomia.

Similarly, Dr. Barton called attention to Mrs. Halprin's swollen lymph nodes. It was important to note that they were present, but Dr. Barton was careful to characterize them further. The reason for doing so is that the different tactile qualities of the lymph nodes are associated with different disease manifestations. "Rubbery" nodes suggest a lymphoid cancer and "hard" suggest either metastatic cancer or a granulomatous infection, while "tender" suggest an acute infection.

What underlies this concern for detail? Obviously, a great deal depends on the quality and quantity of clinical data. Life-threatening and life-saving decisions may be profoundly influenced by an apparently insignificant detail. But beneath the drama of crucial decision making, the concern for data reflects in large measure an appreciation of the nature and problems of clinical information. In this chapter we discuss the sources and structure of the clinical database, the types and characteristics of measurements, and issues concerned with data obtained from clinical studies.

THE CLINICAL ENCOUNTER AS A SOURCE OF DATA

Most clinical data come directly from patients via their recitation of their own history. When a patient's history is not available, the physician is at a tremendous disadvantage, because he or she lacks any way of appreciating the effect of the illness on the individual. Although we are a moderately homogeneous species and produce characteristic responses to a variety of stimuli, everyone reacts somewhat differently to a physiologic insult. Accordingly, the lack of a patient's history can deprive the physician of numerous useful observations.

As a substitute for a personally related history, when the patient is unconscious or incompetent, the physician may question a family member, friend, or someone else in close contact with the patient. The information derived from such sources may be better than nothing, but the more distant the source, the less helpful the information is likely to be.

When patients are able to provide information, the data they supply have a "personal touch." This has both advantages and disadvantages for the physician. The major disadvantage is that the quality of the information may be compromised by the biased recall of the patient. The patient may forget important details or overemphasize some aspects of the history and downplay others. Exposure histories, including chemical contact and food ingestion of even routine medications, such as over-the-counter drugs, are often not volunteered. Intelligent and medically sophisticated individuals (especially physicians) are often terrible historians, because they are quick to formulate their own hypotheses. Patients may wish to avoid embarrassment or escape moral judgment, especially in areas where medical consequences result from socially unacceptable practices. One major advantage is that this coloring often produces insights into the patient's personality, reaction to stress, value structure, priorities, interests, biases, hopes, and fears. Information of this sort is important in both diagnosis and management of the patient's illness.

What the physician most needs from the patient is a clear statement of relevant physical events and the times when they took place. Given this information, the physician can later reconstruct the events into a chronologically ordered sequence of symptoms expressed in the restricted language appropriate to physical and psychological disturbances.

Rarely, if ever, will a patient give an impromptu recitation of all the details that a physician considers pertinent. The physician must round out the patient's account by securing answers to strategic questions. We consider later what makes a question pertinent, but for the moment it is enough to say that the physician must at least be sure to establish an accurate chronology of events.

During the last century, the notion arose that the physician should get the "complete" history from each patient and perform a "complete" physical exam. The impossibility of meeting such a demand hardly needs stressing. Yet the strength of the notion is that it insists that the physician look beyond the details of the present illness and focus on other aspects of the patient that might be relevant to medical evaluation and treatment. This includes such obvious factors as medically significant details of the patient's life prior to the present illness-childhood disorders, immunizations, allergies, operations, and so on. But this also includes such factors as family members with heritable diseases, the patient's finances, personal habits, and living conditions.

To be sure of rounding up any pertinent information that might have been missed, the physician runs through a brief checklist of common complaints referable to each main organ system. This is the review of systems (ROS) that usually comes at the end of the history-taking part of the clinical encounter. The questions asked in the ROS are somewhat arbitrary, but there are only a limited number of complaints referable to a given organ system. For example, ears can hurt or have a discharge. Hearing can be diminished or extraneous noises can be heard. Occasionally, dizziness or unsteady gait is the result of problems with the ears. If one asks all of these questions and receives negative answers, it is unlikely that there are significant problems with the auditory system.

All the elements we have mentioned—the patient's account of the present illness, the physician's questioning, the patient's background, and the ROS—constitute the verbal portion of the evaluation. It is this portion that usually provides the vast bulk of information available to the physician.

The physical examination follows the history taking. It is an ordered sequence of observations that follows much the same pattern as the ROS. However, unlike the ROS, the physical exam is often directed toward the problem at hand in two ways. First, the physician may expand the number of observations of a given organ system when the patient's history suggests a specific category of disorders. Second, the physician may minimize or even eliminate certain segments of an otherwise routine examination if other considerations are more pressing. By and large, a certain set of observations is taught to students as a "complete" screening exam which over time they may modify to their own needs. Unfortunately, neither the questions in ROS nor the physical examination has ever been evaluated for its ability to detect problems that were not evident in the history.

Laboratory results constitute the last data section of the patient-evaluation procedure. Often a standard group of tests are applied to all patients, but both minor abbreviations and extensive expansions of the laboratory database are common. In this respect, deciding what lab tests to perform or omit resembles conducting a physical examination.

Even the very brief description of the clinical encounter we have provided should make it clear that the initial database for patient evaluation cannot be secured by means of a fixed checklist applicable to all patients. The process of securing data is a fluid, dynamic, interactive dialogue between physician and patient. Early attempts to automate patient evaluation required the use of formats that were quite rigid. As a result, investigators discovered that they could deal with only a very narrow category of disorders and, even then, with only a one-dimensional interaction. Such constraints make it clear how difficult it would be to design a history-taking machine that could, for example, successfully deal with both an unidentified individual brought into an emergency room in an unresponsive state and a healthy-appearing person with vague constitutional complaints and a history of psychiatric disease.

For the foreseeable future, skilled physicians remain the best means available for securing and processing clinical data. The patient remains the best source of those data.

THE ACCURACY AND RELIABILITY OF DATA

Some observers have called attention to the differences between data originating with the patient and data produced by the laboratory, and they have proposed dividing all relevant patient information into subjective and objective categories. This proposal has been incorporated in a number of hospital-based training programs in the use of the Subjective-Objective Assessment Plan (SOAP) for charting patients.

The clear implication of the division is that there is a category of data originating from the patient that we cannot trust and a category of data originating from the laboratory that we can. One category is unreliable, and the other we can unhesitatingly utilize.

This is nowhere near the truth. All data, whether derived from people or by the use of machines, have similar parameters that define their usefulness. These parameters are accuracy and reliability. (The terms validity and precision are sometimes used respectively for the same parameters.)

Accuracy

Accuracy is simply how well a datum represents the state it is supposed to be describing. Consider, for example, the hematocrit, the volume of packed red blood cells. As a measurement, it is a reasonably accurate representation of the quantity of red blood cells in a person's blood. At the same time, however, certain characteristics of the red blood cells and the method of obtaining the measurement are going to affect the results. The size and shape of the cells, the viscosity of the serum, the centrifugal force and time of centrifugation, the care in reading the measurement, the accuracy of the scale, and the error in rounding off the value transcribed in the chart are all factors that may influence the result.

Nevertheless, the hematocrit is still a very accurate measurement. The classic example of an accurate or valid measurement is a yardstick. It is a "gold standard" of length, because it conforms to our notions of length and in a quantified manner relates to other physical dimensions, such as weight.

Accuracy (or validity) can be a very elusive goal. For example, the measurement of generalized pain is controversial. Should a patient's self-reporting be accepted? After all it is the patient who is the best determinant of his or her sensations. But even if we use convenient universal endpoints such as "no pain" or "the worst pain possible," how do we know if the endpoints are comparable from one individual to another? In general, accuracy is not measurable in the sense of affording degrees of validity. Experimental psychologists have elaborated criteria for the accuracy or validity of measurements in the attempt to resolve such questions.

Face Validity

Does the concept of the measurement fit the concept of the quantity to be measured? For example, does heaviness reflect one's concept of weight? Does the ability to solve problems in addition and subtraction relate to our notion of competence in arithmetic? By contrast, one might argue that being able to explain proverbs might have little to do with intelligence. In the context of our case, the amylase test has face validity for the diagnosis of pancreatitis, since it is intuitively obvious that the organ that produces the enzyme would be the source of its release when inflamed.

Construct Validity

Does the measurement fit in the conceptual framework of the quantity measured? For example, does heaviness fit into the framework of the physics of gravitational Jaws? An example of good construct validity in medicine is the hemodynamic measurements obtained during cardiac catheterization. These fit in nicely with the physiologic theory behind cardiac contractility. Similarly, echocardiographic measurements of the sort made on Mrs. Halprin agree with principles of cardiac anatomy.

Criterion Validity

Does the measurement correspond to a well-recognized, accurate, verifying norm—a "gold standard"—such as the international standard weights and measures? If gold standards were available for medical tests, we would be on much firmer ground for making conclusions based on tests, but unfortunately they rarely occur. A phonocardiogram, for example, might be considered the criterion to determine the presence of a systolic ejection murmer. Without criterion validity, definitions can often become circular.

Content Validity

Does the measurement adequately incorporate all the dimensions of the quantity being assayed? That is, is it representative? In medicine, we often measure liver function tests. These are assays that measure enzyme activity normally found in the liver in a blood specimen. In fact, they are measures of liver damage, which tends to release these enzymes into the blood stream. Thus, they are more a consequence of inflammation or injury than of function. They lack content validity for liver function.

What emerges from these concepts is the notion that accuracy is necessarily limited, because it is an abstraction from the quantity being measured. A useful analogy is with a map. Any map becomes less and less map-like (and thus less useful) and more and more like the area mapped as it becomes more and more accurate.

In other words, to measure something, we must always single out a feature of the object, then turn this abstraction into a tangible procedure for obtaining the information. Roadmaps show bends in the highway, but they do not indicate breathtaking vistas.

Reliability

The *reliability* or *precision* of a measurement is simply its reproducibility. Suppose, for example, multiple hematocrit determinations were made with a single sample of blood. In a good laboratory, the results will not deviate from each other more than a percentage point and thus are very precise. This means that the measurement is reliable. Most findings from a physical examination are poorly reproducible and depend on the extent of the abnormality and the sophistication of the examiner. Historical data may or may not be reliable, depending on the patient and the examiner.

A systematic error, such as an incorrect scale, could generate a reproducible but inaccurate series of measurements. (In the alternate terminology, the measurements would be precise but invalid.) The use of standard scales and procedures is intended to guard against just such a possibility. A pH meter that is poorly calibrated can give precise but inaccurate results, as can happen with any laboratory measurement. The steps taken to guard against this possibility primarily involve vigilance in checking the instrument against known standards.

It is also possible to imagine measurements that are accurate in the aggregate but not individually precise. A lab technician who was not careful in reading the hematocrit but was unbiased in the reading (that is, read equal numbers of too high and too low values) might arrive at an accurate aggregate value on the basis of imprecise measurements. However, under ordinary conditions, precision is a necessary prerequisite for accuracy. Figure 3.1 illustrates these relationships.

Sophisticated mathematical tools are available for expressing the character and degree of reliability (precision) involved in a given measurement. Statistical textbooks treat the topic thoroughly, but in the next chapter we review the techniques only to the extent necessary to understand the basic concepts, because they figure in our discussion of inference.

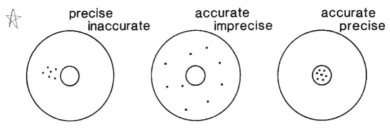

3.1.   Data points that are tightly grouped but off the bull's-eye are precise but inaccurate. Data points that are widely scattered but in the aggregate overlap the bull's-eye are imprecise but accurate (an unusual situation). Data points that are tightly grouped in the bull's-eye are accurate and precise.

The concepts of accuracy and precision apply not only to individual measurements concerning the patient evaluation but also to more general concepts. For example, if we wish to evaluate the activity of Mrs. Halprin's lupus in a quantitative manner, we would need to establish some scale of activity. This scale would have to obey the rules of data, just as individual data points would. We would need to construct the scale in such a way that it had all the types of validity that were mentioned previously, and it would have to be tested in such a way that it was easily reproducible under the conditions in which it would be used.

This kind of scale is all too often absent in patient-based studies. It is the exception that scales of severity or activity of disease have undergone the usual testing procedures that would establish their accuracy and precision. Staging of neoplastic disease is a prime example, as are the functional criteria of the New York Heart Association for severity of heart disease. Many other examples could be mentioned.

By contrast, other scales, such as the Health Assessment Questionnaire

(HAQ) for functional disability for patients with arthritis and the Arthritis Impact Measurement Scale (AIMS) for the same purpose, and more general scales, such as Bush's Index of Well-being, have undergone rigorous evaluation and testing. These, however, are the exception; the rule is that most of the data concerning patients are of unknown accuracy and precision. Thus, the information content is unknown and it is difficult to know how to utilize these data for inferences. A great number of questions in clinical conferences concern the meaning of an individual datum, questions that might be resolved by the formal testing of accuracy and reproducibility.

PATIENT-BASED MEASUREMENTS

Now that we have some understanding of the theoretical aspects of measurement, we can consider how these concepts connect with patient-related data.

We have already noted that there are sources of error in even a very precise and accurate laboratory measurement. The same could easily be said for physical findings. If only one of Mrs. Halprin's ten to twenty physicians felt her spleen and if the spleen was truly palpable, we would have to conclude that the assessment is very imprecise (in the sense that physicians get different results). Its accuracy would also be questioned because of the high proportion of young women with a palpable but not enlarged (and therefore normal) spleen. As a rule, the presence of flagrantly distorted physical findings is commonly appreciated. These physical findings are assessed with precision and accuracy.

Less common findings (such as rare skin lesions) and less flagrant distortions of common findings (such as mild swelling of a joint) are often unreliable because multiple observations by the same or other physicians yield a large distribution of results. These findings may be also inaccurate, in that they are difficult to relate with certainty to a specific pathophysiological situation. This is one reason that experienced clinicians are often called upon to ascertain the presence or absence of abnormal physical findings and their meaning in the context of patient complaints.

Historical data are not commonly viewed in terms of accuracy and precision, but they are also governed by the same rules. A patient who can give a consistent history is giving information of several different types. First is the list of symptoms-sensations. By and large, patients are able and willing to tell physicians about their uncomfortable sensations. Of course, if the patient is unable to communicate for some reason or is untruthful, the accuracy is distorted. But for the most part, symptoms can be deciphered in an accurate and precise manner. Subtle qualitative aspects that have importance in identifying the pathophysiological cause of symptoms are less accurately reported. For example, people sometimes find it difficult to distinguish between sensations that are unpleasant (such as muscle soreness after strenuous-exercise) and ones that are abnormal.

Next is the nonsymptom, factual information. This detail is quite variably reported by patients-some are accurate, some inaccurate; some provide little detail, some too much; and some provide relevant detail, others extraneous information. Thus, in addition to the usual parameters of information, accuracy and precision, relevance constitutes a third parameter. It is not a parameter of the data per se, but of the data's relationship to a particular hypothesis.

The third type of data in the history is chronologic sequence, either of symptoms or of factual information. We separate chronology from other data because it is clearly a phenomenon isolated from the events themselves. Again, some people are excellent in chronologically organizing the sequence of events, while others cannot do this with any accuracy.

The patient history thus contains three relevant types of data: the symptoms, the factual details, and the chronologic ordering of events. In general, patients accurately report symptoms and do so reproducibly. Occasionally, they can be browbeaten by repeated questioning into believing they have a symptom they do not have, or they may be insecure enough about a sensation to report it as a symptom when it is not. (Deciding whether a sensation is abnormal is dealt with in the following chapter.) Factual detail is also usually reported accurately and precisely, but there are often significant errors of omission and commission. Last, chronologic information is quite variably reported, and it is difficult to make generalizations about groups of patients.

The patient does not relate a history in a vacuum. As we mentioned earlier, history taking is an interactive process that involves significant participation by the physician, and experienced clinicians tailor the interaction to meet the needs of the situation. A withdrawn patient needs to be encouraged, and an uninhibited patient needs to be guided. In all cases, accuracy is a quality of the interaction. It depends upon the way the physician interprets what the patient says and reformulates the data. Physicians may wholly discount certain purported events and sensations if there is no corroborating information. More commonly, they seek to clarify any ambiguity and thus establish the degree of accuracy. Precision is only occasionally a problem, although subtle and not-so- subtle changes in emphasis and shadings of meaning are often present on repeated questioning. Mrs. Halprin, for example, recalled being treated with a sulfa drug the second time she was examined, but not the first.

In summary, there are three common sources of patient-based data—the patient who relates a history, the physician who performs a physical examination, and the laboratory that produces the test results. Supplementary factual information is occasionally provided by family, friends, local health departments, places of employment, and so on. Surrogate information for a patient who cannot relate symptoms may be sought from a close relative or friend.

Accuracy and precision are parameters that define the quality of the information. Whether the information is relevant to a given hypothesis is a separate question, which we deal with in Chapter 4 on inference. Historical data may be both accurate and precise and for that reason (and others) are of paramount importance. Physicians distrust working with historical data that were not obtained first hand because they may be less accurate and less precise. Laboratory data are usually very precise but of variable accuracy. Finally, physical findings are often very valuable (and in some circumstances, such as neurologic findings, irreplaceable), but in general are the least accurate and precise of all types of data.

STUDY-DERIVED DATA

The results of empirical studies constitute the other major source of data for inferences in clinical medicine. The design and analysis of clinical studies are the province of epidemiology. The field is relatively young, having developed primarily only in the last three decades, although some of its basic principles were enunciated as early as the eighteenth century. Thus, much of our information on the nature of diseases predates the current notion of the scientific study of disease. This information was obtained from uncontrolled studies. More recently, with the development of epidemiology, the principles of controlled observational and controlled clinical trials have been established. The fundamental aspects of data derived from studies differ little from patient-derived clinical data. Both must be valid (accurate) and reliable (precise). These two types of studies, uncontrolled and controlled, are the focus of this section.

Uncontrolled Studies

Clinical studies performed without an adequate control of a "normal" comparison population are uncontrolled studies. It is perhaps surprising that the vast majority of the "facts" of clinical medicine are a result of uncontrolled clinical observations concerning the signs, symptoms, natural history, and response to therapy of all known disorders. But, in fact, the results of these "unscientific" studies fill the textbooks of medicine. Does this mean that medicine is mostly hearsay? Not at all. Data obtained by careful observation have as a control the expectation of what would happen under normal circumstances. That is, the observations are made in comparison with a hypothetical control group and can be considered legitimate scientific observations.

By contrast, studies with overt control groups have provided important evidence on a relatively small number of issues. One observer has described the controlled observations as anchoring the fabric of medicine, while more cynical individuals have suggested that controlled studies predominantly confirm clinical observations and have contributed little to our overall fund of medical knowledge. Yet there is little doubt that controlled studies have provided scientific data on a variety of controversial issues. The difficulty of making unbiased observations without a control group casts a shadow over the validity of much of the uncontrolled observational database of clinical medicine. Nevertheless, uncontrollable observation remains an indispensable fund of knowledge for the clinician.

All the clinical descriptions of systemic lupus erythematosus were acquired in uncontrolled studies. Only a few clinical trials of therapeutic agents for SLE have been performed, and they have primarily dealt with immunosuppressive drugs. Thus, Dr. Williams's recommendations about Mrs. Halprin's management were based on data from published uncontrolled studies and his personal experiences, which may be considered uncontrolled observations.

Controlled Studies

Controlled studies require the comparison of one group of individuals with another, a subject group and a control group. Subjects and controls may be matched, which means that they are similar in certain specified ways. However, the individuals must also differ in at least one characteristic—the variable or variables of interest in the study. From comparison of the two groups, we learn something about the effect of the differences on the individuals who possess them. For example, patients with systemic lupus erythematosus often have diminished levels of a serum protein system collectively known as a complement. A study comparing patients with lupus with normal individuals could determine how low the levels were in lupus patients, what the range was, and whether the level correlated with disease severity or certain disease manifestations.

A minimum requirement to generate this type of data is two populations of individuals, subjects and controls (e.g., animals, cells, or even the same individuals at two points in time), and two variables (or attributes or characteristics), a dependent variable (e.g., complement levels), usually the outcome of interest, and an independent variable (e.g., the presence of lupus) that is used to define the study group. With multiple comparisons there may be more than one independent or dependent variable. We explore these comparisons in more detail in chapter 4. The conclusions of empirical studies are correlations—*a* relates to *b*, which in turn relates to *c*, and so on. To establish a valid correlation, a study must obey certain rules, which can be briefly summarized.

The Hypothesis

The first rule of study design is that a specific and testable hypothesis must be the root of the investigation. This question that the study seeks to answer will be of the nature that *a* relates (correlates) with *b*, or its stronger cousin that *a.* causes *b.* (See chap. 6 for a discussion of causal relationships.)

The Population

The second aspect of major importance is the identification of the subject or study population. This is not a difficult problem in laboratory studies, because in such experiments the population is usually carefully characterized. Cell types, laboratory animals, and other systems are extensively studied before investigators utilize them in formal experimentation. Clinical studies do not have the luxury of a carefully characterized study population. Thus, it is particularly important to understand how individuals were selected for a study and, on the other side, what type of people were excluded from participation.

Two problems can arise in the selection of a study population. First, the individuals selected may be biased in their responses, either in favor of the hypothesis or against it. In either case, the results cannot be relied upon. For example, if volunteer patients with lupus are enrolled from the clinic and are compared with non-volunteer hospital patients, the study runs the risk of being biased. The clinic volunteers, as a group, are likely to be less sick than the hospital patients, as a group. Accordingly, to avoid bias, steps must be taken to distribute the severely ill and the mildly ill patients equally in the experimental and the control groups. Similar examples abound in the medical literature.

The second problem is one of generalizability of the results. If the study population was unusual, then one could not reliably generalize the results to other groups of patients. This problem often arises in university-based studies, because university hospitals often treat very ill patients. Examples of this difficulty are also not hard to find in the medical literature.

In addition to questions of how the population was selected, the allocation of patients to either the study group or the control group is a major issue. To insure that the groups are comparable, most clinical experiments involve allocating the patients to one of the two groups in a random fashion such as pulling a ticket out of a hat. Ideally this should lead to identical groups, but occasionally, by chance an unequal distribution results in groups that are unequal in some relevant factor, such as age or gender. Thus, clinical studies often present a table of relevant factors and their distribution in the two groups to demonstrate that the two groups were comparable in all relevant factors. In observational studies where nature determines who is a subject and who is a control, there can be no randomization. For example, a study determining whether lupus patients have more coronary disease than normal individuals would have to match the subjects and controls for gender, age, blood pressure, and so forth. Thus, in these studies it is doubly important to ascertain that the observed differences between the affected and the normal individuals are due to the factors the investigators cite and not to some other difference between the groups.

Measurements

To establish correlations, observations and measurements must be made on the study and control populations. These data are used to establish eligibility for the study, to assess baseline characteristics, to characterize the populations, and to quantify the dependent and independent variables. As we said earlier, these measurements should be accurate (valid) and precise (reliable).

Hypotheses are often couched in vague terms, such as severity of illness, survival of patients, or presence of disease. The measurements must both quantify and reify these theoretical concepts. Sometimes one must be satisfied with an easily measured proxy or process variable.

For example, the sedimentation rate of red blood cells is often used to quantify the severity of illness. However, the relationship is quite indirect and elastic. Diseases result in inflammation, which stimulates the liver (by an unknown mechanism) to synthesize and secrete the blood stream proteins, some of which tend to coat the red blood cells. This coating diminishes the electrical repulsion of the cells, allowing them to aggregate and thus sediment faster under gravitational force. This kind of transition from an abstract entity (disease severity) to a physiologic quantifiable phenomenon (sedimentation rate) underlies observational measurements.

To achieve unbiased measurements, clinical trials are often "blinded." That is, the subjects do not know whether they are taking the drug or a placebo (single blind), and the observers do not know who is part of the experimental group and who is a member of the control group (double blind). Analyzing the data without this knowledge is sometimes done (triple blind) and is a further check on the introduction of bias. Observational studies sometimes can be blinded but often cannot be because the difference between the subject group and the control group is too noticeable—like our study of lupus patients and heart disease.

STUDY DESIGN

The issue that most people focus on when they evaluate the validity of a study is design. We have already alluded to two broad categories of studies—experimental and observational. In the former, subjects are manipulated by the investigator, often by receiving a certain therapy. In the latter, people are observed for the occurrence of natural events. These surveys often study the risk factors associated with the production of disease. Clinical trials (double blind) are the prototype clinical experiment. However, it is important to recognize that both case reports and small patient series of diagnostic or therapeutic interventions are experimental studies (usually uncontrolled) as well. These studies use informal comparison groups, such as an expected course of the disorder, based on previous experience or on the natural history of the disease. Again, to draw any conclusions, some sort of comparison is necessary.

Observational Studies and Trials

Surveys create a comparison group by matching rather than by randomizing. A matched population is a group of individuals who are as closely identical to the observed group as possible except for the characteristic of interest, such as exposure to a hazard. This usually involves matching groups for age, gender, ethnic background, and so on. These factors are known as *confounders*, because unless they are accounted for, they can confound the interpretation. If the matching is perfect, then in theory, the only source of the observed difference between the groups is due to the unmatched variable. Both methods, randomization and matching, have limitations, since one can never be certain that all the potential confounders are equivalent in both groups. This problem is virtually nonexistent in laboratory studies, because of the homogeneity of the subject and control populations such as exist in inbred (genetically identical) laboratory animals.

Surveys in the past have documented the relationship of smoking to heart disease, hypertension to stroke, and many other "risk factors" for disease. Whereas experiments (including trials) can only go forward in time, surveys can include phenomena from the past, present, or future. Both experiments and prospective cohort studies (observational studies that follow a group of individuals, a cohort, forward in time) examine subjects initially, then follow them at points in the future. In an experiment, the investigator treats the subject groups and sham treats (placebo) the control group. In a prospective survey, the investigator notes all the relevant information initially, then lets nature take its course. At the end of an experiment, the investigator will relate differences between the randomized treated group and the control group to the intervention. Similarly, the survey investigator will relate what happens to the individuals, such as the development of disease, to differences that were noted at the initial evaluation.

Cross-sectional Studies

Unlike experiments, surveys can look for differences in other time frames. Cross-sectional studies examine populations for correlations that exist at a point in time. Surveys that correlate diet to heart disease or cancer in large populations, such as by countries, are usually cross-sectional. From historical documents, these kinds of studies can examine conditions in the past, such as the relationship between crowding and the incidence of tuberculosis at the tum of the century.

Retrospective Studies

The last type of study we will mention is the case control or the case referent design. In these studies, the investigator identifies cases of a certain disorder and then tries to match them with similar individuals without the disorder. The cases are then examined for a factor or factors that might correlate with the presence of disease. Young women with lupus have been compared with controls for the use of birth control pills, and patients with mesothelioma (a rare type of cancer) have been compared with controls for exposure to asbestos. The relationship between maternal rubella (German measles) and certain congenital defects was first demonstrated by this type of investigation. Many important association s have been identified using this study design. However, it has some problems. Primarily, it is difficult to match cases to controls for all relevant factors.

CORRELATIONS

From all these types of studies, conclusions of the following type are made: "The treated group had four times fewer infections than the placebo group"; "the use of this drug increased the risk of heart disease by twofold"; or "The accidental exposure to this chemical increased the rate of cancer by 3,400 percent." Regardless of what study design was used to acquire the data, the final form of the analysis always involves a comparison or correlation. As we shall see in chapter 4, these comparisons lead to inferences about disease causation, treatment effects, and so on. The crucial question concerning these comparisons is the source the observed differences arise from. There are four possibilities: (1) inherent differences between the groups; (2) differences in the way the groups were studied; (3) random variation; and (4) the hypothesized source of the difference (e.g., the treatment). Possibilities (1) and (2) are problems if the study has a problem in its design. Possibility (3) is a problem if the observed difference could be due to chance, and this possibility is discussed in the next chapter. (4) is what the investigator would like to conclude.

It is to controlled clinical trials that we owe the documentation of the efficacy of many therapeutic interventions. However, it is important to keep in mind that the demonstration of efficacy is not the only relevant consideration in making a decision about a particular therapy. It is also necessary to consider whether a therapeutic effect is worth any associated toxicity, whether the proper outcome measures were used in the clinical trials, and whether the clinical effect was sufficiently large to justify the potential hazards of the therapy.

Medicine is a scientific enterprise, and much of the knowledge base is acquired in controlled studies. Until the 1940s, the idea of a controlled study had not been well formulated, and their use was rare. Now virtually no other type of planned investigation is performed. Physicians must learn the fundamentals of study design and analysis simply to read the articles that report the results of studies. A knowledge of the advantages and deficiencies of controlled studies and of the role they play in weaving the fabric of medical knowledge is of major importance in understanding the character of the clinical process.

RECOMMENDED READING

Chalmers, T.C., H. Smith, Jr., B. Blackburn et al. "A Method for Assessing the Quality of a Randomized Control Trial." Controlled Clinical Trials 2 (1981): 31-49.

Colton, T. Statistics in Medicine. Boston: Little, Brown, 1974. Clinically oriented statistics text.

Der Simonium, R., L. J. Charette, B. McPeek, and F. Mosteller. "Reporting on Methods in Clinical Trials." New England Journal of Medicine 306 (1982): 1332-37. Ellis, B. Basic Concepts of Measurement.London: Cambridge University Press, 1966.

Philosophic approach.

Elston, R. C., and W. D.Johnson. Essentials of Biostatistics. Philadelphia: F. A. Davis, 1987.

Feinstein, A. R. Clinical Epidemiology: The Architecture of Clinical Research. Philadelphia: W. B. Saunders, 1985. Advanced text.

---. Clinimetrics. New Haven, Yale University Press, 1987. Quantification of clinical data.

Feinstein, A. R., B. R. Josephy, and C. K. Wells. "Scientific and Clinical Problems in Indexes of Functional Disability." Annals of Internal Medicine 105 (1986): 413-20. Difficulties with global outcome measures of patient outcome.

Fletcher, R. H., S. W. Fletcher, and E. H. Wagner. Clinical Epidemiology. Baltimore: Williams and Wilkins, 1982. Clinically oriented introduction.

Freedman, G. Primer of Epidemiology. New York: McGraw-Hill, 1974. Introductory text.

Freedman, L., C. Furberg, and D. DeMets. Fundamentals of Clinical Trials. Boston: Wright PSG, 1985. Basic text.

Gaines, P. F., R. J. Mayewski, A. I. Mushlin, and P. Greenland. "Selection and Interpretation of Diagnostic Tests and Procedures." Annals of Internal Medicine 94 (1981): 553-600. Good summary.

Galen, R. S., and S. R. Gambino. Beyond Normality.New York: Wiley, 1975. A clinical laboratory viewpoint.

Kleinbaum, D., L. Kupper, and H. Morgenstern. Epidemiological Research. Belmont, Calif.: Lifetime Learning, 1982. Advanced text.

Kong, A., 0. Barnett, F. Mosteller, and C. Younte. "How Medical Professionals Evaluate Expressions of Probability." New England Journal of Medicine 315 (1986): 740-44. Also related letters, 316,549-51, 1987. How we speak in numbers.

Michael, M., T. Boise, and A. Wilcox.BiomedicalBestiary:AnEpidemiologicalGuide to the Flaws and Fallacies of Medical Literature. Boston: Little, Brown, 1984. Engaging introduction to critical reading.

Murphy, C. A. A Companion to Medical Statistics. Baltimore: Johns Hopkins Univer- sity Press, 1985.

Nagel, E. "Measurement." In A. Danto and S. Morgenbesser, eds., Philosophy of Science. New York: World Publishing, 1960. Philosophy of science approach.

Nunnally, J. Psychometric Theory. New York: McGraw-Hill, 1978. Classic psychology text.

Rothman, K. J. Modern Epidemiology. Boston: Little, Brown, 1986. Sophisticated introduction.

Sackett, D. L., R. B. Haynes, and P. Thgwell. Clinical Epidemiology: A Basic Science for Clinical Medicine. Boston: Little, Brown, 1985.

Weed, L. L. Medical Records, Medical Education and Patient Care. Cleveland: Press of Case Western Reserve University, 1969. Innovative discussion of medical record keeping.

Wulff, H. Rational Diagnosis and Treatment. Oxford: Blackwell, 1976. Discusses measurement in clinical medicine.

CHAPTER 4

Inductive Inference

In the previous chapter, we discussed the major sources and types of clinical data and their characteristics—their accuracy or validity and their precision or reproducibility. We now consider how these data can be used to arrive at defensible conclusions about the state of a patient's health.

The first part of our discussion focuses on the general character of inductive (probabilistic) inference, and this leads us into an examination of some of the basic notions of probability theory and statistics. We then turn to such specific modes of clinical reasoning as inferring normalcy, inferring disease, and diagnostic testing. The chapter concludes with a brief examination of other types of inductive inference that are relevant to clinical practice.

PROBABILITY, PART I: A GENERAL ORIENTATION

As you will recall, Drs. Barton and Williams entertained many diagnoses as they acquired more and more data on Mrs. Halprin. But the diagnostic circle gradually narrowed until fever, pericarditis, and a variety of laboratory findings caused SLE to emerge as the most probable diagnosis. A positive DNA antibody test made the case for SLE overwhelming.

Now the interesting and disturbing thing is that no one can be absolutely certain that Mrs. Halprin has SLE. As Dr. Barton noted, there are no pathognomic features (or "gold standard") of SLE—that is, no features of the disease serve as its definitive conditions. There is no criterion validity. As a result, when SLE is a diagnostic possibility, physicians look for data that make the disease probable and then attempt to raise its probability by testing for additional nonpathognomic features of the disease, such as hypocomplementemia and elevated DNA binding.

One need not turn to elusive disease such as lupus, however, to find physicians faced with uncertainties. Consider Dr. Barton's report that Mrs. Halprin had "spiked a fever to 102°." Even such an apparently straightforward statement is actually the product of a number of background assumptions and inferences. For example, how trustworthy (precise) is the reading? Was the thermometer shaken down, was it in place long enough, was it read correctly, had the patient just drunk something hot? In short, how likely were we to get the same reading if we had retaken her temperature with the same or a different thermometer?

Suppose, as we usually do, that the temperature was taken properly. What about the thermometer itself? Was it biased to register too high or too low? If it was in good working order the day before, can we assume it was working the day Mrs. Halprin's temperature was taken? And what about Mrs. Halprin? How good an indicator of her core temperature was her oral temperature? Did she breathe excessively through her mouth so that her oral temperature was misleading? How did her temperature compare with that of the general population? Is it correct to conclude that, for her, a temperature of 102° F was febrile?

A physician who had serious doubts about any of these questions could take simple steps to allay them. The physician could retake the temperature, use a second thermometer, take the rectal temperature, ask Mrs. Halprin how her temperature varies, and so on. The practical problem of establishing Mrs. Halprin's temperature is not difficult. Yet notice that no matter how many additional steps a physician may take to establish the claim that Mrs. Halprin has a temperature of 102° F and is febrile, it is always possible that this conclusion may be wrong.

The conclusion is one based on an inductive or probabilistic inference. The conclusion is probable (to some degree or other) relative to the evidence, and additional evidence may make the conclusion more probable. Yet, no matter how much evidence is acquired, the conclusion will always fall short of a mathematical certainty.

This is no reason for despair. We all manage to live in a world without certainties, one in which we must deal with imperfect information under conditions in which things we prize are at risk. In this sense, and to some extent, we are all hostages to fortune. What is true in our daily lives is also true in clinical medicine. It is by the use of probabilities that we attempt to minimize our risks and reduce our uncertainties. The fact that we cannot act in full knowledge does not mean we must act in total ignorance.

The role played by probabilistic reasoning in medicine goes far beyond such simple matters as establishing a patient's temperature. The pathologist's diagnosis of a biopsied tissue as malignant is based on an inductive inference. The surgeon's decision to operate for an appendicitis involves weighing the probability of the outcomes resulting from that choice against those of the other options available. Deciding the effectiveness of a particular drug, the choice of surgical procedures, the diagnostic relevance of a particular finding, the preference for medical rather than surgical treatment, the significance of a factor as an indicator of risk – all these and many more decisions like them involve probability estimates.

Probabilities constitute the backbone of inductive inference and decision making under risk, and both processes are essential elements in contemporary clinical medicine. Traditionally, physicians made decisions by drawing on the reserves of accumulated medical experience and relying on intuition and anecdotal information. To a large extent, this is still the case, but now medicine as a scientific discipline has become aware of the significance of analyzed, self-critical experience, and this has encouraged the deliberate use of statistical methods in clinical studies.

We obtain medical probabilities in two ways. First, we estimate probabilities from the data at our disposal. Thus we know from previous experience that SLE is "a relatively common disease," occurring in as many as one out of every thousand women in some populations. We also know from previous experience that there is a high correlation between lupus and elevated DNA binding. This information allows us to estimate both the probability of seeing lupus in a given patient and also the probability of finding elevated DNA binding in patients suspected of having lupus. By using statistical techniques, we can insure the reliability of such information and refine the estimated probabilities based upon it. Because of this, the use of statistical methods has become a sine qua non for acceptable research in clinical medicine.

Second, physicians engage in probabilistic reasoning to arrive at new probabilities from ones that they already have assigned. At the most informal level, we saw Dr. Williams assign a higher probability to lupus once he learned of the elevated DNA binding. However, such reasoning can be made more explicit and formalized by means of the probability calculus. Now that computers have become part of medical practice, programs are available that use inductive methods to calculate diagnostic probabilities.

As these simple examples indicate, it is essential for the contemporary clinician to have a firm grasp of at least the rudiments of probability and statistics. They are too tightly woven into the fabric of current scientific medicine for any physician to remain ignorant of their nature, uses, and limitations.

PROBABILITY, PART II: FOUR CONCEPTS AND A COMPROMISE

We typically talk about the probability of an event as though the meaning of probability were as invariant as the meaning of mass in classical physics. The truth is, there are various concepts of probability. That is, the term probability has several different meanings, and different ways of determining probabilities are required by the various concepts. Thus when Dr. Williams concluded that lupus was a probable diagnosis on the basis of its high prevalence, he was thinking of probabilities in terms of the frequency of cases of lupus in large populations. That is the statistical sense of probability. By contrast, when he concluded on the basis of the evidence before him that it was highly probable that a particular patient, Mrs. Halprin, had lupus, he could not have been thinking of probability in the statistical sense. For that concept of probability does not deal with the relationship between a body of evidence and a single hypothesis.

In this section, we review four common concepts of probability and consider their appropriateness for use in clinical medicine. We show that each has disadvantages associated with it, and we conclude that a compromise notion of probability comes closest to satisfying the needs of medicine and representing its actual practice.

The Logical Concept

Physicians are exposed to the logical concept of probability in their studies of Mendelian genetics. If A is a dominant gene and a is its recessive allele, then crossing an Aa parent with an Aa parent yields offspring of four possible genotypes: AA, Aa, aA, aa. Each of the genotypes AA, Aa, and aA produce phenotypically indistinguishable individuals having the dominant characteristic. Assuming that each genotype is equally likely, as we do in Mendelian genetics, we can conclude that the probability of a given offspring having the dominant character is 3/4, while that of an offspring having the recessive character is 1/4.

On the other hand, suppose an individual is phenotypically dominant. What is the probability that it is of the genotype AA? Since the possibilities are AA, Aa, aA, and each is equally likely, the probability is 1/3.

The conception of probability that our genetic examples illustrate is quite simple. We analyze a chance situation into possibilities that are logically exhaustive, disjoint, and equally likely. The probability of a given outcome is then defined as the ratio of the number of possibilities in which the outcome is realized to the total number of possibilities. Since this approach defines probability in terms of a ratio that is logically determined, it is called a logical concept. The particular version presented here is the earliest and simplest account of probability and is known as the classical or Laplacian approach.

Notice that this account is actually a proposal concerning the meaning of probability claims. As a proposal about meaning, it is open to an obvious conceptual objection: the definition is circular. The phrase "equally likely cases" occurs in the definition and so, in a quite literal sense, the notion of probability is used to define probability. (More recent versions of the logical approach attempt to resolve this difficulty, but such efforts go beyond the scope of our concerns.)

The problem of specifying all possible outcomes makes the logical approach inappropriate for virtually all medical uses. (About the only exception is genetic counseling for diseases that follow Mendelian patterns or heritability.) No physician who gives a patient a 90 percent probability of surviving a surgical procedure can have the classical approach in mind. Nor can the physician's reasoning be sensibly interpreted as based on it. After all, what possibilities could he or she have in mind? It would be nonsense to say the patient will either survive or die and so has a 50150 chance of surviving. The situation the patient is in simply does not resemble one in which we say that we will draw either a red card or a black card from the deck. Nor would it do any better to say the patient either survives without incident, survives with difficulty, or dies. We could always redescribe the situation and increase the number of possibilities, and so we would never be able to get the exhaustive and exclusive list required by the logical concept. But even if we could get a satisfactory list of possibilities, how would we know that each outcome is equally likely? The logical concept is clearly not the understanding of probability that is appropriate for clinical medicine.

The Statistical Concept

Medical researchers conduct many surveys and trials. It is through such studies that we could establish that lupus often flares after the patient has had extended exposure to the rays of the sun. (Dr. Williams considered Mrs. Halprin's visit to the beach relevant to his hypothesis that she had lupus.) Now let us suppose that we know from a reliable study that 15 percent of patients presenting with the features of lupus had had recent high sun exposure. Then we might conclude that the probability that a patient presenting with a lupus flare has had recent sun exposure is 15 percent. Our conclusion, based upon data rather than logical analysis, would indicate that we were using probability in the statistical sense.

Statistical probability, as the example shows, is also calculated as a ratio. The probability of an F being a G is defined as the ratio of the number of Fs that are G to the total number of Gs. If there are infinitely many Gs, then the probability is defined as the limit to which the observed ratios tend. (This is known in statistics as sampling from an infinite population.)

No logical analysis is necessary to apply this concept. We simply make observations of the Gs and keep track of those that are also Fs. If we cannot observe them all, then statistics can aid us in estimating the true probability from our observational data. The statistical concept is obviously one that is well suited for use in conjunction with the statistical methods characteristically employed in contemporary medicine.

The major conceptual difficulty with the statistical concept is that it denies meaning to the assignment of probabilities to single events or hypotheses. Probability assignments are to classes, not to individuals. Thus, questions such as "What is the probability that this patient will die tonight?" and "How likely is that diagnosis?" do not make any scientific sense in this view. We can only legitimately ask, "What proportion of the class of patients like this one will die tonight?"

A question about an individual might have a useful answer if the patient concerned is like a large number of others and so belongs to a class of patients for which we have a good statistical database. We can then reformulate the question about the individual as one about that class. For example, if the patient is in on the first postoperative day after heart transplant, then our question can be rephrased as the answerable question "What proportion of first-postoperative-day heart transplant patients die on the second night?"

Of course, sometimes data are not available to allow for such reformulations. Furthermore, it may not be clear that in moving to a reformulated question, we have chosen the correct comparison class. The physician in our example may well know the transplant statistics but believe that the patient is atypical so that those statistics cannot be reliably used.

The issue involved here is not picayune. We are looking for a concept of probability adequate to explicate the use of probability in medicine. The logical concept did not come close. That statistical concept captures a significant portion of medical usage (especially in clinical studies) but still misses much. Physicians make probability claims all the time, even when they are fully aware that no statistics currently bear on the claim in question. How are we to make sense of this practice?

The Propensity Concept

A designer of dice might appeal to the theories of physics to argue that the dice will land with equal frequency on any of their faces when thrown fairly. Indeed, a relatively straightforward application of the laws of classical mechanics will predict quite accurately the behavior of a cube landing at specific angles on a hard surface.

In general, it is quite possible to use theories to predict the frequency with which a chance mechanism will produce certain outcomes. This has led some students of probability to suggest the following definition: the probability that a given situation will produce a given outcome is the propensity of such situations to produce such outcomes. The propensity in question is taken as the theoretically predicted frequency with which the outcome will occur.

The strength of this view is that it recognizes the possibility that we may have some theoretical basis for determining the chances of a certain outcome before we have acquired any statistical data about the outcome. Thus the designer of a roulette wheel or an automotive engineer can apply physical theories to estimate probabilities in advance of the workings of their actual mechanisms. Similarly, a rheumatologist will often be able to appeal to pharmacology to give a theoretical estimate of the effectiveness of drugs in treating lupus.

The view also allows for the readjustment of estimated probabilities in the light of newly acquired data. If a rheumatologist found that a drug was not as effective in treating lupus as had been predicted, then he or she might revise the hypotheses about the nature of lupus. Theoretical propensity estimates could then be brought into line with observed frequencies. In short, propensities could serve in the absence of statistics, yet not remain unresponsive to them.

The disadvantage of this concept of probability, from the point of view of its appropriateness in clinical medicine, lies in the weakness of medical theories. All too often, medicine simply does not have available to it theories that possess the richness and degree of precision needed to derive propensities. There is reason to hope that as medical theories develop, as the mechanisms involved in biochemical and physiological functioning become better understood, then medicine will be in a stronger position to project probabilities in the absence of statistical data that bear directly on an outcome of concern.

The Subjective Concept

Physicians lacking both the statistics and the theories needed to assign a probability to a particular event are, nevertheless, often able to make a reasonably informed probability estimate based on analogies and relevant scientific data. Similarly, a physician confronted with an unusual turn of events in a common ailment does not need to rely on statistics or theoretical propensities to recognize that critical vital signs show that the patient is unlikely to survive without immediate treatment. The decision to begin treatment is based on the personal or subjective probabilities the physician assigns to the various outcomes he or she believes the patient faces.

The subjective concept of probability accounts quite well for both sorts of cases. It is based on the idea that our degree of belief that an event will occur is reflected in the risks we are willing to run on the basis of our belief. The major theoretical problem in formulating the subjective concept consists in finding a way of calibrating degrees of belief and stating conditions of coherence for them. The problem was solved in this century by L. Savage, B. DeFinetti, and F. P. Ramsey; our discussion employs DeFinetti's approach.

One way of measuring how confident people are that a given event will occur (that a given hypothesis will prove true) is to ask how much they are prepared to risk losing on a bet. Someone with a strong belief will be willing to put up more money or give greater odds than someone with a weaker belief. Thus, if we are willing to set odds of 2 to 1 against Citation winning a race, this means we are willing to pay (say) $2.00 to you if Citation wins, so long as you are willing to pay us $1.00 if he does not. By contrast, if we set the odds at 99 to 1, then we are willing to pay you $99.00 if he wins and you pay us only $1.00 if he does not. Obviously, our confidence that Citation is not going to win is stronger in the second set of odds than in the first.

Another way to look at the situation is to say that there is a combined stake of $3.00 in the first case and $100.00 in the second. If Citation wins, you will receive, respectively, 2/3 and 99/100 of the stake. If we take the odds to reflect our degree of belief (as distinct from yours) that Citation will win, then it must be 1/3 in the first case and 1/100 in the second. In this way, we now have available to us a means of calibrating degrees of belief.

Consider now why coherence becomes important. If in a two-horse race we set the odds against Citation at 2 to 1 and against the other horse at 2 to 1, then you could make money by placing a $1.00 bet on each horse. If Citation wins, you win $2.00 on him and lose $1.00 on the other horse. If the other horse wins, you win $2.00 on him and lose $1.00 on Citation. No matter which horse wins, you have a net gain of $1.00.

You have made what is known as a *Dutch book* against us. Our odds permitted you to win no matter what happened. But if we set the odds at 2 to 1 against Citation and 1 to 2 against the other horse, than neither of us would have a net gain if you took both bets.

Let us suppose you have to set odds against both horses, and you have to accept all bets for or against either horse. If you set the odds in such a way that it is logically impossible to make a Dutch book against you, then your odds for the set of events is said to be *coherent*.

DeFinetti proved that if an agent has a coherent set of odds for a set of events, then the odds can be used to define a probability measure for those events. The numerical measure derived from the odds will be a probability measure in the sense that it satisfies the axioms of a mathematical theory of probability. This condition is one that is generally accepted as definitive of the subjective concept of probability.

The conversion from odds to probability is simple. If your odds against an event e are a to b, then the subjective probability you assign to e is $b/(a + b)$.

Thus odds of 2 to 1 against Citation's winning indicate that the odds maker thinks the chances of Citation's winning are 1/3 and the chances of his not winning are 2/3. Odds of 1 to 2 in favor of Citation's winning convert to a probability of 2/3 for his losing. As this example shows, if the probabilities do not sum to 1, then the odds lead to a Dutch book.

The difficulty with the subjective approach becomes obvious when we recognize that infinitely many distinct sets of odds are coherent in the sense required by DeFinetti. Coherence offers protection only from Dutch books. Yet some coherent sets of odds are objectively better than others. For example, suppose we race a sound Derby prospect against a lame, old nag. If, in all sincerity, you set the odds at 99 to 1 against the Derby prospect and 1 to 99 against the nag, then your odds are coherent. But your belief that the nag has a chance of.99 of winning flies in the face of everything most of us know about horses. Given your ignorance, your chance of losing your money is very high.

In our view, physicians cannot avoid the use of subjective or personal probabilities. Even when statistics are available, the clinician must tailor them to fit the cases at hand. The statistics may show that a drug is effective in 90 percent of cases of a certain kind, but the clinician must determine the probability that it will be effective for this patient. However, it would be bad medical practice to assign a probability of, say, 25 to the effectiveness of the drug for a particular patient unless evidence other than the statistics could be brought into account. If the drug has been tried on this patient before without success, for example, then a probability quite different from.9 might be appropriate. But we cannot condone "off the wall" subjective probability assignments, even if they are coherent.

Some subjectivists have argued that so long as we modify our initial probability estimates with subsequent experience, then the estimates will converge toward those made by others exposed to the same evidence. Thus, defenders of the view that no matter what probability was initially assigned to the diagnosis of lupus in Mrs. Halprin's case, competent observers would converge on the same probability, given the same evidence. This may or may not be so. The issues involved are complicated and controversial, and we can only express our reservations about the subjective view as an adequate account of the way of assigning probabilities.

A Compromise View

One way of modifying the subjective view to make it more suitable as a basis for clinical practice is to place constraints, in addition to coherence, on the odds maker. One source of such constraints might be objective dispositions or propensities expressed as probabilities based on statistical or theoretical considerations.

On this view, a patient has, say, a certain propensity, measured probabilistically, to have a drug reaction. The physician then employs a subjective estimate of the objective propensity, and that estimate is based on whatever relevant statistics, theories, and experiences are available to the physician.

Where statistics are inadequate for a probability assignment to a propensity, then the physician must base the decision on personal estimates of the objective propensities for this patient's responses. Still relevant are such items of background information as statistics about analogous situations, theories, and clinical experience.

This compromise view helps explain how it is possible for two clinicians to be practicing good medicine, even though they differ in their assessments of a patient's chances of recovery or of having a certain disease. For example, suppose Dr. Williams and Dr. Barton had been asked to make a probability estimate of lupus on the basis of their initial examination of Mrs. Halprin. It is quite possible that their estimates would have been significantly different, even though they relied on the same information and the same statistical data. Viewing the same evidence, they might have assigned different weights or different degrees of relevance to it. Consequently, even though the two clinicians disagreed, neither had to be considered wrong at that time. (Of course, additional information or subsequent events may show that one or the other or even both of them were wrong in their estimates.) When the evidence is not overwhelming, then rational people may disagree.

The compromise view also helps explain why clinicians strive to establish objectively informed estimates of probabilities. Such information is crucial to the clinician's effort in making a subjective estimate of propensity in particular cases. Otherwise, the clinician is faced with the task of making a purely personal estimate. Such an estimate may be a very good one, but it lacks the objective basis a probability assignment can provide.

As even this brief review reveals, the foundations of probability and statistics are still very unsettled. Logicians are not certain of what, if anything, we are measuring or how we should measure it when we assess chances and reasons from statistics. However, despite such uncertainties, it cannot be denied that probabilistic reasoning and assessments generally produce successful predictions.

THE INVERSE PROBABILITY LAW

The core of probability theory is the probability calculus. It provides both a method for calculating probabilities and a codification of the laws of probability. These laws hold true whether probability is interpreted logically, statistically, subjectively, or as propensity. Thus many, though not all, students of probability view the probability calculus as a defining condition of probability. A notion that failed to obey its laws would simply not count as a probability measure.

The probability calculus can be encapsulated in a set of explicit axioms from which all other laws of probability can be derived. However, we present neither axioms nor derivations here. We limit our discussion to a theorem of the probability calculus that has very important medical applications--the inverse probability law.

We will use two notations for probability in our subsequent discussion. "Prob( )=X" and "Prob (/)=Y" will stand, respectively, for absolute and conditional probability. If we state that the probability of drawing a face card from a deck is 3/13, then we are giving an absolute probability. By contrast, if we state that the probability of drawing a face card given that the card drawn is a jack or deuce is 1/3, then we are giving a conditional probability. Using our notation we could write these two probabilities:

$$\text{Prob (face card)} = 3/13;$$
$$\text{Prob (face card/jack or deuce)} = 1/2.$$

(Here expressions such as *face card* abbreviate sentences such as *You draw a face card*.)

The inverse probability law may be stated in this way:

$$\text{If Prob } (p) \neq 0 \text{ and Prob } (q) \neq 0, \text{ then}$$
$$\text{Prob } (q/p) = \frac{\text{Prob } (q) \times \text{Prob } (p/q)}{\text{Prob } (p)}.$$

Thus the probability of a diagnosis given a set of symptoms can be calculated from the absolute probability of the diagnosis, the absolute probability of the symptoms, and the probability of the symptoms given that diagnosis.

Recall that after tentatively diagnosing Mrs. Halprin's case as lupus, Dr. Williams sought to raise the probability of the diagnosis by testing for elevated DNA binding. Suppose that prior to the test he assigned a probability of.01 to Mrs. Halprin's having lupus. Suppose, for ease in calculation, that the probability of elevated DNA binding given lupus is.6 and that the absolute probability of elevated DNA binding is.01. Then the probability of Mrs. Halprin's having lupus given positive results from the DNA binding test would be.6 or

$$\frac{.01 \times .6}{.01}.$$

Note that although the probability that Mrs. Halprin has lupus has been increased by a factor of 60, the tests used to clinch the diagnosis have not established it as a mathematical certainty. If we replace.6 in the calculations by.1, then the probability would be raised by a factor of 10 and still remain small (i.e., .1). This should be a warning not to jump to conclusions from nonpathognomic tests that are even 100 percent positive in the presence of a disease. If the disease has a low incidence rate, the probability of that disease might still be quite low.

Let us say, for example, that the ANA test is 95 percent positive in patients with lupus and is 20 percent positive in the general population on nonlupus patients. If the probability of the diagnosis was very low prior to the test, say.01, then the probability after a positive ANA test is

$$\frac{.01 \times .95}{.20} = 0.0475.$$

Thus, even when the test is frequently positive in diseased patients, if it is also positive in other individuals to a relatively high degree, then a positive test may not substantially raise the probability of the diagnosis of the disease.

The absolute probabilities used in the inverse probability formula are known as prior probabilities. In the first lupus example, they are the probabilities of Mrs. Halprin's having lupus prior to the DNA-binding test and the probability that she would have elevated DNA binding under any circumstances. The calculated probability is called the posterior probability, since it is used after the observation is made. The main obstacle to applying the inverse law is the lack of prior probabilities. In medical applications often the incidence of diseases and the frequencies of symptoms for diseases are available, but those of symptoms per se are not.

Bayes' Theorem

An extension of the inverse law called Bayes' theorem helps with this situation. Bayes' theorem reads as follows:

$$\text{If Prob } (p) \neq 0 \text{ and Prob } (q) \neq 0, \text{ then}$$
$$\text{Prob } (q/p) = \frac{\text{Prob } (q) \times \text{Prob } (p/q)}{\text{Prob } (q) \times \text{Prob } (p/q) + \text{Prob } (\text{not } q) \times \text{Prob } (p/\text{not } q)}.$$

We can apply this to the diagnosis-symptoms case by letting D stand for the diagnosis, S for the symptoms, and notD for the statement that the diagnosis is false. Then the Bayes' formula becomes

$$\text{Prob } (D/S) = \frac{\text{Prob } (D) \times \text{Prob } (S/D)}{\text{Prob } (D) \times \text{Prob } (S/D) + \text{Prob } (\text{not } D) \times \text{Prob } (S/\text{not } D).}$$

Here no use is made of the absolute probability of the symptoms, but only of the probability of the symptoms given various conditions.

That is, the probability of a diagnosis of lupus, given Mrs. Halprin's symptoms, is equal to the probability of the diagnosis in the general population (the prevalence) multiplied by the probability of her symptoms, given a diagnosis of lupus, which is then divided by this product plus the probability of Mrs. Halprin's not having lupus (1-prevalence) multiplied by the probability of her symptoms, given the absence of lupus.

It is easy to assign a numerical value to the probability of the disease by using a figure for prevalence, but the other values are difficult to ascertain. For illustration, let us suppose that the probability of lupus for a woman of Mrs. Halprin's age is.001 and that the probability of her nonspecific and somewhat normal findings based on her history and physical examination, given the presence of the disease, is.1. Further, let us suppose that the probability of her symptoms, given the sum of the probabilities of the alternative diagnoses, is also.1. Under these assumptions, the probability of a diagnosis of lupus, given Mrs. Halprin's manifestations is

$$.001 \times .1 = 001(.001 \times .1) + (.999 \times .1)$$

Thus Mrs. Halprin's nonspecific symptoms do not raise the probability of a diagnosis of lupus at all. These are illustrated in figure 4.1.

Let us imagine that0.1 percent of 10,000 people in the population have SLE.

We know from previous studies that only 1I 10of patients with SLE present with symptoms similar to Mrs. Halprin's flulike illness. We also know that flulike illnesses are common in the population, and we estimate their frequency to be

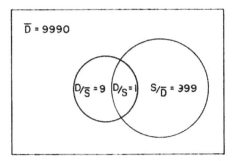

4.1. A Venn diagram illustrating Bayes' theorem. In a population of 10,000 individuals, 9,990 do not have disease (D) and 10 do (D). Of those 10, only one has a "flulike" syndrome (D/S). However, 1,000 individuals have "flulike" illness but 999 do not have SLE (S/D).

1,000 in 10,000 at any given time. We want to determine the probability that Mrs. Halprin has SLE, given her symptoms. That is, we want to solve Bayes' theorem:

$$P\,(D/S) = P\,(S/D)\frac{P(D)}{P(S)}.$$

P(D/S) is the probability of Mrs. Halprin's having SLE, given her symptoms, while *P(S/D)* is the probability of her symptoms, given that she has SLE. *P(D)* is the probability of SLE in the population, and *P(S)* is the probability of symptoms in the population. Using the values given above, we arrive at the solution

$$1/1000 = 1/10 \times \frac{10/10{,}000}{1000/10{,}000}.$$

Thus, from relatively easily obtained data or from estimates, we can calculate the probability that an individual manifesting certain signs and symptoms has a particular disease.

Such calculations also make intuitive sense. If one out of every ten normal individuals has a cold and if flulike symptoms occur as a manifestation of SLE one-tenth of the time, then having these symptoms should not suggest SLE any more than the ordinary frequency of the disease does.

Thus, the presence of flulike symptoms neither raises nor lowers the prior probability of having SLE. It is .1 percent, whether the person has flulike symptoms or not.

We return to Bayes' theorem later in the discussion of testing and review it in detail in chapter 9 in connection with decision making.

Independence

A final probabilistic concept of great importance in medicine is that of independence. Intuitively, to say that lupus is independent of leprosy is to say that one's chances of getting one are not changed once one has the other. This motivates the definition

P is independent of q just in case Prob (p) = Prob (p/q).

When two events are independent, the probability that both occur is the product of their probabilities.

Since one flip of a fair coin is independent of another, the probability of getting three heads in three Hips is (1/2)3 or 118. Similarly, the probability of having both lupus and leprosy is the product of their probabilities. Note that the flulike symptoms and SLE are independent in our previous example.

In medicine, however, independence is uncommon, and calculating conjoint probabilities is rarely easy. Berkson's bias is a clear example of how nonindependence can lead to an incorrect conclusion. It was observed that the frequency of tuberculosis and cancer occurring together in the same patient was greater than would be expected, given the prevalence of the two diseases. This led to the hypothesis that one of the diseases might be causally related to the other. However, as it turned out, the observation of the connection between the diseases was made at a referral center, and the association could be explained by the bias introduced by the referral of more severely ill patients (i.e., ones with both diseases) to the medical center. In this case, the assumption of independence was false, and the association of the two diseases proved accidental. A substantial list of experiments and clinical tests stands discredited by the revelation of false independence assumptions.

Now that we have discussed some of the fundamental concepts of probability theory, we tum to analysis of the important types of probabilistic and statistical reasoning in clinical medicine.

INFERRING NORMALITY AND INFERRING DISEASE

Clinical medicine is an enterprise that aims at promoting the health of patients. This aim gives point and purpose to its activities, and it is with respect to this aim, either directly or indirectly, that data assume their significance. For clinical medicine, data in themselves are of no particular interest or value. It is what can be done with them that is important.

In this section, we consider how data can be used to determine whether a particular finding is a "normal" one and how they can be used to establish the presence of a disease or disorder. Since both types of inference require an understanding of the basic aspects of statistical sampling procedures, it is with this topic that we begin.

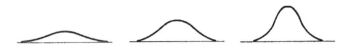

4.2. A random sample from a normally distributed population approaches a bell shape as *n* increases.

Samples and Distributions

In the introduction to the previous chapter, we raised a number of hypothetical doubts about whether we could have any confidence in a thermometer reading indicating that Mrs. Halprin had a temperature of 1 00.4o F. One of those doubts concerned whether we could trust a single measurement (or sample) out of a potentially infinite set of measurements-one thermometer reading.

The reason we are willing to rely on the single reading is that we have a large fund of experience at our disposal that assures us we are not likely to go wrong. We are reasonably certain that if we make repeated temperature measurements on the patient, the outcome will be very close to our original determination. The measurements would most likely form a normal or bell-shaped distribution around a mean value-the so-called sample mean.

As the sample size increases, as we take more and more measurements, the shape of the bell grows tighter and tighter around the sample mean (see fig. 4.2). Furthermore, as the sample size increases, the sample mean comes closer to matching the value of all temperatures taken in a similar fashion under similar circumstances-the population mean (see fig. 4.3). If the sample size grows in number and its mean fails to approach the population mean, this indicates that the sample is biased in some fashion. For example, if the thermometer used to take Mrs. Halprin's temperature was calibrated 1° too low, then as the sample size grew, its mean value would come to center at a point 1o below the population mean.

Statistically, the precision of a measurement is a reflection of the distribution of a class of measurements around the mean. In a normally distributed population, the *standard deviation* is a measurement of precision. It is a way of indicating the range of values associated with about two-thirds of the samples. Two SDs (standard deviation) encompass 95 percent of the sample, and three SDs about 99 percent. As the sample size (n) increases, the SD decreases. The SD of a sample can be determined by the following formula:

$$\sqrt{\frac{\Sigma(x \times \bar{x})^2}{n-1}} \text{ , where}$$

x = observed value;
$\bar{x}$ = mean of observed values;
n = number of observations made.

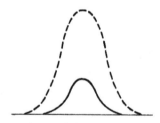

4.3. Sample mean approximates the population mean.

NON–DISEASED INDIVIDUALS

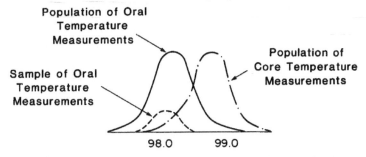

4.4.   Sample mean of oral temperatures approximates the population mean of oral temperatures but underestimates the population mean of core temperatures.

The sample mean provides a better estimate of the population mean than single determinations, in part because individual measurements are more likely to represent outliers. With multiple observations, there is regression to the mean. However, if the measurement is precise (i.e., small standard deviation), such as a temperature determination, then additional measurements are not likely to vary much.

We can state with some confidence that Mrs. Halprin's oral temperature of 100.4° as read from the thermometer is a good indicator of what her oral temperature actually was. But oral temperature is not what we are really interested in. Our concern is with the core temperature, for it is the pathophysiological representative of fever-inducing disorders. We know from empirical studies that oral temperatures tend to be somewhat (a degree or two) lower than core temperatures, although higher than axillary readings. These findings can be represented graphically as in figure 4.4.

The representation shows that the population of oral temperatures and the population of core temperatures are different. The accuracy of the oral temperature as an indicator of the core temperature is quantitatively represented by the distance between the two population means. The precision of the measurement is represented by the width of the bell -shaped curves. The precision affects the degree of overlap, but not the distance between the two peaks. Consequently, even if the oral temperature is perfectly reproducible (a very sharp peak), it will be off target for the core temperature. This is what is meant when we say that a measurement is biased. In our case, the oral temperature is biased one or two degrees below core temperature.

How might we improve the accuracy and precision of the measurement?

Precision is dependent on using a standardized routine for measuring and on the quality of the instrument. Alcohol thermometers are less precise than mercury thermometers, and keen observers are better at reading the level than careless ones. Exacting observers leave the instrument in place longer and get better readings. Electronic thermometers are more precise still.

Similarly, accuracy is improved by picking a temperature source closest to the quantity sought. Rectal is more accurate than oral, and oral is more accurate than skin surface. Still, whatever is done, one is always saddled with some irreducible distance from the quantity sought because of imprecision, inaccuracy, regression to the mean, and sample size.

However, this need not be seen as a counsel of despair. Accuracy as an ideal limit of measurement need not be achieved in order to acquire and employ the kind of data needed for clinical medicine. The use of high technology and specially trained thermometer readers could be used to determine the patient's temperature. But the gain in precision would be so slight and the need for such precision so marginal as to make the investment a bad one.

Normal versus Abnormal

Table 4.1.   Seven Meanings of the Word *Normal* Important in Medicine

Paraphrase	Domains of Use	Preferable Term
1. Having probability density function $f(x) = \frac{1}{\sqrt{\sigma^2 2\pi}} \exp\left[-\frac{1}{2}(\frac{x - \mu}{\sigma})^2 \right]$	Statistics (predicated of a metrical character)	Gaussian
2. Most representative of its class	Descriptive science (biology, etc.)	Average, median, modal
3. Commonly encountered in its class	Descriptive science	Habitual
4. Most suited to survival and reproduction	Genetics, operations research, quality control, etc.	Optimal or "fittest"
5. Carrying no penalty	Clinical medicine	Innocuous or harmless
6. Commonly aspired to	Politics, sociology, etc.	Conventional
7. Most perfect of its class	Metaphysics, aesthetics, morals, etc.	Ideal

Let us suppose then that we have accepted Mrs. Halprin's oral temperature as given by the 100.4° F reading. What are we to make of it? Is it a normal reading or might it reflect the presence of illness or some other phenomenon worth investigating? As E. A. Murphy has observed, the term normal has a variety of meanings, several of which are used in clinical medicine. (See table 4.1.)

Although ultimately we are interested in whether Mrs. Halprin's temperature is indicative of a medical problem, and thus with normality in sense (5), as shown in table 4.1, the first two senses of normality figure centrally in assessing data such as temperature readings. First of all, with a good instrument the distribution of oral temperature readings should form a Gaussian or normal (in sense (1)) distribution, that is, the readings should be randomly distributed about a mean. Furthermore, since the same homeostatic mechanisms control temperature in all human beings, a group of non-diseased people should produce a set of readings that forms a Gaussian distribution of readings around the mean of 98.6° F. Under these conditions, we can be confident that at least 99 percent of oral temperature readings taken from individuals in the group will be within 1°F of 98.6°F. Although this, in itself, says nothing about core temperatures or about the presence of disease, it does tell us there is only a small chance that Mrs. Halprin is one of those normal individuals (normal in sense (3)) whose oral temperature is 100.4° F. Thus, the observation begs for an alternative explanation, and that gives the clinician sufficient reason for further investigation.

It should be emphasized that the probabilistic reasoning applied here was predicated upon the distribution of temperature readings being Gaussian. When data are not distributed randomly about a mean, it may be difficult to conclude anything about the chance of obtaining a particular reading.

Where data do distribute normally about a mean, laboratories commonly issue reports of "normal" or "abnormal" values, according to whether or not the data falls within two standard deviations of the mean. The normal range (two SDs) is established for such tests by administering it to a group of ostensibly healthy individuals. About 95 percent of these individuals will produce results within –two SDs of the mean. Keep in mind, however, that the remaining 5 percent of presumably healthy individuals used to establish the database for the test will produce values that will be counted as "abnormal" on statistical grounds. Knowing this, one can avoid the trap of believing that a technically abnormal test result automatically indicates some pathology.

There are several very good reasons why healthy individuals have abnormal test results: (1) the reading is just one of those unlikely random events; (2) the procedure used to define the normal range excluded a subpopulation (such as the elderly) to which the individual belongs; (3) the procedure for establishing the normal range was an inappropriate indicator of a pathophysiological condition that

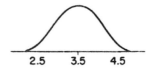

4.5. Distribution of serum potassium concentration in mg/dl in a normal population.

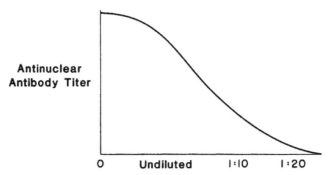

4.6. Distribution of antinuclear antibody titers in a normal population.

this is not just a theoretical argument is illustrated by the frequency of low-titer-positive ANA tests in the normal population. These results are frequently mistaken to indicate the presence of lupus.

Unfortunately, laboratory results are ordinarily not reported with the source and distribution of data from which their normal ranges are determined. A report such as that in figure 4.5 would be quite easy to include. Also it would be especially helpful if non-Gaussian distributions were available. (For example, see fig. 4.6.) Graphs such as these would not only give the clinician an idea of how many "abnormal" results to expect in healthy individuals but also make it much easier for the clinician to decide whether a given result is a strong indication of disease.

Inferring Disease

Many of the tests for the presence of a specific disease-such as sedimentation rate, blood pressure readings, or chemical assays-yield quantitative data, which can be plotted against the number of cases in which the disease is present or absent. For example, if we plot cases of diabetes against blood sugar levels we will obtain two graphs that look something like figure 4.7.

We have combined the graphs by turning one upside down. It is easy to see that the values for subjects who have the disease overlap those for the subjects who do not. (Only rarely can this type of overlap be avoided with a completely perfect test.) This gives rise to a critical question: for which values, if any, in

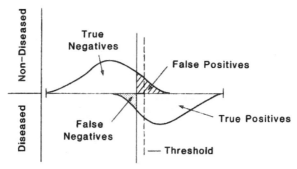

4.7. A hypothetical distribution of values for a test where the result is a continuous variable in diseased and nondiseased individuals. The vertical solid and dashed lines are two alternative thresholds of positive and negative. Moving the threshold to the right diminishes false positives but increases false negatives.

the

overlapping region is it appropriate to conclude that the patient being tested has diabetes (or whatever disease is in question)?

The usual approach to this problem is to select a threshold value and declare all cases on one side of it to be diseased and those on the other side of it to be nondiseased. We have indicated one threshold on our graph with a solid vertical line. Any threshold will divide the population into four classes:

True positives, who have the disease and are counted as having it by the test;
True negatives, who do not have the disease and are not counted as having it by the test;
False positives, who do not have the disease but are counted as having it by the test;
False negatives, who do have the disease but are not counted as having it by the test.

Obviously, both false positives (false alarms) and false negatives (false reassurances) (misses) are undesirable, but their seriousness will vary with the disease, the test, and the nature of follow-up tests and treatment. For example, false positives from a skin test for TB are not very serious, since the response to a positive skin test is perhaps only to order a chest x-ray. On the other hand, if a positive result on a test were to lead to brain surgery, then false positives would be quite serious. On the false negative side, one needs to consider the seriousness of missing a case of the disease. Missing a case of TB is quite serious, so we want to minimize the false negative rate. On the other hand, if a disease is self-limiting or has no cure or is not communicable, missing cases of it may not be of great consequence.

If we raise the threshold for the test to count as positive, we decrease the number of false positives, which simultaneously increases the number of false negatives. (We have indicated this in fig. 4.7 with a broken vertical line.) If we lower the threshold, the effect is the opposite. Thus, we can adjust one rate only at the expense of the other. (In other words, as we will see below, there is a trade-off between sensitivity and specificity.) In the case of the TB skin test, although decreasing the false negative rate causes the false positive rate to increase, this may be appropriate. A missed TB case is far more serious than a false alarm.

The analysis we have given so far leads to some other useful concepts concerning diagnostic tests.

Sensitivity and Specificity

During the case presentation Dr. Williams remarked that when four of the eleven American Rheumatism Association criteria (for lupus) are satisfied, "the result is 96 percent sensitive and specific for SLE."(See chap.7 for a fuller discussion of SLE and chap. 3 for more on clinical data.) We are now in a position to explain this remark in terms of the concepts we have developed so far.

When a test has a low false negative rate-misses few true cases of the disease-it is called a (highly) sensitive test. Since a sensitive test misses few cases of the disease it tests, the ratio of its correct positive results to the actual number of cases will be high. Thus the sensitivity of a test is defined as

$$\text{Sensitivity} = \frac{\text{True Positives}}{\text{All Cases of the Disease}}$$
$$= \frac{\text{True Positives}}{\text{True Positives} + \text{False Negatives}}.$$

Thus satisfying four of the eleven criteria, being 96 percent sensitive, is a test that misses only 4 percent of lupus cases.

When a test has a low false positive rate, it is said to be a (highly) specific test for the disease in question. The ratio of its correct negative results to the actual nondiseased cases will be high. So the specificity of a test is defined as

$$\text{Specificity} = \frac{\text{True Negatives}}{\text{All NonDiseased Cases}}$$
$$= \frac{\text{True Negatives}}{\text{True Negatives} + \text{False Positives}}$$

Thus the test of satisfying four of the eleven criteria, also being 96 percent specific for lupus, will lead to a false diagnosis of lupus in only 4 percent of patients tested.

Other useful ratios include the following two:

$$\text{False Alarm Rate} = \frac{\text{False Positives}}{\text{All NonDiseased Cases}},$$

the converse of specificity.

$$\text{False Reassurance Rate} = \frac{\text{False Negatives}}{\text{All Diseased Cases}},$$

the converse of sensitivity.

We can also express all four notions in the terms of conditional probability. Thus

Sensitivity = Prob(Positive/Diseased);
Specificity = Prob(Negative/Nondiseased);
False Alarm Rate = Prob(Positive/Nondiseased);
False Reassurance Rate = Prob(Negative/Diseased).

Furthermore, we can relate these values through Bayes' theorem. Thus the positive predictive value of a test, that is, the probability of the disease given a positive test result, is

$$\text{Prob}(D(\text{iseased})/\text{Pos}(\text{itive})) = \frac{\text{Prob}(D)\text{Prob}(Pos/D)}{\text{Prob}(Pos)}$$
$$= \frac{\text{Prob}(D)\text{Prob}(Pos/D)}{\text{Prob}(D)\text{Prob}(Pos/D) + \text{Prob}(\text{not}D)\text{Prob}(Pos/\text{not}D)}$$
$$= \frac{\text{Prob}(D) \times \text{Sensitivity}}{\text{Prob}(D) \times \text{Sensitivity} + \text{Prob}(\text{not}D) \times \text{False Alarm Rate}}$$
$$\text{or}$$
$$1 - \text{specificity}$$

Figure 4.7 illustrates this trade-off between sensitivity and specificity. As the threshold moves to the left, sensitivity increases; as the threshold moves to the right, specificity increases. A convenient way of representing this trade-off is the receiver operating characteristic curve (ROC), which plots sensitivity (true positive rate) against I minus specificity (false positive rate). A test with no information content is a straight line at a 45° angle from the origin. Most tests are bowed up and to the left, as in figure 4.8.

The optimal operation point can be calculated from this expression:

$$\frac{p(D-)}{p(D+)} \cdot \frac{(C_{fp} - C_{tn})}{(C_{fn} - C_{tp})}.$$

$p(D-)$ = probability a disease is absent; $p(D+)$ = probability a disease is present; C_{fp} = cost (i.e., utility) of a false positive; C_{tn} = cost of a true negative; C_{fn} = cost of a false negative; C_{tp} = cost of a true positive. That is, the optimal point for a given test is inversely proportional to the prevalence of disease. Thus, the optimum ratio of true positives to false positives for a disease with low prevalence is high or further down and to the left. The opposite is true for a disease with high prevalence. Notice that, all things being equal, if the cost (utility) of a false positive result is high, the optimal operating point is also further down and to the left. Screening for AIDS in the general population is an example of the above characteristics: low prevalence and high cost (psychologic) of a false positive.

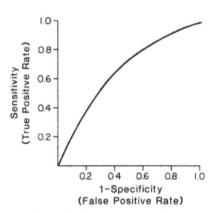

4.8.   The receiver-operator curve (ROC) for a hypothetical test.

Sometimes the cost of a test is incommensurate with its value. For example, a test may be valuable to diagnose a nonfatal disease, but it may very rarely cause death. Such instances have been very troublesome to decision analysts and critics of decision analysis. There is a methodology for evaluating test utility that does not depend on developing commensurate cost dimensions, but it utilizes information theory and is beyond the scope of this book.

Different tests can be compared on the same ROC graph. Each test is represented by a single curve, and the one that is further up and toward the left is a better discriminator of diseased versus nondiseased individuals. Of course, one should keep in mind that <u>the performance of a test under ideal circumstances (efficacy) may diverge substantially from its performance in the real world (efficiency).</u>

Although epidemiologists are likely to be concerned with the distribution of positive and negative results in diseased and nondiseased populations (and thus with the sensitivity and specificity of a test), practicing clinicians want to know how likely it is that a patient is diseased given a positive test. They are concerned with the predictive values of a test. Unfortunately, these values must be approached with an important caveat. A test's predictive value will vary with the prior probability of the disease, unlike its sensitivity and specificity.

In practical terms this means that the predictive value of the test will vary according to the prevalence of disease in the subpopulation of patients being examined. For example, if we use the TB skin test, which is highly sensitive, in screening an ordinary cross section of the population, the probability that a given individual has the disease given a positive test is considerably less than that for an individual selected from a population in which TB is rampant, say immigrants from Southeast Asia.

A sensitive but not specific test for SLE is the antinuclear antibody (ANA)

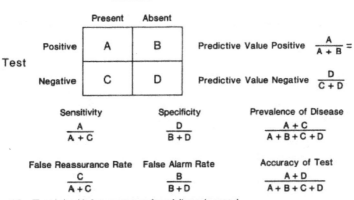

4.9. The relationship between test results and disease in general.

test. The ANA test is positive in 95 percent of patients with lupus, but it is also frequently positive in other diseases. Its specificity is not more than 80 percent.

By contrast, the double-stranded DNA-binding test is virtually never positive in patients who do not have lupus. It has a specificity of 99 percent. However, the test is frequently negative in patients with lupus. Its sensitivity is 60 percent. Thus, the test is specific but not sensitive. Their relationships are represented in figures 4.9, 4.10, and 4.11.

The Value of Clinical Testing

When Mrs. Halprin first entered the hospital, she was given a battery of tests aimed at determining the nature of her disease and its extent. As the discussion between her physicians indicated, this was no matter of ordering a hodgepodge of vaguely relevant tests and weighing the results against each other. That naive approach is unacceptable for at least three reasons.

First, there is a plethora of tests available for many diagnostic entities. It is neither practical nor sensible for a physician to order anything like the whole range of possible tests merely for the purpose of generating additional data that may be of use. In addition, serious doubts about the relative efficacy of many tests make their use without a clear end in view doubly unwise. Second, there has been a dramatic increase in the number of invasive tests that have associated with them well-defined rates of morbidity and mortality. The use of such tests obviously demands a careful evaluation of their risks and benefits. Third, the increase in surveillance of medical practice by the government and third-party insurers provides a strong motive to employ only tests that are of demonstrable diagnostic usefulness.

Generally speaking, the value of a diagnostic test depends on the relationship between the characteristics of the test, the purpose the test is supposed to serve, the pretest probability of disease, the safety and efficacy of therapy, and the costs of correct and incorrect diagnoses. This can be seen most clearly by considering the five most common circumstances in which tests are considered appropriate.

Screening for Multiple Diseases

The usual battery of admissions tests, such as the blood and urine tests given to Mrs. Halprin, for the most part screen for a broad range of disorders. They are highly sensitive tests that usually give abnormal readings when the patient is ill. However, most are not specific-they flag illness without identifying it, and they may yield a significant percentage of false positives. Thus liver function tests will indicate whether a liver is diseased but may not distinguish cirrhosis from hepatitis. The commonly screened disorders are ones that are highly prevalent. It does not make sense to screen for rare diseases because even if one uses a highly sensitive test its predictive value will be low due to the small value of Prob(D).

Case Finding

Once Dr. Williams had evolved some diagnostic hypotheses, it made sense to search for single diseases. Again the team used highly sensitive tests, such as the antinuclear antibody test for SLE. These tests are known to register positively in the presence of these specific diseases but may also give positive results due to other factors. As before, it does not pay to use such screening tests if the disorder has a low prior probability for the patient being tested. The low value of Prob(D) pulls down the predictive value of the test. Thus it is difficult to screen for rare genetic disorders, such as phenylketonuria or Lesch-Nyhan disease, even when tests very sensitive for them are available. Finally, any screening test employed with a large number of patients should be low in both cost and morbidity.

Excluding Disease

Certain forms of screening are an attempt to exclude disease in high-risk populations. Stool Hemoccult and sigmoidoscopy examinations in men over age fifty are forms of screening that require high sensitivity (few false positives), but also reasonably high specificity. A false positive may require an expensive follow-up procedure, and because screening involves a large number of individuals, the cost may be considerable.

Confirming a Diagnosis

Tests with a high degree of specificity are useful in confirming a diagnosis. That is why Dr. Williams's team ordered the DNA antibody test. Highly specific tests tend to be more costly than screening tests, if for no reason other than they are less frequently performed. Also many, such as biopsies or angiograms, are risky. Thus they come later in the diagnostic process, when, owing to a greater confidence in the tentative diagnosis, both physicians and patients are more willing to tolerate their negative features.

Histologic evaluations of biopsy material are perhaps the tests most commonly used for diagnostic confirmation. These tests are considered highly specific, but they also involve high costs and often high patient risk. It is also important to note that histologic diagnoses lack the degree of criterion validity they once had. They are no longer the "gold standard" they were considered to be. This change has been the result of well-documented observer variability in histopathologic diagnoses, a discordance between clinical syndrome defined by patient outcome and histologic syndrome, and the need for pathologists to determine subtle differences using only small amounts of tissue. Once it was the pathologist who was assumed to have all the answers, but we now know that there is more to confirming a diagnosis than pathologic findings.

In general, if the disease is serious and good therapy is available and if false positive test results are not very harmful, then the test should be constructed to maximize sensitivity. By contrast, if the treatment is costly or marginally beneficial and if false positive diagnoses are harmful, then the test should maximize specificity.

Tests for Prognosis

While most tests come into existence for diagnostic purposes, they frequently become established as useful predictors of either disease outcome or disease activity. Tests that correlate with prognosis are helpful in informing the patient about his or her condition, but they also help the clinician with management. More complete knowledge of patient outcome provides a basis for significant changes in medication and ancillary services.

Mrs. Halprin's prognosis was presumed to be good when a kidney biopsy showed that she had only mild renal disease. Thus, the clinical team had a basis for deciding to treat her with low-dose prednisone and hydroxychloroquine.

Management Tests

Some tests are primarily performed as an adjunct to patient management. For example, the results of coronary angiography and various other radiologic procedures are often used to aid in deciding whether to intervene surgically, whether or not the results have diagnostic or prognostic importance.

It is important to bear in mind the purpose of a test when ordering it or when evaluating its results. However, it is equally important to remember that a test ordered for one purpose may also serve other purposes, depending upon the clinical circumstances.

Bayes' Theorem and Sequential Testing

In modern medical practice, it is quite common to administer a battery of tests to generate a diagnostic conclusion. Some authors, in attempting to find the "logic of diagnosis," have analyzed this process by means of Bayes' theorem. The analysis usually proceeds on the assumption that the tests are administered sequentially, which is usually preferable to simultaneous testing. To illustrate, we can let T_1, T_2, and so on stand for positive findings from each successive test. Using the inverse probability law here for simplicity, Prob(D/T_1) is calculated from the prior probability of disease Prob(D) by

$$\text{Prob}(D/T_1) = \frac{\text{Prob}(D) \times \text{Prob}(T_1/D)}{\text{Prob}(T_1)}.$$

Then, Prob(D/T_2) is obtained by replacing Prob(D) by Prob(D/T_1) and applying the formula

$$\text{Prob}(D/T_2) = \frac{\text{Prob}(D/T_1) \times \text{Prob}(T_2/D)}{\text{Prob}(T_2)},$$

with the process continuing until the tests are exhausted or an arbitrary point of "confirmation" is reached.

There is a serious problem with this type of analysis however. Responses to clinical tests are frequently probabilistically dependent. Thus, given that the first test has been positive, it may be more likely that the second will be also. Consequently, the denominator in the last formula may be too small and the resulting probability, as a consequence, too large. If this problem arises in a long series of tests, then the final probability, calculated via the inverse probability law or the more complicated Bayes' theorem, is certain to be greatly exaggerated. Unfortunately, there is no way short of empirical studies to evaluate the degree of independence among clinical tests or the effect of administering them in different orders. A more sophisticated analysis is clearly needed.

It is also worth noting that the whole matter of serial and parallel testing is more complex than we have indicated. Because parallel testing saves time, it may seem to be more efficient. But sequential testing requires fewer tests per accurate diagnosis, so in this sense it is more efficient. Obviously, a simple appeal to "efficiency" is not adequate to resolve conflicts between the two approaches.

Testing Statistical Hypotheses

Clinical investigators such as Dr. Williams are likely to carry out studies of factors relevant to the diseases they treat. In evaluating and reporting their results, they will be expected to use modern statistical techniques. Statistics is the science of making inferences about populations using observations on samples from that population. Specifically, statistics allows one to quantitate the effect of random variation on the conclusions derived from measurements on a sample. Biostatistics should be thought of as embedded in the more general field of study design and analysis, which includes such other issues as confounding and bias. We cannot hope to include even the semblance of a comprehensive discussion of those techniques here, but we can usefully introduce one of the basic ideas, that of rejecting the null hypothesis.

Let us suppose we suspect that patients with SLE are more likely to be anemic than other patients and want to test the hypothesis that this (or any other diagnostic or therapeutic association) is the case. We can certainly specify certain blood test results as criteria for anemia and proceed to test as many of our SLE patients as we can. It might even be safe to assume that our patients form an unbiased sample, which we will assume for the rest of the discussion. Let us also suppose that we have run the test and have found that in our sample of twenty-five SLE patients, thirteen are anemic (according to our test for anemia). Since this is only a small sample of the total population of SLE patients, how can we conclude anything about that larger population? Using the technique of testing the null hypothesis, we might be able to conclude that the results obtained from our sample would be quite unlikely if anemia were not associated with SLE. That conclusion might be enough to justify further research into the association between SLE and anemia.

The hypothesis we want to test is that SLE patients are more likely to have anemia. The null hypothesis, in this case, is that the incidence of anemia in SLE patients is the same as it is in ordinary people. For the sake of this example, let us assume we already know that the probability of an ordinary person being anemic is.2. We can then use probability theory to calculate the mean and standard deviation of the distribution of test results for anemia to be obtained from twenty-five random samples drawn from a population of ordinary people.

This distribution will vary according to the probability of being anemic.

Thus, if the probability of anemia is high, then most random samples should contain a large proportion of anemics. If, as in our example, the probability is low, then most of the samples will contain a small proportion of anemics. If the null hypothesis is true, then random samples of SLE patients should follow the same distribution of random samples as ordinary people. Thus, we should expect a small proportion of our sample to be anemic. Since, in fact, over 50 percent of our sample proved to be anemic, the null hypothesis is probably false and should be rejected.

Table 4.2. Two-by-Two Table for SLE and Anemia

Anemia	SLE +	SLE −	Total
+	13	5	18
−	12	20	32
Total	25	25	50

That is the basic idea behind testing the null hypothesis. However, the matter is usually put much more precisely, with talk about "most samples" being replaced by information about how many standard deviation samples of a given proportion fall from the mean. The convention in hypothesis testing is to select either two or three standard deviations as specifying the range of "most samples." If we use two SDs, then by "most of the samples" we mean approximately 95 percent, and if we use three SDs, then by "most of the samples" we mean 99 percent. We can calculate the SD for samples of size 25 when the mean is .2. This is .08. Thus, there is only a 5 percent (i.e., 100 - 95) chance that the proportion of anemics in a random sample of twenty-five ordinary patients will exceed .36 and only a I percent chance that it will exceed .44. Since the proportion of anemics in our sample is more than 50 percent, it would be quite unexpected if the null hypothesis were true (i.e., < I percent chance), whether we interpret "most samples" as 2SDs or 3SDs within the mean.

In statistical parlance, our results are statistically significant at the .05 and .01 levels. By contrast, suppose that only ten of the twenty-five patients sampled were anemic. The results would then be significant at the .05 level but not at the .OJ level. Finally, if only eight were anemic, then the results would not be counted as significant at either level. Given current conventions, we would not be justified in rejecting the null hypothesis. We run the risk of failing to reject the null hypothesis when it is in fact false, because of too small a sample size (Type II error).

Instead of using proportions, we can use actual numbers and visualize testing the null hypothesis in terms of a 2 x 2 table. Our original sample contained twenty-five patients with SLE, and thirteen of them are anemic. We now select twenty-five controls who are matched for age and gender and, true to form, have a .2 prevalence of anemia. We can represent this information in table 4.2.

Testing for statistical significance basically involves predicting what numbers should appear in the boxes by using the numbers in the margins. If

the fourfold table is labeled as in table 4.3, Then χ^2 is calculated from
$\dfrac{(ad - bc)^2 (a + b + c + d)}{(a + b) (c + d) (b + d) (a + c)}$ and produces the result 5.5, which converts to
a probability $.01 < p < .05$.

Table 4.3.   Two-by-Two: Statistical Form

a	b	$a+b$
c	d	$c+d$
$a+c$	$b+d$	$a+b+c+d$

Another useful notion connected with the 2 x 2 table is the odds ratio $\dfrac{a \cdot d}{b \cdot c}$, which in our case is 4.3. Thus a person with SLE is 4.3 times more likely than normal to have anemia. The odds ratio and its cousin, the risk ratio are used as measures of effect in inferences about causation.

Some qualifications should be mentioned in connection with testing the null hypothesis. First, the standard deviation is a function of sample size; as the sample size increases, the bell curve tightens and the standard deviation becomes smaller. Thus, percentages that are not statistically significant for small samples can become so as the sample size grows larger. For example, if our sample size increased to one hundred, then the SD would be .04. In this case, a sample of one hundred containing 40 percent anemics would count as significant both at the .05 and .01 levels. Second, we reject the null hypothesis because the results are unlikely, given the truth. However, they are not incompatible with its truth. Thus, rejecting the null hypothesis does not prove the other hypothesis is true. The result tells us only that it is worth investigating the other hypothesis further. Third, since the values of the standard deviation vary with both the mean and the sample size, we could reject the null hypothesis too hastily by simultaneously using a large sample and a less stringent significance level. As we saw, 40 percent became significant at the .01 level when we increased the sample size from twenty-five to one-hundred. Indeed, with large samples the test we have sketched may be inappropriately sensitive, in the sense of regarding as "significant" sample means that differ by "negligibly" small amounts from the mean postulated by the null hypothesis (type I error).

We can again illustrate this conclusion by a 2×2 table (table 4.4). In hypothesis testing, we make claims about the truth or falsity of the null hypothesis that there is no difference between what we observe and what we expect.

Type I errors are false positive claims or rejecting the null hypothesis too readily.

Type II errors are false negative claims or accepting the null hypothesis too readily.

Of course there are means for examining many hypotheses at once. For example, we determine whether there is a statistically significant association of SLE with age, gender, race, socioeconomic status, and soon. These techniques are known as multivariate analysis and are beyond the scope of this discussion.

Table 4.4. Testing the Null Hypothesis

Statistical Claim	Reality	
	T	F
T	TP	FP
F	FN	TN

However, all techniques rest on the fundamental notion of the null hypothesis.

There is much more to statistics than tests for significance and much more to significance testing than we have been able to present here. Nevertheless, we have indicated some of the ways in which statistics can play a critical role in evaluating clinical experience.

OTHER TYPES OF INDUCTIVE INFERENCE

In addition to using statistical techniques to carry out probabilistic inference, clinicians use a number of other forms of inductive reasoning. These remain more or less at the level of common sense, since inductive logic as a science is nowhere nearly as developed as statistics. Despite this, we believe these forms deserve mention, even if only briefly.

The Statistical Syllogism

At one point Dr. Williams reasoned as follows: the kidneys of a high percentage of patients with SLE are damaged; Mrs. Halprin has SLE; thus it is quite probable that her kidneys have been damaged. He might have put the matter more exactly. For example: 80 percent of patients with SLE have damage kidneys; Mrs. Halprin has SLE; thus the probability that she has damaged kidneys is .8. More generally, the statistical syllogism, as this form of inference is called, takes the form

$$X\% \text{ of } As \text{ are } B;$$
$$\text{thus, this } A \text{ is a } B \text{ with probability } p.$$

The inference often makes good sense, but it is not without its pitfalls. First, other forms of the inference applicable to the very same case can lead to contradictory conclusions. For instance, a high proportion of patients with normal EKGs do not have coronary artery disease, whereas a high proportion of patients with radiating chest pains do have coronary artery disease, and the same patient may suffer from radiating chest pains and have a normal EKG (the pains being due to an injury, say). Thus, two applications of the statistical syllogism could yield the conclusions that it is both highly probable and highly improbable that the patient suffers from coronary insufficiency! Second, the relationship between the numerical proportion of As that are Bs used in the premise and the probability number used in the conclusion is not entirely clear. If about half the As are Bs and the population of As is small, it may not be appropriate to conclude anything about a particular A. Despite our lack of understanding of its limits and reliability, the statistical syllogism is often as useful as it is pervasive.

Analogical Reasoning

When we infer that a patient will respond to a certain drug because that patient is similar to other patients of the same age, gender, height, weight, medical history, severity of disease (or whatever else we deem appropriate), we are reasoning by analogy. Similarly, we apply analogical reasoning when we predict that a process taking place in a laboratory animal (with relevant similarity to humans) is likely to take place or to follow a similar course in humans. Again, we apply this sort of reasoning when we conclude that one as yet poorly understood human disease is likely to be amenable to a treatment similar to that used in treating a well-understood disease. Analogical reasoning is thus deeply woven into the fabric of medical thought.

Despite this, this form of reasoning is even less understood and less reliable than the statistical syllogism. The inference goes:

$$A \text{ is similar to } B \text{ in respects } X, Y, Z, W, \ldots;$$
$$B \text{ is an } F.$$
$$\text{Thus, it is probable that } A \text{ is an } F.$$

A strengthened form of the inference would add a further premise to the effect that A and B are not dissimilar in any relevant respects. Yet, this inference form gives us no indication of how probable it is that A is an F; nor does it tell us how that probability varies with the number and variety of ways in which A and B are similar. Common sense tells us that the probability increases as the number of "relevant" similarities between the two increases. But how is relevance determined? A statistically significant proportion of rats contracted bladder cancer in the famous studies on saccharin. Were the similarities between their circumstances and those of humans sufficiently similar to warrant the conclusion that humans under ordinary exposure to saccharin have a greater risk of getting bladder cancer? We will not hazard an answer. But we can point out that the debate has focused upon the quality of the analogy between the rats in the study and humans. Not only are there questions concerning the biological similarities between the two, there are also questions concerning the high dosage levels given to the rats. One side argues that the dissimilarities between the two are not relevant (because, say, previous models of human diseases in rats have proved to be reliable). The other side argues the opposite.

Animal models of lupus include certain strains of rabbits and mice with features of autoimmune disease. Therapeutic interventions are often tested in these animal models before they are made available to patients, even for experimental trials. In these sorts of cases, we argue by analogy that if the treatment was effective in the animals, then it is likely to be effective in humans.

It is unfortunate that we do not have a better understanding of analogical reasoning, because it plays a major role in both medical research and practice. (See chap. 6 for a discussion of analogical reasoning and models.)

Enumerative Induction

Suppose physicians sent to care for a newly discovered tribe of people find that each of the several hundred patients they have observed is infected with a certain intestinal parasite. The physicians are likely to conclude that the next number of the tribe they examine will be infected also (alternatively, that all members are infected). Our physicians use enumerative induction, a probabilistic inference taking the form

The *As a, b, c, d, e, f,* ... are *B*s;
Thus, it is probable that this *A* is a *B*.
(It is probable that all *As* are *B*s.)

Although such reasoning often makes good sense, the difficulties with it are readily apparent. Let us expand upon our example. Our physicians, it happens, have examined only members of the tribe who drink from a certain spring in which the infecting parasites thrive. Furthermore, most of the other members are at sea on an extended pilgrimage to another island. They use a different water source and, consequently, are not infected. Our physicians know none of this, but when they find it out, they will retract their conclusions about the incidence of the infection in this tribe.

The statistical syllogism, analogical argument, and enumerative induction are among our favorite forms of inference. Yet what are we to conclude from our rehearsal of their weaknesses? Some might urge that we foreswear them entirely, but we recommend a moderate course. Let us recognize the inferences as useful devices for drawing tentative conclusions that are then to be supported by additional evidence. The physicians in our last example were certainly right to entertain the hypothesis that all tribal members were infected by the parasite, but they should have then looked for additional evidence to test it. Likewise, the saccharin studies certainly justify a program of research aimed at directly determining the effects of saccharin on humans. To adopt such a program is by no means to endorse the truth or even the high probability of the hypothesis that saccharin increases the incidence of cancer in human users. It is merely to take the next sensible step. Similarly, a drug shown to be effective in animal models of lupus deserves clinical testing.

The Problem of Induction

The considerations we have just entertained lead easily to the famous and venerable philosophical problem introduced by the eighteenth-century philosopher David Hume. Known as the problem of induction, it applies not just to the forms of inferences considered above but to all forms of probabilistic inference. The short of it is given in this question: Given that a probabilistic inference can never yield its conclusion with total certainty, how can it ever be rational to accept conclusions obtained by such methods? We cannot attempt to give a satisfactory answer to this question in a book of this sort. An entire treatise on inductive logic might not produce one, since even today there is not unanimity among philosophers and statisticians concerning the foundations of inductive inference.

To avoid giving any answer at all, we will offer this: Return to the example of the physicians encountering parasites in the members of the newly discovered tribe. Given the evidence, what could have been a more rational alternative to accepting tentatively the hypothesis that the parasite is endemic to the tribe? If the physicians accept only those conclusions that they can establish with utter certainty, there will be few interesting conclusions at all for them to draw. Virtually none of the conclusions will formulate new information about the tribe. Perhaps the physicians should have accepted some other hypothesis compatible with the evidence, for in this particular example the hypothesis accepted was wrong.

But this example is more the exception than the rule. Thus it would appear that using probabilistic inference is the only rational alternative we have. So let us use induction, and let us encourage statisticians and inductive logicians to try to understand its limitations more fully. Then we will be in a better position to assess the risks of applying it in particular instances.

Before leaving the problem of induction we should point out a circularity to our own answer, because it illustrates the kind of problem that has plagued many of the other philosophical attempts to deal with Hume's problem. Notice we have argued that the parasite example is "more the exception than the rule." But how do we know this? The only way we can know it is from our previous experience with inductive inference. But this is presumably only a sample of the entire experience that humans (and other reasoning beings) will have with inductive inference. Thus, in concluding from our own limited experience with induction that the parasite example is only an exception (or that induction does have a reasonable degree of reliability to it) we are using induction itself!

The problem of induction and the inadequacies of contemporary inductive logic become more apparent when induction is contrasted with deductive inference. This form of inference also plays a central role in medical inference. Let us turn to it now.

RECOMMENDED READING

Atkinson, P. The Concept of Evidence. Oxford: Oxford University Press, 1983. Col- lected essays on the logic of discovery and confirmation.

Blois, M. S. Information and Medicine. Berkeley: University of California Press, 1984.

Chernoff, H.,and L. Moses. Elementary Decision Theory. New York: Wiley, 1974. This mathematics text introduces both Bayesian and non-Bayesian approaches to statistics. Feinstein, A. R. Clinical Judgment. 1967. Reprint. Melbourne, Fla.: Krieger, 1974.

This book contains valuable discussion of the use of statistics in medicine.

---. "Clinical Biostatistics: XXXIX. The Haze of Bayes, the Ariel Palaces of Decision Analysis, and the Computerized Ouija Board." Clinical Pharmacological Theory 21 (1977): 482-96. This highly critical article attacks the use of Bayes' theorem and decision analysis in clinical contexts.

Griner, P. F., R. J. Mayewski, A. I. Mushlin, and P. Greenland. "Selection and Interpretation of Diagnostic Tests and Procedures." Annals of Internal Medicine 94 (1981): 553-600.

Galen, R. S., and S. R.Gambino. Beyond Normality. New York:Wiley, 1975.Bayesian approach to lab testing.

Giere, R. Understanding Scientific Reasoning. New York: Holt, Rinehart and Winston, 1979. This excellent introduction to the nature of scientific theories and reasoning focuses on the use of probability and statistics in science.

Goodman, N. Fact, Fiction and Forecast. 3d ed. Indianapolis: Hackett, 1979. This book contains a proposal for dissolving the problem of induction, as well as arguments against the possibility of an objective logic.

Hacking, I. Logic of Statistical Inference. New York: Cambridge University Press, 1965. More formal attempt to analyze statistical inference using logic.

Hogarth, R. Judgement and Choice. New York: Wiley, 1980. Easily understood text on the psychology of decision making.

Kahneman, D., P. Slovic, and A. Tversky. Judgment under Uncertainty: Heuristics and Biases. New York:Cambridge University Press, 1982. Collected papers on the psychology of judgment.

Kyburg, H. Epistemology and Inference. Minneapolis: University of Minnesota Press, 1983. This book contains some very good high-level discussion on the concept of probability and its interpretations.

Metz, C. E. "ROC Methodology in Radiologic Imaging." Investigative Radiology 21 (1986): 720-33.

Murphy, E. A. The Logic of Medicine. Baltimore: Johns Hopkins University Press, 1976. In the tradition of Feinstein's Clinical Judgment, this book has several insightful chapters on statistics and medicine.

Raz, J. Practical Reasoning. Oxford: Oxford University Press, 1978. Philosophy of everyday logic.

Resnik, M. D. Choices. Minneapolis: University of Minnesota Press, 1986. This introduction to decision theory presents logical foundations for decision analysis.

Savage, L. Foundations of Statistics. New York: Dover, 1972. Classic subjectivist account.

Skyrms, B. Choice and Chance. 3d ed. Belmont, Calif.:Wadsworth Publishing, 1986. This is a good logical and philosophical introduction to inductive inference, the problem of induction and probability, and its interpretations.

Wulff, A. Rational Diagnosis and Treatment. Oxford: Blackwell, 1976. Clear discussion of Bayesian inference.

CHAPTER 5

Deductive Inference

The rules and structures of deductive logic provide the skeletal framework of medicine. They supply the principles needed to organize and articulate theories, laws, observations, generalizations, statistical data, and the other forms of information that constitute the substantive body of medical thinking. They also supply the patterns of reasoning and modes of thinking that permit us to move from observation to observation and to focus the appropriate generalizations on a particular case.

The major aim of this chapter is to provide some sense of the role and significance of deductive logic in clinical medicine. We begin with a brief examination of the way in which deductive patterns of reasoning are often tacitly employed. Then we turn to a more detailed examination of the role of deduction in medicine. We introduce some of the technical concepts of logic and present some specific rules of deduction that are of particular importance in medicine. The chapter ends with a discussion of the use of deduction in diagnosis.

THE HIDDEN ROLE OF DEDUCTION

Anyone beginning the study of linguistics may be surprised to learn that whenever we speak, our utterances can be analyzed into morphemes and phonemes. A similar surprise may be in store for those who are introduced to logic. Whether we are aware of it or not, we often employ the modes of analysis and patterns of reasoning characteristic of deductive logic in instances that, on the surface, seem quite simple and straightforward.

Consider, for example, the remark that Dr. Williams made in discussing Mrs. Halprin's diagnosis: "The liver function tests neither exclude nor confirm the diagnosis of viral hepatitis prodrome." Implicit in this remark is the logical claim that the data obtained from the liver tests are logically compatible with both the truth and falsity of the diagnosis of hepatitis –that the test results cut neither way. Of course, Dr. Williams expected the members of the clinical team to grasp this implicit claim without his having to spell it out for them.

Similarly, during the several times that those on the team reasoned hypothetically, they tacitly employed a pattern of deductive reasoning. Dr. Barton explained one of her decisions in this way: "I thought viral hepatitis prodrome was possible so I ordered liver function tests, hepatitis antigen, prothrombin titer, and an assay for immune complexes."

Dr. Barton, like Dr. Williams, did not spell out all the details. We can reconstruct her reasoning as a pattern that starts with the assumption that Mrs. Halprin had viral hepatitis prodrome. From this assumption, plus additional background information, Dr. Barton reasoned, "If the prodrome is present, then the tests may show certain characteristic results." She then ordered the tests in the hope of confirming or excluding the assumed diagnosis.

Nonhypothetical, straight deduction was employed by Dr. Williams when he ruled out various strategies for dealing with Mrs. Halprin's illness. He told the clinical team:

> One general rule is that physicians do not like to perform more than one therapeutic modality at the same time, unless either they are a physiological sensible combination or the patient is in the rapid evolution of an irreversible process. For future management, one would like to know whether the current decline is due to the indomethacin or not, and as a separate issue whether the patient's nephritis responds to steroids or not. [Strategy (2) of stopping indomethacin and starting high-dose steroids will prevent us from resolving those issues.] Therefore, I would be against strategy (2), unless she was rapidly losing all kidney function and needing dialysis.

The bracketed sentence makes Dr. Williams's reasoning explicit. Strategy (2) would lead to X; X is not now acceptable; therefore, strategy (2) is not now acceptable. Notice that Dr. Williams also relied implicitly on his belief that a rapid loss of kidney function would constitute the "evolution of an irreversible process," a condition that would justify employing multiple therapies.

This scattering of examples shows that physicians use logic whenever they are engaged in medical reasoning. In this sense, then, they can be said to "know" logic. But this does not mean that, if asked, they would all be able to articulate a set of rules that they follow when reasoning. Very few native speakers of English would be able to give a complete list of all the morphemes of the language, but in the sense that we all use them, we all "know" them.

There is a paradoxical asymmetry between the place of inductive logic (i.e., probability and statistics) and deductive logic in medicine. Contemporary physicians must have at least a rudimentary grasp of probability theory and statistics to be able to appraise most of the research published in medical journals. For this reason, statistics courses are a standard part of medical education.

By contrast, it is generally believed that physicians know how to reason deductively with sufficient acuity to meet the needs of medical practice and research. This is not a point of view we wish to challenge .The truth is, the uses of deduction in medicine are generally quite simple and do not require a sophisticated understanding of the nature of logical systems and all their formal apparatus. So far as we are concerned, there is no pressing need to incorporate the study of logic into the already crowded medical curriculum.

At the same time, we do not wish to minimize the significance of deductive logic. Indeed, it is such a central feature of medical reasoning that a failure to discuss it here would be tantamount to telling the story of the Iliad without mentioning Achilles. The very fact that the centrality of deduction in medical thinking is generally unrecognized makes it all the more important that we not dismiss it with a nod.

SOME GENERAL FEATURES OF DEDUCTIVE LOGIC

It is impossible to appreciate the role of deductive logic in medicine without knowing something about the character of logic itself. In this section, we introduce some of the basic concepts of logic and then consider the use made of deduction in prediction and explanation.

Arguments

Scientists, mathematicians, lawyers, and philosophers are used to defending their positions by presenting *arguments* for them. An argument is a piece of reasoned discourse in which a statement is put forward and other statements are offered as reasons or evidence in support of it. The statement itself is the *conclusion* of the argument, and the statements offered in support of it are the *premises*.

The methodology of mathematics places great emphasis on the rigor and style of its arguments. To a lesser extent, other disciplines emulate the standards set by mathematics. However, arguments in medicine are rarely as stylized as those in mathematics. Typically, premises are often taken for granted or left unstated. (In the jargon of logic, they are *implicit*.) For example, Dr. Barton reported to Dr. Williams that "I thought disseminated gonococcal infection was possible so I cultured her cervix, rectum, and pharynx." As it stands, this explanation is not an argument, but it is easy to see how it can be turned into an argument when an implicit premise is made explicit:

Explicit 1   Disseminated gonococcal infection was a diagnostic possibility.

Implicit 2.   When such a possibility is present, it is proper to culture the cervix, rectum, and pharynx.

Implicit 3.   I follow proper procedures.

Conclusion.   Therefore, I cultured the cervix, rectum, and pharynx.

As we mentioned earlier, we are all by nature and experience subtle reasoners, and we generally do not have to have everything spelled out for us. We work within a context in which background information is shared and taken for granted. Consequently, most arguments are presented in only truncated forms. It is only when we attempt to follow the rigorous models of deductive reasoning that we recognize the need to be complete and thorough and to make explicit everything that we are taking for granted.

Being explicit has its advantages, of course. Once someone who has offered us an argument has made explicit all the premises, we are in a much better position to understand the force of the argument. Furthermore, and perhaps more important, we are in a better position to raise questions or challenge premises that we may find doubtful. (As shown in chap. 9, one of the most valuable aspects of decision analysis is that it also forces us to make explicit underlying assumption.)

Deductive and Inductive Arguments

Logicians distinguish between two major methods of argumentation –two types of arguments. The distinction is made on the basis of the relationship between the premises of the argument and its conclusion. If one uses deductive methods, then one attempts to construct arguments with conclusions that follow necessarily from their premises. Metaphorically speaking, the conclusion of a deductive argument is already contained in the premises. If the premises are accepted, then the conclusion must be accepted as well.

By contrast, if one uses inductive methods, one attempts to construct arguments with conclusions that are probable with respect to the premises. That is, the premises supply reasons for the conclusion, but since the conclusion is not already contained in the premises, it is possible for the premises to be correct while the conclusion is wrong. The premises do not guarantee the conclusion of an inductive argument. They merely support it to some degree or other.

Of course, we would all prefer to deal with certainties rather than probabilities. Unfortunately, in most instances in medicine and science, sufficient information for correct deductive arguments from acceptable premises is lacking. We must then rely on inductive inferences from premises accepted as true. This is the sort of reasoning we discussed in the last chapter. As we saw there, it is inductive argument that does the main work in medical reasoning.

Validity

Deductive logic is concerned with arguments that yield their conclusions with certainty. In technical terms, these are called valid arguments. A valid argument is usually characterized as one in which it is impossible for the conclusion to be false while all the premises are true. Here is a trivial, stylized example that illustrates the idea:

> No one is dead if the vital signs are normal.
> Jones's vital signs are normal.
> Hence, Jones is not dead.

Obviously, the two premises cannot both be true and the conclusion false. It is in this sense that the truth of the premises can be said to guarantee the truth of the conclusion .This is sure to be clear to anyone who understands the example.

An argument is valid if, and only if, its conclusion is appropriately related to its premises—that is, if, and only if, the joint truth of the premises requires the conclusion to be true also.

Notice that this concept of validity permits a valid argument to have a false conclusion, if at least one of its premises is false. It also permits a valid argument with one or more false premises to have a true conclusion. It excludes only the case in which all premises are true and the conclusion is false.

Arguments that are both valid and have true premises are referred to as sound arguments in logic. At first sight, it might seem as though there is no reason for science and medicine to be concerned with anything but sound arguments. However, as we will see below, arguments that are not sound also have their uses. Because deductive logic focuses on the relationship between the premises and conclusions of arguments, logic can often be used as a method for determining truth.

First, if one starts from premises that are not just hypothetically assumed "for the sake of argument" but are known to be true, then arguing validly from them will lead to true conclusions. Thus logic has the capacity to produce new and unrecognized truths from familiar ones. (In a sense, the truths were already there, but they were hidden away in the thicket of premises.) It is this use of deduction that permits us to reach new conclusions on the basis of known theories and accepted facts.

Second, logic can tell us what else must be true, if we assume that certain statements are true. This is the idea that lies behind the empirical testing of hypotheses. To test a hypothesis, we assume the truth of the hypothesis, plus background assumptions, then construct a valid argument. The argument tells us that such and such "is to be expected," and we then look to see if such and such can be found. (We talk about more of the details of this process in chap. 6.) It is this procedure that is followed in deriving diagnostic or prognostic predictions from diagnostic hypotheses –for example, predicting EKG changes in the case of suspected myocardial infarction. This is also the same procedure followed in what is sometimes called *heuristic reasoning.*

Third, logic can be used to show that a statement is false by showing that a valid argument from it leads to another statement that is obviously false. "All people with headaches have clubbed fingers" is easily shown to be false by examining a patient with a headache who does not display clubbed fingers. Since a valid argument with a false conclusion must have one or more false premises, we then know to go back and check our initial assumptions.

Finally, logic can be used to show that one or more of a group of statements must be false by showing that the group as a whole is inconsistent. Excluding a diagnosis because it is incompatible with other findings or reordering tests because the data "don't make sense" are the most common uses of this method.

In short, a number of significant uses of deductive logic in medicine do not involve sound arguments. Perhaps in a perfect world, all our arguments would be sound ones. But operating as we do in a world of confusion and uncertainty, the methods of deductive logic are just one more set of tools that assist us in coping with the problems presented to us.

It is important to note, at least in passing, that each of the methods employing deductive reasoning that we have discussed has a probabilistic analogue. Thus, we often accept a diagnosis because it is probably true, given what we believe, and we often reject a diagnosis because it is unlikely to be true, given our data. Similar parallels hold for the other three methods.

Deduction and Logical Form

Almost three thousand years ago, early logicians recognized that the validity of an argument was independent of its subject matter. This meant that a good method of reasoning in one field could be easily transferred to another. Logic, like mathematics, was freed from particular cases, and the opportunity to develop general criteria for recognizing good arguments became possible. An argument could be recognized as valid because of its form, no matter what the argument was about.

Consider the following bit of diagnostic dialogue: "You will recall that our two diagnoses were strep throat and infectious mononucleosis. Well, the throat culture was negative so the patient must have mono." We can cut out the inessentials of the dialogue and reconstruct the argument in this way:

> The patient has strep throat or mononucleosis.
> The patient does not have strep throat.
> Thus, the patient has mononucleosis.

The argument is clearly valid-granted the premises, the conclusion follows. It remains valid if we replace strep throat and mononucleosis with mumps and measles, with rheumatic fever and systemic lupus erythematosus, or with a poodle and a setter. Indeed, the argument remains valid whenever we have two alternatives and one of them is ruled out.

Schematically; we can represent the argument in this way:

> (1) A or B.
> (2) B is not the case.
> (3) Thus, A.

In going from our initial argument to a schematic representation, we have passed from an argument to an argument form. We now have a representation of not just one argument, but of indefinitely many arguments. The premises and conclusions of those arguments may concern various subject matters.

Consider any argument of this form. If both premises are true, then statement B must be false, otherwise premise (2) could not be true. But then premise could not be true unless A is true. However, A is also the conclusion. Thus, the argument must be valid: if both its premises are true, the conclusion must also be true.

As this example shows, in passing from arguments to argument forms we have a means for establishing the validity of an indefinite number of arguments. Once we have established a form as valid, we can then establish particular arguments as valid by showing that they have the form of a valid argument.

We can also use argument forms to establish invalidity. Consider this argument:

> A necessary condition for Mrs. Halprin's having lupus is that she
>   fulfill four out of the eleven ARA criteria.
> She fulfills four out of the eleven criteria.
> Thus, Mrs. Halprin has lupus.

With respect to Mrs. Halprin's case, all these statements are true. Moreover, the presence of conditions that satisfy the four criteria are strong evidence for the diagnosis of lupus. Yet the evidence is inductive, and the argument above is not a valid deductive argument.

One way of recognizing this is to examine its form:

(1) B is a necessary condition for A.
(2) B.
(3) Thus, A.

An argument is valid if, and only if, it is impossible for its premises to be true while its conclusion is false. Thus, if all arguments of the above form were valid, there could be no instance of it in which (1) and (2) were true while (3) was false.

But there can be such instances. Here is an argument with the same form that is obviously invalid:

(1) The presence of oxygen is a necessary condition for fire.
(2) Oxygen was present at the top of the Washington Monument on January 1, 1987.
(3) Thus, there was a fire at the top of the Washington Monument on January 1, 1987.

Clearly, (1) and (2) can be true while (3) is false.

Moving from arguments to argument forms gives us a hold on both validity and invalidity and explains both the universal and skeletal nature of logic. Since logic turns out to be a matter of form only, the nature of the material fleshing out the form is irrelevant. For this reason, logic can be used to structure and organize any discipline.

The history of logic can be viewed as a quest for the best ways to represent the logical form of arguments. The Greek logicians, particularly Aristotle, made a remarkable start in this endeavor. Aristotle's theory of the syllogism captured a wide variety of simple arguments in which validity turns on the use of quantifiers like all, some, no, and so on. Thus an argument like

No one with a temperature of 110° F can survive.
Some people have had temperatures of 110° F.
Thus, some people have failed to survive.

is valid by virtue of the relations expressed by the sentences containing "no one" and "some people." Aristotle and his successors developed a catalog of valid forms for this sort of argument and a set of algorithms for checking validity.

The ancient Greek Stoics took another approach and concentrated on arguments in which validity depends on the ways in which the sentences are related by connectives like *if. .. then. .., either. .. or. .., not*, and so on. The argument discussed at the beginning of this section ("The patient has strep throat or mononucleosis," etc.) is an example of an argument of this sort.

Neither of the two schools of logic ever developed rules that could prove the validity of obviously valid arguments that employ both quantifiers and statement connectives, such as this one:

> Anyone who goes to medical school works hard.
> If everyone works hard, then no one is happy.
> Thus, if everyone goes to medical school, then no one is happy.

With only a few minor advances, logic as a discipline remained virtually stagnant until 1879. It was then that the German mathematician Gottlob Frege invented a new representational scheme in which the logical form of both compound statements and quantificational statements could be expressed.

Frege's insight was to recognize that statements like "All whales are mammals" can be paraphrased as "Given anything, if it is a whale, then it is a mammal." This, in turn, could be paraphrased as "given anything x, if x is a whale, then x is a mammal." This technique of rewriting sentences makes an explicit connection between *if* and *all* and thus between the approaches of both Aristotle and the Stoics.

Frege also extended both logics and introduced special symbols to abbreviate logical forms. Contemporary logic has kept Frege's basic idea but has introduced a new system of notation. Thus, the sentence about whales is now represented as $(x)(x)(Wx \supset Mx)$. The "(x)" is read as "for every x" and the horseshoe "$\supset$" expresses the "if.., then..." connection between the two component simple sentences.

Frege's logic turned out to be adequate to account for the validity of all mathematical reasoning. This impressive fact, plus a revival of interest in the foundations of mathematics, directed a lot of mathematical talent toward the analysis of deduction. Today, a flourishing branch of mathematics—mathematical logic—has grown directly out of Frege's work.

A BUDGET OF RULES

It is neither appropriate nor necessary to present a complete system of deductive logic here. Furthermore, as we mentioned earlier, deductive conclusions are typically arrived at in medicine without the deliberate or self-conscious use of any rules at all. Nevertheless, it is useful to become aware of some of the more common rules that are implicitly followed. Such awareness makes it possible to be more critical in evaluating and understanding modes of reasoning that are frequent in medicine.

We limit our consideration to rules belonging to the logic of compound statements. This so-called propositional logic is restricted, as we mentioned earlier, to dealing with arguments whose validity depends on the way in which the components of compound statements are related to one another by such connectives as *or* or *if..., then....* We do not discuss any of the rules of quantificational logic.

Rules of logic are not, in some way, imposed from the outside. The rules are, in effect, abstracted from arguments that we antecedently recognize as valid arguments. Like the rules of grammar, the rules of logic have their roots in actual practice, even though once made explicit they may then come to influence practice. (A similar nonnative-descriptive interaction arises in decision analysis, as we see in chap. 9.)

The rules we consider are stated in terms of the forms of the statements to which a rule applies. Thus we can determine whether an inference conforms to a rule if we simply check to see whether the inference conforms to the pattern of the rule. This means that even computers can check inferences for conformity to the rules of logic, so long as the inferences are written in an appropriate computer language. This fundamental fact about the rules of modem deductive logic has made it possible to design programs for carrying out deductive reasoning. Such programs are a crucial part of some approaches to computerized diagnostics.

Modus Ponens

Perhaps the most basic and simplest rule of logical deduction is the one that bears the traditional name modus ponens. It can be stated in this way Given two statements of the form "if A, then B" and "A," we may conclude "B." For example:

> If Mrs. Halprin has lupus, she is at risk for renal failure. $A \supset B$
> Mrs. Halprin has lupus. A

> Thus, she is at risk for renal failure.   *B*

Modus Tollens

Modus tollens is perhaps the second simplest and most common rule followed in all reasoning. The pattern expressed in the rule is one in which we work from denial to denial. It can be stated in this way: Given two statements of the form "If *A*, then *B*," and "*B* is not the case," we may conclude "*A* is not the case." For example:

> If Mrs. Halprin has hepatitis, then her liver function tests will be abnormal.
> Her liver function tests are normal.
> Therefore, she does not have hepatitis.

The Disjunctive Syllogism

We have already met the disjunctive syllogism in earlier examples. It can be stated this way: Given two statements of the form "A or B" and "A is not the case," then one may conclude "B." For example:

> Mrs. Halprin has hepatitis prodome or SLE.   *A* or *B*
> She does not have hepatitis prodome.   —*A*
> Therefore, she has SLE.   *B*

The importance of this rule in clinical reasoning is difficult to over-emphasize. It is this rule that underlies the procedure of establishing a diagnosis by systematically eliminating alternative possibilities. It is possible to think of making a diagnosis as considering all the alternatives ("either *A* or *B* or *C* or *D*....") that are exclusive, then eliminating all but one. This is called diagnosis by exclusion. To think in these terms involves an element of idealization, for it is assumed .that the possibilities are mutually exclusive and exhaustive, but nevertheless the logical rule behind the actual process is the disjunctive syllogism.

We do not present any proofs for the validity of these rules, even in an informal way. We hope that the rules appear to be just expressions of common sense and that the validity of such arguments will be seen as intuitively obvious. In special and very limited circumstances, the rules can lead to the sorts of internal inconsistencies we call paradoxes. However, for the vast majority of instances formal logic captures what we all would agree is proper or correct reasoning.

Fallacies Associated with the Rules

A fallacy is a bad argument that so closely resembles a good argument that it can easily be mistaken for one. Each of the three rules we have presented has a fallacy associated with it-an invalid argument that resembles the valid argument expressed in the rule.

The invalid argument that accompanies modus ponens is known as the fallacy of affirming the consequent. (The "consequent" is the sentence that follows the then in an *if...*, *then...* statement. The sentence after the *if* is the "antecedent.") The fallacy is committed by asserting that because the consequent is true, then the antecedent is true also. So instead of arguing (validly) "if *A*, then *B*," and "*A*," therefore, "*B*," one argues (invalidly) "if *A*, then *B*," and "*B*," therefore "*A*." Here is an example of the fallacy:

> If Simpson has essential hypertension, his blood pressure
>   will be high. $A \supset B$
> His blood pressure is high. $\underline{ B }$
> Therefore, Simpson has essential hypertension. A

We recognize the fallacy in simple cases such as this, because we know there are many causes of high blood pressure. In instances in which our ignorance is greater, we may be much more tempted to affirm the antecedent, just because the facts allow us to affirm the consequent.

The fallacy of denying the antecedent is a slip that occurs with respect to modus tollens. It results from arguing that because the antecedent if false, then the consequent is also false. That is, instead of arguing (validly) that "if *A*, then *B*," and "*B* is not the case," therefore, "*A* is not the case," one argues (invalidly) "if A, then *B*," and "*A* is not the case," therefore, "*B* is not the case."

Here is a straightforward and quite plausible illustration of the fallacy at work:

> If Mrs. Halprin has hepatitis prodrome, then her liver
>   function tests will be abnormal. $A \supset B$
> Mrs. Halprin does not have hepatitis prodrome. $\underline{ {-}A}$
> Therefore, her liver function tests should be normal. B

The premises in this argument may all be true. Nevertheless, it is invalid. Mrs. Halprin may have suffered liver damage from causes other than hepatitis prodome.

The fallacy of unexhausted alternatives accompanies the disjunctive syllogism. This is not a fallacy connected with the form of the argument, as in the other two cases. It is a fallacy connected with matters of fact. We may validly argue that "Mrs. Halprin has either lupus or hepatitis. She does not have hepatitis. Therefore, she has lupus." But this may not be a sound argument. That is, the first premise may not be true, because the two diseases named may not exhaust the alternatives. In such a case, eliminating hepatitis does not thereby demonstrate that Mrs. Halprin has lupus.

The danger associated with the use of the disjunctive syllogism is quite real in medicine. Sets of findings are associated with so many diagnostic possibilities that it is exceedingly difficult to be sure that alternatives have not been overlooked. The repeated use of the disjunctive syllogism to eliminate possibilities is one means of guarding against the danger of the fallacy. That is, one can argue "Either X or Y; not-X; therefore Y," and "Either Y or Z; not-Y; therefore, Z," and so on. Yet, in the final analysis, it is whether all the diagnostic possibilities have been considered that determines whether or not one has argued fallaciously.

Chains of Inferences

The rules we have discussed are not adequate to construct all possible valid arguments. Yet the addition of a very few more rules produces a set that is adequate for all mathematical deductions. The reason that so few suffice for so much is that the rules may be used to form lengthy chains of inferences. In such chains, statements deduced from the initial premises can be used to deduce additional statements. These statements, in tum, can be used to deduce even more, and in this way, the class of statements available for use in further deductions grows ever larger.

A chain of inferences is easy enough to illustrate by starting with a set of statements taken as premises and examining some of the consequences that follow from them. To make the case a realistic one, imagine that Mrs. Halprin has myocarditis and we are considering a myocardial biopsy.

Premise 1. If Mrs. Halprin has SLE, then she satisfies the ARA criteria.

Premise 2. If Mrs. Halprin satisfies the ARA criteria, then she will not show Aschoff bodies on myocardial biopsy.

Premise 3. Either she will show Aschoff bodies or she will have Libman-Sachs endocarditis.

Premise 4. If she has Libman-Sachs endocarditis, then she will show hematoxylin bodies on biopsy.

Premise 5. Mrs. Halprin has SLE.

(Conclusion) 1. Mrs. Halprin satisfies the ARA criteria.
2. She will not show Aschoff bodies on myocardial biopsy.
3.She will have Libman-Sachs endocarditis.
4.Biopsy will show hematoxylin bodies.

(Aschoff bodies are inflammatory lesions of the endocardium seen in acute rheumatic fever. Libman-Sachs endocarditis consists of inflammatory changes in the heart seen in SLE. Hematoxylin bodies are degenerated cell nuclei found on tissue biopsy in SLE and in white blood cells as the LE phenomenon.)
    Using letters to stand for component sentences and relying on the rules we introduced earlier, we can represent the above argument in the following abstract way.

Premise 1. If A, then B. Premise 2. If B, then not-C. Premise 3. Either C or D. Premise 4. If D, then F. Premise 5. A

(Conclusion)1.B
2. not-C
3. D
4. F

Premise 1, premise 5, modus ponens
Premise 2, line 1, modus ponens
Premise 3, line 2, disjunctive syllogism
Premise 4, line 3, modus ponens

It is easy enough to imagine other trains of reasoning fitting into this abstract pattern in which the concern is with confirming or eliminating diagnostic possibilities by referring to physical findings. The machinery of logic cranks out the results no matter what subject matter may be fed into the premises. For the most part, the role of deduction in clinical medicine goes unrecognized. We do what we do in reasoning, without necessarily being aware that we are following rules or employing valid arguments. Yet understanding and studying the process of reasoning can have genuine benefits. Not least, we may be able to improve the way we reason.

Logic, used explicitly and critically, now plays a significant role in programs of research that promise to alter the practice of clinical medicine .The attempt to develop computer models and programs to assist (or even perform) clinical diagnosis is a clear example of the application of deductive logic in medicine. An early model of diagnostic reasoning, developed by R. R. Ledley and L. B. Lusted, was based on the elementary logic of classes. (A similar logic forms the core of the model of diagnostic reasoning we present in chap.8.) This model was the forerunner of an increasing number of efforts to develop additional models and programs. For example, the concepts of elementary class logic were also used by Feinstein to explicate the process of causal reasoning in clinical medicine. So-called alternative logics, ones that invalidate some of the inferences allowed by the standard rules while validating others not allowed, have recently been mentioned by some clinicians as providing a useful framework for dealing with clinical matters. In our discussion of computerized diagnosis, we return to these matters.

The following chapter concerns the testing of hypotheses and theories, the relationship between Jaws and theories, and the nature of scientific explanation and prediction. In exploring these topics, we illustrate in quite a concrete way the essential role of deductive logic in science and medicine.

RECOMMENDED READING

General Introductions to Deductive and Inductive Logic

Copi, I.Introduction to Logic. 7th ed. New York: Macmillan, 1986. For the past thirty years this text has led the field of "freshman" logic books. It contains a general introductory survey of logic and the philosophy of science.

Quine, W. V. 0. Methods of Logic. 4th ed. Cambridge, Mass.: Harvard University Press, 1982. This classic text by America's leading philosopher-logician is the most difficult of the books listed in this section, but it also contains more material than the others.

Suppes, P. Introduction to Logic. New York: D. Van Nostrand, 1957. A good text that falls between Copi and Quine in rigor and sophistication.

Advanced Texts

Boolos, G., and R. Jeffrey. Computability and Logic. 2d ed. Cambridge: Cambridge University Press, 1981.Covers the major results of mathematical logic, including the limitation theorems of Godel, Skolem, and Church-Turing. The most accessible to nonmathematicians, but still a difficult and demanding book.

Haack, S. Deviant Logic. Cambridge: Cambridge University Press, 1975. A very clear philosophical discussion of alternative logics and the reasons for using them.

Hughes, G. H., and M. J. Cresswell. An Introduction to Modal Logic. London: Methuen, 1968. A good introduction to the logic of possibility and necessity.

Mccawley, J. D. Everything that Linguists Have Always Wanted to Know about Logic (But Were Ashamed to Ask). Chicago: University of Chicago Press, 1981. Written by an eminent linguist, this book can serve as an introduction to both standard symbolic logic and alternative logics.

Mendelson, E. Introduction to Mathematical Logic. 2d ed. New York: Van Nostrand Reinhold, 1964. Covers material in Boolos and Jeffrey, 1981, but less accessible to nonmathemati cians.

Shoenfield, J. R. Mathematical Logic. Reading, Mass.: Addison-Wesley, 1967. Covers material in Boolos and Jeffrey 1981, but less accessible to nonmathematicians.

Applications to Logic in Medicine

Feinstein, A. R. ClinicalJudgment. 1967. Reprint. Melbourne, Fla .: Krieger, 1974. A classic attempt to use rigorous mathematical and philosophical methods in medicine, this book contains an application of class logic to the characterizations of diseases.

Ledley, R. R., and L. B. Lusted. "Reasoning Foundations of Medical Diagnosis." Science 130 (1959): 9-21. The first use of logic to construct a model of diagnostic reasoning.

Murphy, E. A. The logic of Medicine. Baltimore: Johns Hopkins University Press, 1976. A critical-thinking approach to medicine written by an eminent biostatistician and epidemiologist.

Wulff, H. Rational Diagnosis and Treatment. Oxford: Blackwell, 1976. A clear and accessible discussion of critical thinking in medicine.

Computerized Logic

Clancy, W. J., and E. H. Shortliffe. Readings in Medical Artificial Intelligence. Reading, Mass.: Addison-Wesley, 1984. A collection of important papers.

Wos, L., R. Overbeek, E. Lusk, and J. Boyle.Automated Reasoning: Introduction and Applications. Englewood Cliffs, N .J.: Prentice-Hall, 1984. A text on symbolic logic and the computer implementation of algorithms for carrying out deductions in symbolic logic.

CHAPTER 6   *Hypotheses, Laws, and Theories*

To mention a particular patient—say, our Mrs. Halprin—in connection with theories seems quite inappropriate. Mrs. Hairpin is concrete and individual, while theories are abstract and general. The patient seems real and undeniable, while the theories seem to be mere inventions and open to doubt. Theories appear to be quite remote from the distress and suffering of Mrs. Halprin, and being remote, they seem irrelevant.

Granted such perceptions, it is no wonder that beginning medical students chafe at having to spend years of their time mastering the theories of the basic sciences, rather than immediately and fully devoting themselves to demands of patient care. And yet, apparently paradoxically, those same students when they become practicing physicians may lament not knowing even more basic theories than they were required to learn.

What makes the paradox only apparent and not real is the fact that theories are not so remote and unconnected with the practice of clinical medicine as they might appear. The outstanding feature of contemporary medicine is that it is scientific medicine. Not only is medicine scientific in its methods and some of its ambitions, but it is scientific in its substance. Clinical medicine employs or embodies fundamental biological and biochemical theories. Most important, these theories are not used for decoration or for invoking the magic of science (as they are in some forms of quackery). Rather, the theories are an essential ingredient in the composition of contemporary medical practice.

In addition to the fundamental theories of science, medicine has developed its own special theories. The recognition of discrete diseases, the elucidation of the mechanisms of their operation, and the understanding of the consequences following from various modes of intervention are just some of the characteristic concerns of medicine that are bound up with the formulation of relatively specific theories.

Far from being irrelevant to the suffering of Mrs. Halprin, theories are essential to understanding and dealing with it. The observations made of Mrs. Halprin, the identification of her illness, and the initiation and modification of her therapy were all actions performed by her physicians against the backdrop of scientific and medical theories. Theories are the lenses through which the physicians viewed Mrs. Halprin and brought her disorder into focus. Without theories, medicine is hardly more than a blind fumbling in the dark.

But what are theories? Exactly what roles do they play in medicine? Furthermore, where do we get our confidence in theories? Why are we willing to accept some while rejecting others? How are theories related to prediction? How are they related to explanation?

These are the questions we address in this chapter. They are related ones, and picking up the string at any point leads into the whole tangle. But to avoid confusion, it is most sensible to begin with a discussion of the questions that are most basic or most elementary in the logical sense, namely, with explanations and theories.

We begin by defining the term theory as used in science. This serves to limit our concerns to theories considered as sets of principles used to explain and predict. It also gives us a motive for going on to characterize principles and laws and describe the role they play in explanation and prediction. We present two models for the explanation of events and explain how causal explanations, though they appear to employ no laws, are actually ones that satisfy one of our models. We then show how grounded predictions can be regarded as essentially the same as explanations.

We turn to considering the ways in which hypotheses, as candidate laws, are tested and either accepted or rejected. We illustrate the role that auxiliary assumptions play in testing and show how the acceptance or rejection of a hypothesis is never something that occurs in isolation from other laws or conditions.

At this point, the way is then clear for us to turn attention away from laws and focus on theories. We analyze the logical structure of theories, examine the criteria that must be satisfied for the explanation of a law by a theory, and consider what is involved in testing theories. Afterward, we look briefly at the role that models and analogies play in applying and developing theories.

In the final section, we present some of the objections to the analysis of science and medicine that we have developed. We conclude by briefly outlining the characterization of the nature of the scientific enterprise offered by Thomas Kuhn in The Structure of Scientific Revolutions.

THEORY DEFINED

"What is a theory?" is not a question as hard to answer as jesting Pilate's "What is truth?" Indeed, one difficulty with our question is that there are so many accepted answers, not that there is none. That is, the term theory is used in several distinct and legitimate ways in science and medicine, and an explanatory catalog of those uses would fill many pages.

We will limit ourselves to the concept of the theory that suggests understanding, reliability, and grounded belief. Theory in this sense is bound up with experimental tests of hypotheses, explanatory power, predictive success, and confirmed assertions. How a theory may come to have such features or enter into such relationships is something we must consider in detail.

We define theory as a group of related principles that can be employed to explain and predict phenomena occurring within a certain restricted domain. Thus, Newtonian mechanics is a theory in this sense, and so is population genetics (selection theory), atomic theory, the germ theory of disease, the theory of particulate inheritance, phlogiston theory, the humoral theory of disease, the antibody-antigen theory of immunology, quantum mechanics, the wave theory of light, the Lamarckian theory of evolutionary change, and soon. Some of the theories mentioned here as examples are now rejected as false.

Nevertheless, according to our definition, they may still be considered theories. What leads to the rejection of a theory and what might lead us to consider a theory false are matters separate from the question of whether something is a theory.

The theories we are concerned with are empirical theories –as distinct, perhaps, from logical or mathematical theories or even theological theories. Roughly speaking, empirical theories are ones whose acceptance or rejection is conditioned by observation and evidence. That is, a theory is empirical when our willingness to accept it or reject it is at least partly a function of such matters as the outcome of predictions based on the theory.

Principles

Our definition of theory is stated in a way that refers to principles. A principle, for our purposes, may be considered a statement or other expression (including mathematical ones) that is logically general. That is, if an expression can be fit into the logical form "For all instances satisfying description X, then description Y is satisfied," then the expression is logically general. Statements such as "DNA replicates semiconservatively," "$s = \frac{1}{2}gt^2$," and "glucose + 2 ADP +2 HPO^{2-}_4 + 2 oxidized NAD$\rightarrow$ 2 pyruvic acid + 2 ATP = 2 reduced NAD" are all logically general ones.

It is clearly not the case that all logically general expressions are also principles. No one would want to say, for example, that "All patients in Boston Central Hospital have a detectable pulse" is a principle, even if it is true. More than logical generality is required to make a statement into a principle.

Exactly what additional features a principle must possess is an issue that has not been fully resolved. But at least two more requirements seem reasonable. First, the statement must be about a potentially (if not actually) unlimited class. This means that a statement mentioning individuals (Mrs. Halprin, Boston Central Hospital, etc.) cannot be a principle, even if it is general in its logical form.

Second, the statement must be one that is asserted to hold for all space and time. Thus, a statement that is a generalization about what is true of a certain geographical area or certain period of time cannot be a principle. A statement about the behavior of sodium in the nineteenth century or in France is obviously not a candidate for being a principle, although each might provide evidence in support of a principle that is truly general.

These two additional features help capture what we expect of the principles of a scientific theory. We expect them to be logically general, but more than this, we expect them to be unrestricted or universal in their applicability. The principles of geometrical optics should hold for Saturn as well as for Seattle. Similarly, the statement that lupus is an autoimmune disease is one that is asserted to hold for all patients with lupus, no matter when or where.

Notice that the features of logical generality and universal applicability are also ones that we expect even probabilistic principles to satisfy. They are, after all, generalizations to the effect that under specified circumstances, an additional characteristic is to be expected with a certain degree of probability. Thus, the principles of population genetics are probabilistic, but they are also unrestrictedly universal, in that they apply to all genetic systems possessing certain reproductive characteristics.

Principles and Laws

There is no clear-cut distinction between principles and laws. All principles are laws, but there is some reason to say that not all laws are principles. Generally, and somewhat intuitively, we might say that we regard principles as in some way more basic or fundamental or more general than laws.

On this view, "The renal manifestations of lupus are the consequence of immune-complex deposition" is a law, whereas "All organ-system involvement in lupus is immune-complex mediated" is really a principle. The second deals with all organ systems, and so the first can be derived from it. Thus, the first is a special case of the second, and this makes it less general. (Neither may be true.)

But this distinction requires that we be able to compare one formulation with some other in order to decide which is relatively more general or basic. As a result, what counts as a principle, as distinct from a law, is relative to other formulations that are available at the time. While it is true that we do often distinguish laws from principles in this way, there is nothing fundamental about the distinction. It is not necessarily "better" in any sense to be a principle than to be a law.

Given that there is no basic difference between laws and principles, we are free to reformulate our definition of theory. A theory, we can say, is a group of related principles or laws that are employed to explain and predict phenomena occurring within a certain domain.

This slight modification of our original definition recognizes a significant aspect of actual practice in medicine and science. It acknowledges the possibility that the laws considered to be a theory and used to explain and predict may themselves be explained in terms of a higher-level theory or more general set of laws. Thus, the modified definition recognizes the hierarchical relations that sometimes exist among a group of theories. We discuss such relations in more detail later on. For the moment, it is enough to rely on the sense of a hierarchy that we have when we think of the relations among quantum mechanics (at the top), then chemical-bonding theory, biochemistry, cell metabolism and dynamics, immunologic physiology, autoimmune theories, and generalizations about SLE.

THE EXPLANATION AND PREDICTION OF EVENTS

We look to theories to provide us with explanations of events that we find puzzling or, for some reason or other, significant. High-level theories are rarely brought to bear directly on the explanation of events. Rather, events are typically explained via lower-level laws, then we rely on the higher-level theories to explain those laws. (For example, in calculating reflection and refraction angles, we are not likely to rely on the laws of quantum mechanics. Instead, we would employ the principles of classical optics.)

Eventually, we shall want to discuss the structure of theories and the ways in which theories can be said to explain lower-level laws. However, it is more illuminating of the role of theories in science to begin with the explanation of events.

Nomological-Deductive Explanation

Mrs. Halprin has pericarditis—the sac surrounding her heart is inflamed. One explanation for this phenomenon is that Mrs. Halprin has immune complexes circulating in her blood. These often lodge in the small blood vessels of the lining tissue of visceral organs, where they produce inflammation.

There are many details and aspects left out of this very simple account: What sort of immune complexes are involved? Where do they lodge to generate the tissue reaction? What are the biochemical mechanisms of the tissue reaction? And soon. Nevertheless, we have an explanation for the pericarditis if we know merely that it is caused by the presence of immune complexes. It may not be a detailed explanation nor a complete explanation, but it is an explanation.

We can formulate the explanation in this way:

Whenever immune complexes are present in the pericardium in significant quantity, then pericarditis occurs.

Mrs. Halprin has immune complexes present in her pericardium in significant quantity.

Mrs. Halprin has pericarditis.

Explanations of this sort are known as nomological-deductive explanations. The nomological in the name means that the explanation contains a law or laws; the deductive refers to the relationship between the law and the initial conditions and the event to be explained.

This model of explanation can be represented by the following abstract scheme:

$L_1 \ldots L_n$ **(Laws)**
$I_1 \ldots I_n$ **(Initial Conditions)**

E *(Explanandum)*

The sentences above the line are known as the explanans (that which explains), and the sentence below the line is called the *explanandum* (that which is explained).

In the explanation of events, the explanans is made up of two sorts of components: (1) at least one law; (2) statements of the relevant initial conditions. The explanandum consists of a statement describing the event.

The following criteria are ones that must be satisfied before we are prepared to accept the explanation as a good one:

1. *The explanans must be true.* That is, the laws must be confirmed sufficiently for us to at least accept them as true. Strictly speaking, we are never in a position to say whether any universal generalization is true—even if it is a very simple one like "All copper conducts electricity" and we know

of no contrary instances. Put in a negative way, this first requirement tells us that we must not make use of a law we know to be false. Obviously, an explanation that rests on a false law is no explanation at all.

The sentences in the explanans that are not laws are descriptions of what are sometimes called initial conditions. That is, they provide the information about the circumstances under which the event occurred and make it appropriate to apply the law or laws to the event. In laws that are mathematically expressed, for example, the initial conditions supply the values of the relevant variables (such as mass, speed, molecular weight, viscosity, presence and amounts of specific nutrients, etc.).

The sentences describing the initial conditions are, unlike the laws, not universal sentences. Practically speaking, this means we are prepared to say they are true if they correctly represent the salient features of the situation.

2. *The explanandum must be true.* That is, the event we are concerned with explaining must be correctly described by the sentence. It must be true that Mrs. Halprin has pericarditis if this is what we are concerned with explaining. Otherwise, obviously, no explanation is possible. It is, after all, impossible to explain why something occurred if, as a matter of fact, it did not occur.

(It is worth noticing here something we discuss in more detail later on, namely, the event that we are concerned with in explanation is the event as described in a certain way. Since the same event can be given alternative descriptions—some more detailed than others or some in a vocabulary that differs from the vocabulary of other descriptions-it is important to recognize that our criteria are only ones for an explanation of the event.)

3. The *explanandum* must be a logical consequence of the explanans.

According to the nomological model, an explanation is (logically speaking) an argument. It is an argument to the effect that the event to be explained is not a wholly unique occurrence. Rather, it can be made understandable or intelligible by recognizing that it is part of a general pattern. The law (or laws) in the explanans expresses the pattern, and the initial conditions indicate that this pattern is the appropriate one for this instance. Consequently, deriving the description of the event from the explanans is a way of demonstrating that the event falls into the general pattern.

To return to our example, if it is true that Mrs. Halprin has pericarditis, and if it is true that she has deposits of immune complexes in her pericardium, and if it is true that whenever immune complexes are present in the pericardium in such a quantity then pericarditis occurs, then we have explained Mrs. Halprin's pericarditis.

Causal Explanations as Nomological-Deductive

To explain an event either in ordinary life or in science and medicine is often to tell what caused the event. Thus we say such things as "The explosion occurred because somebody left the gas on," "The chicks ran for cover because the hawk-shape is a releasing mechanism," and "An immune complex diathesis is the cause of Mrs. Halprin's pericarditis."

Such explanations appear to involve no laws. The event is explained merely by mentioning its cause. No logically general sentences seem to be involved, for the causal sentence ("*X* caused *Y*") is apparently only about individual events and circumstances.

However, despite appearances, causal explanations are, in fact, merely incomplete or implicit versions of nomological-deductive explanations. Their explanatory force depends upon an implicit reference to a causal law. Although the law may be unstated in cases in which a causal ascription is made, in a legitimate causal explanation it must always be possible to make the law explicit.

To understand why causal explanations that employ causal sentences are just incomplete nomological-deductive explanations requires that we touch on the analysis of causality. Of course, this is a vexed topic about which a great deal has been written. Fortunately, for our purposes a complete analysis is not required.

It is generally accepted that a causal relationship is one in which there is an invariant or constant connection between events of two kinds. Furthermore, the relationship is of such a kind that the occurrence of one event, under stated conditions, is followed by the occurrence of the second event. Thus the following scheme expresses the claim that there is a causal relationship between events of types *A* and *B*:

Whenever *A* occurs (under conditions *C*), then *B* occurs.

Generalizations of this form, if true, are usually acknowledged as causal laws. Evidence supporting their truth consists in observations and experimental manipulations of the factors (variables) in particular situations. The usual difficulty is to separate genuine causal connections from those that are merely correlational or otherwise "accidental." It is to resolve this difficulty that a variety of experimental techniques has been developed. However, this is not the place to discuss them.

In terms of this analysis, cause is sufficient condition. Thus a causal sentence like "An immune-complex diathesis is the cause of Mrs. Halprin's pericarditis" gains its explanatory power from its implicit assertion that an immune-complex diathesis (under the appropriate conditions) is a sufficient condition for producing pericarditis. Since a statement to this effect is a causal law, we can say that the causal sentence gains its force from a causal law.

If we make the causal law specific and if we provide a description of Mrs. Halprin's circumstances, we end up with an account that fits neatly into the nomological-deductive pattern:

> Whenever an immune-complex diathesis occurs in the pericardium, pericarditis results.
> Mrs. Halprin has an immune-complex diathesis in her pericardium.
>
> _____
>
> Mrs. Halprin has pericarditis.

The main point to notice here is that even when we explain an event by mentioning its cause, we are still relying upon laws. Although a causal sentence is about a particular event, it succeeds in being explanatory only because of its connection with a generalization about events of the same kind.

Causes and Conditions

The interpretation of cause as sufficient condition is in close keeping with the use made of the concept in ordinary life and medicine. We talk about fever or stomach cramps, for example, as being events that may have several possible causes. (The same is true of Mrs. Halprin's pericarditis.) In this sense of cause, then, what we mean is that several sets of conditions are separately sufficient to produce the event that we are concerned with. The problem in each case is to identify the conditions that are the cause in that instance.

Cause as sufficient condition is far from being the only interpretation current in medicine and science, not to mention ordinary affairs. It is worth taking a moment to sketch out three alternative interpretations.

Cause as Necessary and Sufficient Conditions

To say that a condition or set of conditions C is necessary and sufficient for the occurrence of an event of type E is to say that the following general statement is true: Whenever C occurs, then E occurs, and whenever C does not occur, then E does not occur. This is the most rigorous interpretation of a causal relationship, and to establish laws that express such a relationship is regarded by many as one of the goals of clinical medicine. Laws of this sort make it possible to infer that a particular causal event must have occurred, just on the basis of the observed outcome.

The existence of a physical sign that is pathognomic for a certain disease is generally recognized by virtue of the fact that the causal relationship between the disease and the sign can be expressed in terms of the invariant relationship represented by necessary and sufficient conditions. Very few examples of this kind are found in medicine.

Cause as a Necessary Condition

To say that a condition of type C is necessary for the occurrence of an event of type E is to assert the truth of the following generalization: E never occurs in the absence of C.

The concept of cause as necessary condition is encountered in medicine most frequently in ascribing a disease-causing role to particular agents. The polio virus, for example, is the cause of polio—in the sense of being the necessary condition for the disease. Other factors in addition to the presence of the virus are required for the disease to occur, and while many of them can be specified, it is not presently possible to list all the conditions that are necessary and sufficient (or even sufficient) for the occurrence of the disease. Still, the disease is never present unless the polio virus is also present. Hence, it makes both practical and scientific sense to identify the characteristic virus as the cause of the disease.

More is involved in identifying a factor as the cause of an event, even when it is a necessary condition. Not all necessary conditions are regarded as causes. For example, the presence of free oxygen is a necessary condition for respiration, hence for cellular metabolism, hence for polio. Yet it would be absurd to call the presence of oxygen the cause of polio—or even a cause of polio. Such conditions we typically regard as trivial in an explanatory sense, for they constitute the relatively constant background conditions. Usually, it is the factors that are unusual or that vary from case to case that we examine in order to find the "cause."

Cause as a Significant Condition

Exposure to ultraviolet light (perhaps as one of the components of sunlight) is generally thought to be one of the factors precipitating a flare of SLE. In this sense, then, Mrs. Halprin's exposure to intensive sunlight over a substantial period of time might be said to have caused the flare of her disease.

In saying this, however, no one would want to be taken as suggesting that exposure to sunlight is, by itself, either a necessary or a sufficient condition for the disease. A universal generalization connecting sunlight with the disease would be rejected as false by any clinician. How then are we to understand ascribing a causal role to sunlight?

The fact is that we frequently identify a single factor as a cause without intending to mean that it is the "whole" cause or even that it is a necessary condition. Rather, what we mean is that the factor is a condition that belongs to a set of conditions that is either sufficient or necessary and sufficient for the occurrence of events of the sort we are concerned with.

Let us put the point more schematically. Suppose we accept the following generalization as true:

Whenever C *(A, B, F, G)*, then E.

That is, whenever C is satisfied (whenever conditions *A, B, F, G* are present), then an event of type E occurs. Since C is a set of conditions that are (let's assume) jointly sufficient for the occurrence of E, we might refer to one member of the set as the cause of E without thereby intending to suggest that that member is itself a sufficient condition for the occurrence of E.

This mode of ascribing causes is familiar from cases in which we are concerned with assigning responsibility. Suppose someone leaves an unlighted gas burner turned on in a lab, gas accumulates, and another person coming into the lab flips the light switch. The flow of electricity across the poles ignites the gas, and there is an explosion.

What was the cause of the explosion? Strictly, it was the whole set of conditions that were present: the accumulation of methane in a certain concentration, the presence of oxygen in the atmosphere, the introduction of a heat source, and so on. But what we are likely to say is that the person who left the gas turned on caused the explosion-the gas was the cause of the explosion. Or we might say that the person who turned on the light caused the explosion—the electricity initiated the combustion.

Thus the factor that we identify as "the" cause is one that we consider to be significant according to some point of view. Often this factor is the last condition that completes a set of conditions that are sufficient-perhaps, for example, the exposure of Mrs. Halprin to sunlight. Such a "triggering" event is often considered of great importance to medicine. It is used to support such contrary-to-fact (counterfactual) claims as "Mrs. Halprin would not have developed SLE had she not exposed herself to UV radiation." Such counterfactuals, in turn, are sometimes used as a basis for generalizations about preventive measures. Consequently, anyone displaying signs that indicate the presence of predisposing factors for a certain disease may be advised to avoid actions or circumstances that are likely to complete a set of conditions and so trigger the full-blown manifestations of a disease.

Sometimes the factor (or factors) we identify as "the" cause of a disease is a standing condition(s) that predisposes someone to develop a particular disease or to develop its most serious signs. For example, individuals with sickle cell trait are ordinarily asymptomatic, but they may show clinical manifestations of the disease at high altitudes or under other conditions of low oxygen pressure. "The" cause of the abdominal or limb pain that may develop might well be said to be the abnormal hemoglobin.

There is no doubt a variety of other implicit criteria connected with particular interests (prevention, treatment, etc.) or point of view that lead us to identify factors of a particular kind as the cause of the event we are concerned with. This mode of identification is only a recognition of a relative significance and is never intended to be construed as a commitment to the belief that the identified factor is itself a sufficient or necessary and sufficient condition for the occurrence of the event.

Nomological-Statistical Explanations

The world is a very complicated place, and we are not always sure exactly how it works. Sometimes the best we can do is find out how it frequently works. That is, when we are not able to establish laws that represent causal connections between events, we can sometimes turn the darkness into a shade of gray by finding probabilistic or statistical connections.

Statistical laws are statements to the effect that the probability is Y that an event of kind F is also one that will be followed by kind G. Or put more schematically:

$$P(G, F) = Y.$$

Statistical laws that have a form like this are established by collecting data that represent the frequency with which F and G are associated. (See chap. 4 for a discussion of alternative concepts of probability and the role of probabilistic reasoning in medicine.)

There are, of course, elaborate mechanisms involved in analyzing data. But behind all the statistical machinery is the simple fact that statistical laws are established in virtually the same way as "All emeralds are green" is established. We come to believe that emeralds are green by finding one emerald, then another and another, and so on. We come to believe statistical laws by considering the results of one set of tests, then another and another, and so on.

At first sight, it may seem that statistical laws are not really laws. For one thing (looking back at the criteria we discussed earlier), they do not seem to be universal in form. They talk about the probability of such and such, rather than mentioning what always happens.

But this is a misleading way to think about statistical laws. They are universal in form, and they do talk about what always happens. What always happens is that events of kind G are associated with events of kind F with probability Y. That is, the law is a generalization to the effect that there is an invariant probability relation between G and F. So we could formulate them, if we wanted to make this explicit, by saying that "Whenever an event of kind G occurs, there is always a probability of Y that an event of kind F will occur."

Of course, there is still an essential difference between probabilistic laws and others. The invariant relationship they express is still a probability relationship. This unblinking fact has its consequences for explanation. Consider an example. Suppose Mrs. Halprin had subacute bacterial endocarditis (SBE) and was given an antibiotic by her physician and recovers. How are we to explain her recovery?

Obviously, she recovered because of the antibiotic. But we do not have a general law that says "Whenever a person with SBE is given an antibiotic, then he or she will recover." As a matter of fact, some people recover and some do not, and we do not have an adequate understanding of why this is so.

All that can be asserted in cases like Mrs. Halprin's is that administering an antibiotic results in a cure in a high percentage of cases. We might say that there is a statistical probability of .8 that the SBE will disappear. So if Mrs. Halprin recovers from her SBE, we can say that this is what we expected (with a probability of .8) to happen.

The explanans in a nomological-statistical explanation consists of a statistical law plus statements of the initial conditions. The explanans does not logically imply the explanandum, as in deductive-nomological explanation. Rather, it establishes that the explanandum event was probable to a certain degree.

Consider how we might explain Mrs. Halprin's recovery. To avoid awkward phrasings, we use the following abbreviations:

h = Mrs. Halprin;
B = an individual has SBE;
R = an individual recovers;
P = an antibiotic is administered;
p = probability;
d = a number.

$p(R, B$ and $P) = d.$
B_h and $P_h,$
$$\overline{\qquad\qquad} \quad (d)$$
R_h

The explanans provides us with a reason to believe that Mrs. Halprin recovered because of the antibiotic. It is quite possible that she recovered for other reasons. Perhaps other factors unknown to us were at work. Nevertheless, at the time we want her recovery explained, this may be the best we can do. We at least have some evidence to believe that the recovery was due to the drug she was given.

Some statistical explanations seem to be only stopgap measures. Depending upon how we look at the situation, they are only expressions of our ignorance or, at best, of our limited knowledge. What we would really like to know about antibiotics, for example, is why, when they are given to patients with SBE, some recover while others do not. This very fact inclines us to additional inquiry. We want to be able to replace the statistical connections with causal ones. We want to be able to say why Mrs. Halprin recovered but Mr. Zemfel did not.

Statistical correlations are both the salvation and the curse of the social sciences. Psychology, sociology, and economics could hardly have advanced beyond pure speculation and good guesswork without the artillery provided by statistical methods. Similarly, medical epidemiology would have had little luck identifying the factors connected with frequently occurring illnesses without the tools of statistics.

Whether the subject is social or medical events, the hope in all cases is to replace the statistical connections with causal laws. Basically this has meant discovering the mechanisms through which associated factors produce the outcome they do. When we acquire understanding, then it also becomes possible to see why those factors have causal consequences in some instances but not in others. When we understand exactly how the ingredients in cigarette smoke result in damage to the heart, then the closer we come to replacing the statistical correlation of cigarette smoking and heart disease with causal laws. Medicine and the social sciences employ statistical laws because they must.

A statistical law is better than none at all, but investigators always keep before them the goal of replacing those laws with an understanding of causal mechanisms. But we must keep in mind that, so far as our best theories can tell us, some of the fundamental laws of nature are inherently probabilistic. We have no way of knowing exactly when an electron is going to change its orbital location, nor do we know exactly where it is to be found in a sphere surrounding the nucleus of an atom. We can, however, assign a probability value to its location. The basic physical processes of quantum mechanics are ones that require probabilistic laws for their understanding. And so far as we can tell, that is just the way the world is. Laws expressing invariant, nonprobabilistic regularities simply do not seem possible.

Statistical explanations, like nomological-deductive explanations, do their job by connecting an event with some other event or circumstance. Laws are the devices by which the connection is made. Thus, probabilistic laws also express patterns of regularities, and explanation is achieved by the demonstration that the explanandum event fits into that pattern. A probabilistic pattern may not be as satisfying or as useful as a causal pattern, but even a flickering candle is better than total darkness.

Prediction

The nomological models of explanation are also models for prediction. In fact, the logical structure of prediction is, according to the model, identical with that of explanation. The only difference is that of the time of the occurrence of the event: if the inference is made before the occurrence of the event, the sentence describing the event is a predictive one; if the inference is made after the event has occurred, the sentence is an explanandum sentence.

The reasoning behind what is usually called the symmetry of explanation and prediction is straightforward and persuasive. If explanation consists in knowing the laws and the initial conditions, then it is possible to see the event to be explained as fitting into the pattern expressed by the laws. That way we can be said to understand why that event occurred. By contrast, if we know in advance both the laws and the initial conditions, then we can see that the event will occur. Thus, the same considerations that allow us to understand the event after it has happened would have permitted us to anticipate the event had we possessed the information before its occurrence.

The same line of reasoning holds for probabilistic predictions. If we possess probabilistic laws that tell us that, under certain conditions, a particular event is likely to occur with a particular degree of probability, then when those conditions are present we are warranted in concluding that the event is likely to occur to just that degree.

This general analysis of prediction is intended to hold only for what are sometimes called rationally grounded predictions. That is, the analysis is limited to predictions that are justified by laws and theories. There are other senses of prediction that are not captured by this construal. Most generally, to make a prediction is only to offer a claim about some state of affairs that is either expected to obtain in the future or is presently unknown. If the person making the prediction offers it only as a guess or a hunch or on the basis of unanalyzed and unarticulated "experience," we may be willing to accept the prediction, even to the extent of acting on it, but it is quite different from a prediction that is rationally grounded by means of established laws. Medicine, in particular, may often have to be satisfied with such predictions. Subjective probability estimates of the sort we discussed in chapter 4 may also serve as predictions. For example, Dr. Williams thought Mrs. Halprin had lupus before he received the lab data that clinched that diagnosis. His belief (and prediction) was based on his assessment of the information available to him at that time. Clinical experience and clinical judgment often serve as a basis for prediction.

Events and Descriptions

We speak of events in an easy and familiar way as though we were always quite clear about what is an event and what is not. A bomb explodes, an airplane crashes, Mrs. Halprin's white cell count goes up-these are all events. But what about Mrs. Halprin falls ill, Mrs. Halprin has SLE, Mrs. Halprin's T-cells are malfunctioning? Surely these are events also, but in some way they seem to be overlapping, nonexclusive, or constituently related events. Some may be the same events as others or parts of the same events. How are we to understand this?

Events are complex, spatiotemporal chunks of the world. As such, they can be described in many ways. Some descriptions may be quite precise, while others are highly general. The more general descriptions will determine a class that is more inclusive than the more precise ones. If we describe Mrs. Halprin as ill, then we have assigned the event to a class much broader than the class associated with the description "Mrs. Halprin has SLE."

We speak loosely of explaining and predicting "events," but what we ordinarily mean by this is explaining and predicting an event under a certain description. Thus we may be able to explain why Mrs. Halprin is ill by referring to generalizations that connect such events as an increase in her white cell count and an increase in her body temperature, while at the same time we may not be able to explain why she has SLE.

Our laws and theories provide explanations for events as those events are described in the terms (quite literally) of the laws and theories. For this reason our dissatisfaction with laws and theories in medicine and science frequently stems from the fact that the explanations they give us are under descriptions of too high a level of generality. We are concerned about why Mrs. Halprin is ill, but we are even more concerned with why she is ill in precisely the way that she is—why, that is, she manifests the features we identify as SLE. That explanations involve descriptions makes it clear why progress in medicine and science frequently consists of establishing generalizations and theories that employ more refined descriptions than those available at a preceding time. Similarly, the need for descriptions makes it clear why progress may consist in demonstrating that a previously existing theory with more refined descriptions can be applied to a range of phenomena previously covered by a theory with less-refined descriptions. Thus, the recognition of SLE as an immunologic disease made it possible to redescribe in biochemical terms the phenomena constituting it. The result was to produce an understanding that was, in a sense, "deeper" and more detailed.

(Incidentally, one of the reasons we value quantitative results in science and medicine is that the mathematics involved allows us to provide descriptions of a high degree of refinement. It makes it possible to replace quantitatively vague phrases like *elevated temperature* and *insufficient coronary output* with ones that are exact. This, in turn, opens the way to establish generalizations that supply us with a more detailed understanding of the events or processes that are of concern to us.)

To sum up, when we speak of explaining or predicting events, this is only a shorthand way of talking. It is the explanation or prediction of events of a certain description that is our real concern. The shorthand is unobjectionable, but it must not blind us to the fact that the explanation of an event may be a perfectly good explanation and yet not satisfy us. It may fail to do so because we are not satisfied with the level of description under which the event is explained or, what is often the same thing, because we wish to have an explanation in terms of a particular (deeper or more fundamental) theory.

ESTABLISHING LAWS: TESTING, CONFIRMING, AND REJECTING HYPOTHESIS

We have talked about the use of laws and generalizations in explanation and merely taken for granted that we have available one or more appropriate laws. Similarly, we have talked about theories that explain laws and taken it for granted that we have available a set of basic principles we can employ to satisfy the nomological-deductive requirements of explanation.

Now let us step back from these assumptions and ask how laws and theories become established in the first place. Our concern is not with the partially psychological questions of how laws and theories are thought up or invented or discovered. Rather, our question is about the ways in which they come to merit our belief and win our endorsement. We can approach this question most directly and clearly by considering the way in which rather simple generalizations are established. This will lay the groundwork for considering how more complicated networks of generalizations and principles—theories— gain their warrant.

Testing Hypotheses

The kind of test regarded as most significant is that of predictive success or failure, although other factors also govern the ultimate fate of a hypothesis. SLE has become the classic instance of an autoimmune disease, and the sorts of factors that are involved in testing, rejecting, and confirming hypotheses and theories can be illustrated by considering briefly a few examples from the development of immunological theory and its relationship with SLE. Considering these examples will also help make it clear how theories played a role in decisions that were made in diagnosing the treating Mrs. Halprin.

The central concern of immunology as a scientific discipline is with the long-recognized fact that the body detects the presence of foreign substances and responds to them. The basic problem thus becomes the discovery and elucidation of the mechanisms that produce the response. A knowledge of these mechanisms and the means by which they are activated make it possible to recognize autoimmune diseases such as SLE, to devise laboratory tests to assist in their diagnosis, and to test the effectiveness of therapies.

It has been known since roughly the end of the nineteenth century that antigens, foreign material, trigger a sequence of cellular events that produce antibodies, protein molecules that combine specifically with each antigen. Lymphocytes known as B-cells synthesize and secrete antibodies. Other lymphocytes known as T-cells play a role in collaboration with B-cells but also can attack foreign substances by marshaling other effective cells.

But how does it happen that lymphocytes produce antibodies that are specific for a given antigen? The first significant hypothesis to explain this phenomenon was proposed around the beginning of this century by Paul Ehrlich. Ehrlich postulated that lymphocytes had side chains that were the antibodies. The set of side chains constituted the set of possible antibodies the cell could produce. When an antigen reacted with a side chain, the cell began producing the specific antibody by increasing the number of appropriate side chains.

Ehrlich's hypothesis predicted that, in the presence of a specific antigen, all but one type of side chain would disappear, while those being produced by the cell would show up in increased numbers in the blood serum. This turned out in large measure to be the case. The substances in the serum that were considered mysterious during a disease process were identified as specific types of antibodies. It was held that the serum of those with pneumonia, for example, contained a substance distinct from the substance found in the serum of those with tuberculosis. Both substances, according to the hypothesis, were the side chains that the different antigens induced the cells to produce.

Thus, Ehrlich's prediction turned out to be correct. It squared with the facts uncovered by investigation into the character of the mysterious "substances" that had already been detected in the serum of disease sufferers. The prediction, we can say, confirmed Ehrlich's hypothesis.

In general, we can say that a hypothesis is confirmed when it is used in making a prediction and the prediction turns out to be correct. Successful prediction does not prove the hypothesis is correct, however. It is both logically and practically possible to make a successful prediction on the basis of a hypothesis that is known on other grounds to be false. Nevertheless, a successful predictive outcome does provide us with strong evidence for believing that a hypothesis is true. And, obviously, additional correct predictions provide additional evidence in support of the hypothesis.

Confirming Auxiliary Assumptions

Ehrlich's side-chain hypothesis was confirmed by the results of future investigations, for what the hypothesis predicted would be so turned out to be so. But we must not overlook the fact that Ehrlich's hypothesis did not stand alone. The prediction was based on the hypothesis and a set of additional assumptions.

It is very hard in any particular case to spell out just what additional assumptions are being made. The same is true of Ehrlich's hypothesis. Here, however, are some of the more obvious ones:

- Antigens and side chains become connected by means of some mechanism or other.
- Lymphocytes possess mechanisms to shed unneeded side chains and to produce copies of needed ones.

- Antigens are distinct from one another.
- Lymphocytes have appropriate side chains for every antigen.
- The laws of chemical and physical theory (the ones current at the time) are correct.

These assumptions are usually referred to as auxiliary assumptions. When they are taken into account, what is actually confirmed by a successful prediction is the entire set of premises from which predictions are derived. This includes the hypothesis, but it also includes much more. Success of predictions based on the side-chain hypothesis also confirmed the belief that, for example, antigens could in some way lock onto the side chains of lymphocytes.

Ultimately, then, what the successful prediction confirmed was a whole network of claims about the immune response. The observations or facts that make the predictions true are the strands that tie the network to the world. Much more is involved in even this relatively simple case of hypothesis testing than the hypothesis itself. This is invariably the case in all scientific and medical inquiry. The network that includes the hypothesis might also include quite specific initial conditions, but it may also include additional principles from some other theory. These may or may not be made explicit.

In summary, we can say: (1) a hypothesis is confirmed when it is used as the basis for a successful prediction; (2) a prediction is successful when it is in agreement with observed facts; (3) when a prediction confirms a hypothesis, it also confirms the auxiliary assumptions that also played a role in making the prediction; (4) the following deductive model represents the basis of rational prediction:

H (hypothesis)
$A_1 \ldots A_n$ (auxiliary assumptions)

P (prediction)

We have talked about confirmation occurring when the prediction derived from the premises that include the hypothesis turns out to agree with observations. But what happens when the hypothesis is incorrect? When it does not square with the facts? That is what we must consider next.

Rejecting Hypotheses

Ehrlich's side-chain hypothesis was well supported by its predictions. In addition, it pointed the way toward the development of specific research programs by raising questions about the immune response that had not been raised before. Thus, it led to investigations designed to distinguish among antigens, to identify the mechanisms by which the cell produces antibodies, to identify the mechanisms by which antigens induce the productions of antibodies by attaching to the side chains, and so on.

The downfall of the hypothesis was the result of doubts about the truth of one of its auxiliary assumptions. Ehrlich assumed that for every antigen there would be a preexisting side chain attached to the lymphocytes. Karl Landsteiner produced a body of evidence that made this assumption quite implausible. In a series of experiments, Landsteiner tested the ability of modified forms of organic compounds to induce antibody production. For example, he discovered that he could produce antibodies specific for nitrobenzene, then after modifying the molecule, antibodies against dinitrobenzene. Indeed, it seemed that there was no end to the list of organic compounds that would elicit a specific antibody response. Thus, it seemed highly unlikely that a cell would have side chains specific for any possible antigen. By the 1940s, Ehrlich's side-chain hypothesis was abandoned by most investigators.

In the simplest form of falsifying a hypothesis, a prediction turns out to be false. This, in turn, falsifies the hypothesis from which it was derived. The valid argument form modus tollens represents this relationship.

If *P*, then *Q*
not-*Q*

---

not-*P*

Because of its relation to the argument form, the rejection of a hypothesis because of a predictive failure is called modus tollens falsification.

In practice, what is really falsified is the set of assumptions that includes the hypothesis. The side-chain hypothesis was rejected not because there was a clear predictive failure, but because one of the auxiliary assumptions was false. Since predictions, including successful ones, were based on the entire set of assumptions, the demonstration that one of them was false meant that the set of claims constituting the explanation of the immune response could not be correct.

The response might have been to attempt to save the side-chain hypothesis by devising some way in which side-chains could respond to an apparently endless array of antigens. However, in fact, research took another turn and other models of the responses were devised.

SLE and Current Hypotheses

Autoimmune diseases like SLE are associated with the response of an organism's immune system to its own cells. How such a breakdown in self-tolerance occurs is not known. At the present time, however, several hypotheses are under investigation and each can claim some support from experimental and clinical evidence.

The Alteration of Self-Component

According to the alteration of self-component hypothesis, the immune system begins to produce antibodies against self-components when those components become changed so as to be unrecognizable. Viral material may become incorporated into the cell membrane or a virus may cause a cell to form an abnormal membrane. These altered cells are then no longer recognized as belonging to "self" and so become the target of antibodies.

The Exposure of Hidden Antigens

The exposure of hidden antigens hypothesis suggests that since materials within cells do not encounter lymphocytes during the immunologically unresponsive period of embryonic development, later exposure by infection or trauma may cause the lymphocytes to react to them as foreign substances. Similarly, antigens hidden within the folded chains of proteins may be brought into reactive positions if the proteins are denatured.

The Mutation of Lymphocytes

According to the mutation of lymphocytes hypothesis, mutation of lymphocytes is a constant process, and some of the mutations will react with self-components tolerated by the ordinary lymphocyte population. If the mutants are not themselves eliminated, as they may not be in a defective immune system, then they will increase in number.

T-Cell Defects

The defective T-cell hypothesis holds that B-cells always have the ability to react with self but are kept from doing so by a suppressor function of T-cells. If mutation or viral infection alters the T-cells so that this function is lost, B-cells produce autoantibodies.

It is against the background of these hypotheses that some of the laboratory tests were ordered in an attempt to arrive at a diagnosis of Mrs. Halprin's illness. In particular, tests for antinuclear antibodies were considered particularly relevant by Dr. Williams. Antibodies to double-stranded DNA are found almost uniquely in SLE, and a test for their presence is regarded as good practice when SLE is suspected.

Although none of these hypotheses can be regarded as so well supported that we can exclude the others, this is not such an important fact from the clinical standpoint. The hypotheses provide direction in diagnostic inquiry, and diagnostic inquiry, in turn, provides information that can be used to support one (or more) of the hypotheses in contrast with the others. For example, investigators studying SLE are more likely to favor the defective T-cell hypothesis, simply because it can account for the fact that in patients affected with lupus it is possible to find autoantibodies for almost every body constituent. In this respect, then, observation supports this hypothesis more than it supports, say, the exposure of hidden antigens hypothesis.

THE LOGICAL STRUCTURE OF THEORIES

For most theories in science and medicine, it is virtually impossible to identify fully and correctly the principles and laws that might be said to constitute the theory. To a considerable extent this is because the enterprises of inquiry, experiment, explanation, prediction, observation, and so on all take place in a context in which it is difficult to separate theories from one another. One theory (e.g., one from immunology) often makes use of principles (e.g., atomic bonding) borrowed from another. Similarly, it is often impossible to say just what consists of general background information common to every theory (e.g., the solubility of organic salts in water) and what belongs to the theory proper. Finally, even a single theory may exist in several variant forms so that to speak of "the" theory of such and such may be both incorrect and misleading.

Such a logically and conceptually messy situation is typical of theories that are involved in ongoing research and application in medicine and science. The theories that are the clearest and most easily formulated are those that are, in a sense, wrapped up and finished. Classical mechanics in physics, for example, is a theory that is relatively easy to specify. It consists, essentially, of Newton's laws of motion and universal gravitation. Other laws and generalizations about phenomena that can be understood in terms of point masses and forces acting upon them can be regarded as special application of these basic principles. Similarly, classical Mendelian genetics can be construed as a theory that consists of a set of principles concerning the ways in which entities known as "genes" are distributed and expressed in reproductive generations. Explanations and predictions of the appearance of certain traits can be secured by appealing to the principles.

Such "finished" theories can serve as examples of some of the outstanding features of what we look for or want from successful theories. By relying on them as reference points, we can develop abstract and somewhat idealized models of theories. These models are not so much actual descriptions of real theories as they are expressions of criteria that we believe that theories ought to satisfy. In this sense, then, the models are normative ones (since they express standards), but they are also descriptive ones (since they are based on what we consider to be successful theories).

Components of Theories

Theories, according to our original definition, are sets of principles or basic laws that can be employed for the purposes of explanation and prediction .If we think of a "completed" or "finished" theory in an abstract and somewhat idealized way, it can be construed as an axiom system. That is, the theory can be represented as having the same kind of logical structure as that which we associate with Euclidean geometry or any other complete mathematical theory. The theory as an axiom system can be analyzed into three components: axioms, correspondence rules, and theorems.

Axioms

The principles of a theory are the basic laws that make the theory what it is. They are the ultimate basis for explanation for the phenomena that fall within the scope of the theory. In an empirical theory (such as those in medicine and science), the principles are not simply "given" or assumed. Rather, they are supported, both directly and indirectly, by observational evidence and are open to falsification and rejection.

Logically speaking, when principles serve as axioms, then laws belonging to the theory that are narrower in scope or represent restricted applications are explained by demonstrating them to be the deductive consequents of the principles. (See chap. 5 for a more detailed account.)

Rules of Correspondence

The principles of a theory usually contain terms that cannot be applied to observational phenomena in a direct, straightforward way. The concepts and terms of the theory have an abstract character, and they also have a certain "open" character. Thus, it is necessary to connect terms like electrolytic balance, gene, and mass with others that apply more directly to phenomena.

In practice, this means making use of empirical principles or generalizations (sometimes called operational definitions or bridge principles) that establish connections between statements about theoretical phenomena and observed phenomena. Theories of molecular genetics, for example, must (implicitly or explicitly) establish a relationship between the behavior of DNA codons and phenomena that are attributed to the action of "genes."

Theorems

In an axiomatic deductive system, statements that are deductively derived from the axioms by logical rules are theorems of the system. In the construing of theories as axiom systems, the theorems of the axioms are the lower-level laws. These laws are explained by the principles of the theory when (with the help of the correspondence rules) they are derived from them.

In addition to the components of theories that we have named, we might also say that deductive rules of inference and formation rules (to determine what counts as a legitimate "formula" in the system) need to be added. But since these can be regarded as elements belonging to any axiomatic deductive system, we need not list them as separate components.

The Explanation of Laws

The account of the structure of theories that we have outlined can be summarized in the following scheme:

$$P_1 \ldots P_n \quad \text{(Principles)}$$
$$CR_1 \ldots CR_n \quad \text{(Correspondence rules)}$$

$$\overline{L_1 \ldots L_n \quad \text{(Laws)}}$$

From this point of view, the laws belonging to the theory are experimental laws that can be established antecedent to the formulation of the theory (or at least independent of the theory). The role of the theory is to explain the laws, and this it does by showing that they are the deductive consequents of the principles of the theory.

Consider as an example the gene rearrangement theory of immunology. The theory explains antibody response to antigens (the generation of diversity) by maintaining that lymphocytes possess the genetic material that codes for the entire array of antibody specificities. The empirical law (confirmed generalization) that antigens trigger an antibody response by the clonal expansion of a lymphocyte possessing the specificity appropriate for the antigen can, with some added information, be derived from the gene arrangement theory. Thus, the phenomena covered by the law can be regarded as special instances of the principles of gene rearrangement.

The account of the explanation of laws provided by this model is similar to the account provided of the explanation of events. The model is a nomological-deductive one—explanation is achieved by the deduction of that which is to be explained from a set of one or more laws.

Accordingly, the specific criteria for explanation that must be satisfied are also similar:

1. The theoretical principles (the axioms of the formulation) must be true.
2. The explanandum sentence (the experimental law) must be a deductive consequent of the explanans (the set of principles).
3. The principles that play a role in the explanation must be empirical ones. That is, they must be open to falsification and not be merely disguised definitions or ad hoc assumptions.
4. The correspondence rules must be true. Since the correspondence rules establish a relationship between sentences that contain theoretical terms and those that contain observational terms, they have the status of empirical generalizations. (Generalizations about the "gene for" a particular biochemical product must hold also for generalizations about a particular codon.)

ESTABLISHING THEORIES: TESTING, CONFIRMING, AND REJECTING THEORIES

Theories, as we have said, are sets of principles or basic laws that are employed for purposes of explanation and prediction. A theory can be appealed to for justifying a prediction or for grounding an explanation—the nomological models give an account of these functions. But since no theory can be considered self-justifying or self-evidently true, a basic question necessary to settle about any theory is why it should command belief. That is, where does a theory get its own warrant? How is a theory justified? Or if a theory is not justified, then what are the grounds or reasons for rejecting it?

Fortunately, the answers to these questions can be given in very short compass. Our previous discussion of testing and confirming hypotheses introduced most of the issues, and what can be said about hypotheses can be said, for the most part, about theories as well.

Testing Theories

Theories are tested by their deductive consequences. That is, predictions derived from a theory are tested against relevant observations and data. A prediction that turns out to be correct increases our confidence in the theory. As with a hypothesis, it is the set of assumptions (the laws or principles) from which the prediction was derived that is confirmed by a successful prediction.

Theories make predictions about individual events only via laws (plus initial conditions). But theories also predict laws. That is, general statements about classes or types of events can be derived from the principles that constitute a theory. (As we mentioned earlier, for example, the clonal expansion laws can be derived from the gene rearrangement theory.) In accordance with the nomological-deductive model, such a theory explains the law that is derived. Notice, however, that this also has consequences for confirmation. If a theory is successful in explaining an established law (an accepted hypothesis), this provides us with grounds for believing that the theory is correct. Just as our confidence in a hypothesis is increased by the range, variety, and number of successful predictions derived from it, so our confidence in a theory is increased when the theory is shown to be broad and encompassing in a similar way. The theories of classical and molecular genetics, the synthetic theory of evolution, and the theory of quanta are supported by the successful generalizations that can be derived from them (or at least, based on them).

Thus, success in explaining laws (both in number and variety) is one of the marks we look for in evaluating a theory. We expect a "good" theory to be one that is broad in scope, strong in explanatory power, and suggestive of future lines of development.

Direct and Indirect Confirmation

A theory is directly confirmed by the already established laws that can be derived from it. But those laws themselves are supported by the successful predictions that are based on them and by other relevant data. This means, then, that the predictions and data directly supporting the laws provide indirect support for the principles from which the laws are derived. Furthermore, as we mentioned earlier, hypotheses that are candidates for laws are indirectly supported by the principles from which they are derived.

The result, as we described it in our discussion of confirming hypotheses, is a network of laws, principles, evidence, and predictions. It is the network as a whole that is supported. Evidence for a theory is transmitted into support for derived laws and successfully supported laws. These laws, in turn, transmit their direct support as indirect support for the theoretical principles.

Thus, theoretical principles that seem to float freely in some high abstract realm are actually anchored to the world by experimental laws, which are themselves directly tied to observations. In this way an observation as basically trivial as the white-eye of a fruit fly can support apparently remote principles of genetics.

It should not be forgotten that theories themselves may form a hierarchy of generality. Theories at a "lower" level may be explained by (derived from) principles that are more general. When this can be done, then the direct and indirect evidential support of both theories comes to be shared by each.

When relationships of the sort we have been discussing are recognized, it are ever tested, accepted, or rejected in total isolation. Every item is just one piece of what investigators hope is a single grand design. Consequently, it is ordinarily a virtual impossibility to alter one part of the design without introducing alterations in some-if not all-parts of the remaining pattern.

Rejecting Theories

Theories, according to the nomological-deductive model, are rejected when they are falsified. They are falsified by the same kind of modus tollens procedure involved in falsifying a hypothesis. That is, when a prediction based on the theory turns out to be incorrect, then the principles of the theory on which the prediction was based cannot all be regarded as correct. At least one of them must be considered false. (We are assuming, of course, that nothing is wrong with the test conditions.)

Strictly speaking, a falsified theory must be rejected. After all, it has been shown to involve at least one false law or principle. Thus it loses all claim to our endorsement, for we can no longer rely on it to supply us with reliable predictions and grounded explanations.

In practice, of course, matters are rarely so simple. Investigators typically attempt to find ways of saving a theory that has proved to be successful in the past and that is supported by other predictions and by a range and variety of direct and indirect evidence. One possible response is to introduce an ad hoc hypothesis as part of a reformulated theory that is otherwise identical with the original theory. The classic example of the use of ad hoc hypotheses is the addition of epicycles to the Ptolemaic theory to make observations of planetary motion square with the theory's principles that all orbits are perfect circles and the earth is at the center of the solar system.

The modification of theories by the addition of ad hoc hypotheses is generally considered to be, in itself, an inadmissible way of rescuing a theory from falsification. However, as in most scientific matters, the line between legitimate and illegitimate modifications is often difficult to draw. The use of hypotheses that are testable and can be supported by independent evidence is, in fact, a legitimate maneuver. It is one of the ways in which theories respond to the observable data.

Logically speaking, a theory can be regarded as no more than a complicated hypothesis for the purpose of testing. As in testing a hypothesis, it is the predictive results that are of most significance. If the theory predicts a law that is already well established or if the theory is used to predict an event that occurs in the expected way, then our confidence in the theory is increased. On the other hand, an unsuccessful prediction based on a theory (other things being equal) falsifies the theory. We must then either reject the theory as it is formulated or attempt to find a new formulation that will be successful.

THEORIES AND MODELS

Science in general and medicine in particular make considerable use of models in attempting to understand phenomena. The kinetic theory of gases is characteristically explained in terms of the ping-pong model and classical mechanics in terms of the billiard ball model. In clinical medicine, frequent reference is made to the electrical circuit model of brain function, the bellows model of lung mechanics, and the hydraulic pump model of the cardiovascular system. What are models and how are they related to theories?

Theoretical and Simulating Models

The term *model* is used in a great variety of ways in ordinary language: model student, model airplane, model K-5A, artist's model, architectural model, and so on. The term itself is so suggestive that it has been appropriated by the sciences, where it is also used in a variety of ways. Some of these ways simply contradict each other. Consequently, when one speaks of a model in science or medicine, it is not at all clear what is intended by the term. To find out, one must simply look and see what is meant.

In the view of some scientists and philosophers of science, a model is a necessary part of a theory—the Ping-Pong ball model is necessary for the application of the gas laws. Furthermore, for many scientists and social scientists, the term *model* is identical in meaning with *theory*. To have a model of a piece of social behavior is to have a theory about that behavior. Models in science can be divided into two major types: *theoretical models* and *simulating models.*

Theoretical models are those employed to develop and explain the fundamental ideas and concepts of a theory. The planetary model of the atom is a prime example of a theoretical model. Niels Bohr used the familiar and well-understood idea of the planets revolving about the sun to represent relationships expressed in experimental data. In addition, his model opened the way for raising questions about the behavior of the model system, behavior that pointed toward additional laws and experiments. In a sense, a theoretical model is a metaphor ("the atomic nucleus is like a sun, and electrons are like planets"), and its appropriateness is judged in terms of its coherence with the basic theory and the data. It is also judged in terms of its fruitfulness in suggesting ways in which the theory can be developed and extended.

Scientists use theoretical models to describe aspects of the scientific reality with which they deal. By and large they expect us to take them as realistic representations. Molecular biologists, for example, think of their models as exhibiting genuine molecular structures. But the word *structure* should be emphasized, for no molecular biologist thinks that molecular bonds are literally sticks or lines.

Simulating models, by contrast, are used to test and develop theories in domains that are clearly distinct from the domain of the model. In medicine, perhaps the most important simulating models are those involving animals and laboratory cultures, for they have played major roles in acquiring an understanding of disease processes and the effects of new therapies. Artificial intelligence—the computer simulation of intelligent behavior–has provided many simulating models in recent years, and computer models of diagnosis are currently being actively developed and refined.

Simulating models, like theoretical models, work by being analogous to the subject they model. The difference between the two types is a matter of the function they serve. Medical scientists make no claim that rats have anatomies or physiologies that are sufficiently identical to ours to serve as representations of them. They claim only that rats share enough relevant similarities to permit us to test hypotheses that, because of ethical, legal, or time constraints, cannot be tested directly on humans. Such tests show only that humans probably (or, perhaps, only might) respond similarly. Unfortunately, there are no a priori means for determining which predictions based upon a nonhuman model will prove true of humans as well. The applicability of a simulating model is ultimately a matter of our experience with it.

Some Models and Analogies in Medicine

Two animal models have played an important role in developing our understanding of systemic lupus erythematosus. In the 1960s a number of investigators studied the effects of injecting bovine serum albumin into rabbits. The rabbits developed one-shot serum sickness, so called because of its similarity to the disorder affecting people injected with serum from another person or animal. After a delay of several days, the rabbit's immune system forms antibodies to the foreign protein, the complement level falls, and a clearing of the foreign protein from the blood ensues. At the same time, there is also evidence of kidney inflammation, in addition to the systemic illness. When foreign proteins are no longer present in the blood, the disease remits. The rabbit's immune-complex disease bears several obvious and important similarities to SLE. The second model consists in the spontaneous occurrence of a multisystem disorder in the offspring of New Zealand white mice bred with New Zealand black mice. This disorder has the features of chronic immune-complex disease.

Both models have led to many hypotheses about SLE. The first showed, for example, that an immune-complex disorder like SLE can result in kidney damage. The second allowed scientists to test certain toxic drugs, such as cyclophosphamide, which are used in treating SLE. Both models strengthened the theory that SLE is associated with the presence of immune complexes in the blood of affected patients. These substances cause injury to various tissues, and the tissue damage is manifested in the signs and symptoms of SLE.

The relationship between the theory of SLE and its models has been reciprocal. Predictions made using the theory have been tested in the models, and observations made using the models have led to revisions of the theory. For example, after a theoretical understanding of the role of chemicals such as prostaglandins in the inflammatory response of SLE had been achieved, scientists tried to experimentally alter prostaglandin metabolism in the NZB/NZW mice. Conversely, the observation that these mice suffer from a chronic viral infection led to an intensive search for such viruses in humans afflicted with SLE, and it raised the probability of the hypothesis that incompletely sup- pressed chronic infections can lead to immunologic diseases.

More important, despite the many indications that lupus is an autoimmune disorder, compelling evidence is still lacking. Thus the existence of such evidence in the mice model not only confirmed the theory, but also let it be applied, together with general immunologic theory, to predict correctly that suppressor cells would be defective or deficient in lupus patients. (Suppressor cells are lymphocytes that dampen the immune response.)

Simulating models are never identical with the subject matter they model. Accordingly, there will always be dissimilarities (disanalogies) as well as similarities (analogies).For example, in the mice model of SLE, the mice often die of types of cancer with rates that are not reflected in SLE patients. Furthermore, the disorder in the mice models involves the presence of viral antigen, yet no analogous antigens have been found in SLE patients. Because of the dissimilarities between the model and what is modeled, there is always room to doubt that what is established as true of the model will also hold true of the subject modeled.

Reasoning from models generally involves arguing by analogy. That is, we claim that because the model and the thing it models are similar in certain relevant respects and because one has a certain property, then it follows that probably so does the other. (See the discussion in chap. 4.) This form of reasoning is pervasive in clinical medicine. Physicians argue that because one patient responded to a certain drug in a given way, so will another patient who is similar to the first. Or they look for risk factors for diseases, assuming that if they can find the relevant similarities between patients who have had the disease, then they can predict who is likely to get it. Sometimes the correlations they observe can be given theoretical explanations. More often than not, one must take them as mere correlations awaiting future explanation.

The shortcomings of reasoning from models and reasoning by analogy raise serious questions about their propriety. So we will now address the questions briefly.

Reasoning via Models and Analogies

Our concern is with simulating models. (For a discussion of the formal features of analogical reasoning, see chap. 4.) With regard to these models, the distinction between the model and the thing that it models is readily acknowledged. The same distinction is controversial when applied to theoretical models, but that need not detain us. Their primary use is for description and not for inferring properties of entities distinct from themselves, and so they stand and fall with the theories of which they are part. How then can we infer from a simulating model to the thing it models or conversely? How can we conclude anything about SLE in humans from inherited disorders in mice or conversely?

In approaching this question we must distinguish two theoretical contexts in which our reasoning might take place. In the first context both the model and its image fall under the same general theory. For example, suppose that it has been established as a matter of general histologic theory that a given concentration of an acid will cause an irritation on human skin if and only if it has the same effect on the naked skin of a rabbit. Then rabbits can be used as test models for cosmetics or topical drugs containing the acid in question. Given the theory in question, one can deduce the effects on humans from the results of the experiments with rabbits.

Similar remarks apply to clinical situations in which observations involving a group of test patients are used together with a background theory to draw conclusions about another patient. In physics and chemistry, for example, it is common to carry out special experiments to determine the values of universal constants, which are then used in all other calculations in which they are needed. Such an extrapolation from a single experiment is, of course, underwritten by general physical and chemical theory.

Using animal models to experimentally test or extend a general biological theory follows the same logic. It is a matter of straightforward deduction: the theory tells us that what happens in this particular experiment will occur in all other cases of the same kind (baring anomalies and other problems associated with the experiment itself); we observe that a certain thing has occurred in the experiment and conclude that it will occur in all other situations of the same type.

Unfortunately, the second theoretical context is much weaker inferentially and much more common in medicine. This is where we do not know of any general background theory of the kind presupposed by the first form of reasoning. We know of some similarities between the model and its image, but we also know of important differences between them, and worse, we know that there is much we do not know about the two. Then we must reason by analogy. As we noted in chapter 4 on inductive reasoning, reasoning by analogy is a form of probabilistic reasoning that is not well understood by contemporary logicians and statisticians. In particular, there are no currently available means for determining the degree of probability various features of a model or its analogue confer on conclusions drawn from one to the other. Nor do we have methods for determining which shared features are significant or relevant and which disanalogies may be discounted. Since the use of models and analogical reasoning is so pervasive in clinical and research medicine, it is unfortunate that we cannot quantitate degree of analogy. On the practical side, it warns us to approach this form of reasoning with caution and to seek to substantiate the conclusions it yields by independent means.

OBJECTIONS AND ALTERNATIVES

The analysis of the character of scientific laws, theories, and hypotheses that we have presented is one that unquestionably illuminates various aspects of the nature of science and medicine. However, the general point of view that lies behind the analysis is one that has been challenged in several respects in recent years. Here we briefly examine some of the objections that have been raised to the general analysis and present some of the basic features attributed to science by Thomas Kuhn in his influential book, The Structure of Scientific Revolutions.

Some Objections to the Analysis

Few philosophers of science are prepared to endorse the normative status of the models of explanation, hypothesis testing, and theory structure presented earlier. The models are considered either too restrictive, too encompassing, or as resting on false assumptions about the character of legitimate science. Consequently, according to the critics, the models provide an unrealistic, misleading, and essentially false picture of scientific theories and explanations.

Without attempting to be either detailed or complete, here are some of the more important objections that have been raised:

1. Most current theories do not satisfy the formal requirements of an axiomatic system. Only "dead" or completed theories can be represented in this way. By suggesting that all theories ought to resemble this ideal, the analysis is misleading and unilluminating.

2. The criteria for scientific explanations can be satisfied without producing genuine explanations. For example, geometric optics and the physical assumption that light travels in straight lines will allow us to determine how high a building is, but it does not explain why the building has that height. Thus, the claim that the model constitutes necessary and sufficient conditions for explanation is incorrect.

3. Some scientific theories, such as the synthetic theory of evolution, provide legitimate explanations, although they have little or no predictive power. Without justification, the formal models would brand such theories as second rate.

4. Hypotheses that are experimentally falsified are not always rejected. Sometimes they are retained and used to guide research, even though they are

known to be defective. Thus, taking the criterion of falsification as requiring theory rejection would probably hamper the process of scientific research.

5. The analysis assumes that "facts" exist independent of theories, but the observations we make and the reports we give are always in terms of some particular theory. The nonphysician who observes Mrs. Halprin is simply not going to see what the physician sees.

These objections are serious ones, but we will make no effort to evaluate them here. If they are accepted as correct, one might say that they adequately demonstrate the false and misleading character of the analysis of science. However, one might also say that, at the most, they show only that the scientific enterprise is more complicated than the models suggest. Thus, the models might be regarded as nothing more than a first approximation of actual scientific practice. As such, they may still serve as useful guidelines or goals, even if we are not prepared to endorse them as strict standards that ought always to be followed.

The Kuhnian Alternative: The Paradigm View of Science

Thomas Kuhn's The Structure of Scientific Revolutions does, indeed, concern scientific revolutions. But more than this, it offers a view about the nature of science that is based upon the history of scientific change, a view that is apparently significantly different from the nomological view.

According to Kuhn, the standard image of science (the image that is the basis of the nomological view) is drawn mostly from the study of finished scientific achievements. Science textbooks represent the content of science as embodied in observations, laws, and theories and describe the techniques used in gathering data and expressing them in theories. The implication of this view is that science develops by a process of accumulation that is rational and logical. Older theories are replaced by better theories, and a theory is better when it has not been falsified and is better confirmed by the data.

Kuhn is wholly concerned with replacing this standard image of science with one that is based on the "historical integrity" of science. Even theories that we now consider wrong, he claims, were not less scientific in their own time. What we consider "science" must include beliefs that are incompatible with those we now hold, and this in itself makes the "accumulative" view of science doubtful.

The paradigm view that Kuhn offers as an alternative to the standard or "accumulative" image of science is based on three basic concepts: paradigm, normal science, and revolution. We explain each of these briefly, and from this the paradigm view of science should emerge.

Paradigm

A paradigm is a network of concepts, theories, methods, and basic beliefs that has been successfully used to solve concrete scientific problems. The humoral theory of disease is one paradigm, the germ theory another. Aristotelian mechanics is one paradigm, Newtonian mechanics another. Behaviorist psychology is one paradigm, Freudian psychology another.

A paradigm is accepted by a scientific community when it can supply solutions to problems, and these solutions can be used as examples or models for solving other problems. Mendelian genetics, for example, showed how it was possible to predict accurately the distribution of certain traits in successive generations. Solutions worked out for pea plants served as models for solving other trait-distribution problems. Furthermore, the paradigm became elaborated and developed so that it could be used to solve new problems-ones about partial dominance, the nature of the "unit" of inheritance, and the material basis of inheritance.

Furthermore, paradigms also determine what kinds of problems are relevant or important, and what will count as a real scientific solution-as distinguished from a guess or speculation. A paradigm also determines what things exist (such as forces, genes, mutations, proteins, codons, etc.) and what we observe when investigating certain phenomena. Thus, paradigms tell us both what there is to see and what we are seeing.

Normal Science

Normal science is ordinary, everyday science. It is what most scientists spend most of their time doing. It is an activity that takes place when a scientific community accepts a paradigm as the basis for its operation. The community then works to get nature to fit the paradigm. It articulates and develops the paradigm, formulating theories, laws, and concepts, developing new techniques of measurement and new means of experiment, in an effort to extend them to cover as many phenomena as possible.

A paradigm becomes accepted by a scientific community when the paradigm has shown itself to be successful in solving at least some problems. This success encourages the attempt to employ the paradigm to solve additional problems of the same type and to extend the paradigm to new areas. The paradigm is thus not accepted by fiat or on the basis of authority alone, although once adopted it may come to have a force and authority that is almost impossible to resist. In the beginning, at least, it is the problem-solving power of the paradigm that secures adherence.

Normal science is basically a "puzzle-solving" activity. The puzzle is always how to understand phenomena by fitting them into the paradigm. Normal science does not seek out new and strange phenomena that do not fit the paradigm. In fact, phenomena that do not fit into an accepted paradigm may simply be ignored, said to be a problem for some other area of science, or be dismissed as unreal.

Revolution

Revolution is the rapid and discontinuous shift from one paradigm to another. It takes place when an old paradigm runs up against too many puzzles that it cannot solve, and no one has been able to think up ways of modifying it so that it will be adequate. The paradigm is still used, to the extent possible, but it has clearly broken down and is a source of doubt and dissatisfaction. The only way to get back to normal science, back to business as usual, is by getting a new paradigm.

The new paradigm must, in effect, solve the old puzzles and the new ones as well. Or more accurately, it must be superior in puzzle-solving effectiveness. More of the world must fit into its boxes, and the aspects that caused trouble to the previous paradigm must-for some reason or another-disappear.

The most obvious examples of large-scale revolutionary changes are the replacement of the creationist view of species with the evolutionary view, and the triumph of relativity theory and quantum theory over classical mechanics. But revolutions may take place on a smaller scale. The identification of DNA as the genetic material and the working out of its structure was a revolution that effectively replaced both classical and fine-structure genetics as the basic paradigm of inheritance. In immunology, gene rearrangement theory replaced somatic mutation theory as an account of the generation of diversity.

Revolution involves a discrete break—an old paradigm is rejected and a new one is accepted. When this happens, phenomena are seen in the new way. Thus, as Kuhn says, to change paradigms is like making a gestalt switch. At one moment you are looking at a figure that you see as a duck, and at the next moment, you see the figure as a rabbit. Similarly, what is seen at one time as a humoral imbalance is seen at another time as a bacterial infection.

When paradigms change, nothing remains as before. Even "facts" change. No one needs to be concerned with explaining the "fact" that bloodletting has a therapeutic effect, if the paradigm in which that "fact" is recognized is no longer accepted. If flu is caused by a virus infection, then there is no need to account for how getting wet and cold causes flu.

The history of science, in Kuhn's view, is the history of scientific revolutions. It is the history of discrete breaks, of times when a dominant paradigm collapses, is rejected, and is replaced.

A mature science is a science that has adopted a single paradigm. When that has come about, then normal science proceeds to apply, elaborate, and extend the paradigm. But at some periods of history, more than one paradigm may be in competition. It was this way before quantum mechanics replaced classical mechanics, before evolutionary biology replaced creationism and Lamarckism. It is this way today in many areas of science, particularly in psychology and sociology.

Since paradigms determine the way people see the world, those who hold different paradigms will not be able to agree on facts, concepts, laws, problems, solutions, or anything else. Furthermore, since the concepts of a paradigm determine observations -since there are no neutral or paradigm-free observations -there is no way to "translate" one paradigm into another. Paradigms are incommensurable.

As a result, paradigms are both incompatible and incomparable. We cannot look through green glasses and pink glasses at the same time—we have to make a choice. We have to be able to see the ambiguous gestalt figure either as a duck or as a rabbit -we cannot see it as both at the same time.

The paradigm view makes it clear why scientists often talk past one another. They do so because they hold different paradigms, and without a shared basis, they cannot even disagree over the "facts" and their significance. Appealing to the facts has no power, because facts are paradigm-dependent.

The paradigm view also helps us see why those who hold older theories are only very reluctantly converted to new ones. They have become accustomed to seeing the world in terms of the older paradigm, and it is their definition of reality. Moreover, their professional careers as researchers have been con-ducted in accordance with the paradigm they accepted at the beginning of their work. To throw over that paradigm and to accept one incommensurable with it is to acknowledge that the work they have done is without enduring significance. Accordingly, they will have both a personal and professional loyalty to the older paradigm and be unwilling to surrender their allegiance to it.

Finally, the paradigm view makes it obvious why the accumulative view of science cannot be the correct one. Science can be accumulative only if it is possible to establish more and more neutral facts over time. But facts are not neutral. They are paradigm-dependent. Hence, every change in a paradigm is, in effect, a reconceptualization of the world and the things that are in it. Succeeding paradigms may be more successful than their predecessors (in the sense that they solve more problems), but they do not build upon their predecessors.

Philosophers of science have raised serious objections to Kuhn's analysis. For example, some have pointed out that if paradigms are incommensurable, there is no way to say one is better than the other. Thus, changing paradigms would have to be regarded as an arbitrary action. Similarly, if paradigms cannot be compared, how can science be said to make progress?

Most students of the philosophy of science are prepared to admit that many of the strictures urged against the standard nomological-deductive, accumulative view of science are genuine weaknesses, but they are not prepared to admit that the Kuhnian paradigm analysis is wholly correct. Much effort has been spent in recent years in attempting to provide an analysis of science that combines aspects of both views.

Science does seem to involve paradigms, but at the same time there seem to be aims and values that are not unique to particular paradigms. For example, accuracy in measurement is always valued; so too is simplicity and an intolerance for ad hoc theory-saving hypotheses. All paradigms seem to be committed to explanations that are, in a sense, atomistic. That is, explanations that explain phenomena by appealing to the workings of underlying fundamental mechanisms are valued.

Furthermore, the paradigm view fails to supply a detailed account of the ways in which hypotheses and theories are tested, confirmed, and rejected. Such a logical analysis can clearly be of value in deciding just what is to count as satisfactory scientific practice. The nomological account may go too far in offering its models as defining legitimate scientific practice as all and only those formulations that satisfy the models. Nonetheless, the models may well have normative force and heuristic value.

√5. Perhaps, then, there is a middle ground between the nomological analysis and the paradigm analysis. At the moment, it is too early to say exactly what it is, for even if it has been discovered, it remains relatively uncharted.

It seems appropriate to end this chapter by raising the question "What does all this philosophy of science have to do with Mrs. Halprin and with clinical medicine?" The nonintellectual answer is that it has nothing to do with either. It is quite possible to practice medicine on the basis of empirical rules and procedures that ignore both medicine's scientific component and its conceptual background. This is the sort of "cookbook" medicine characteristic of ill- educated practitioners during the last century.

However, to give this answer is to ignore the fact that medicine is an intellectual discipline as well as a practical art or skill. As an intellectual discipline, it engages in inquiry, formulates and tests hypotheses, offers explanations, confirms theories, and directs practice in accordance with scientific theories and principles. In addition, scientific theories are an essential part of the matrix of contemporary medicine.

Because this is so, an understanding of the character of medicine requires an understanding of the character of science. It may well be that no one, in fact, formulates explanations in medicine that explicitly conform to the nomological-deductive model. However, the fact that good explanations can be recast in the form of the model allows the model to serve as a standard for judging the quality and adequacy of proposed explanations. Familiarity with the model, in turn, informs even the physician in practice of the sort of standards that good science requires.

Such considerations may affect Mrs. Halprin's care in a direct fashion. The use of plasmapheresis developed out of an understanding of the role of immune complexes in the pathogenesis of tissue damage in SLE. The more recent attempts to use radiation therapy in refractory cases of SLE derive from a knowledge that lymphocytes participating in the immune response are particularly sensitive to x-radiation.

Failure to see that Mrs. Halprin is at the focal point of an immensely complicated conceptual and scientific process is failure to grasp the character of contemporary medicine. Immunologic and biochemical theories determine the way in which the disease processes affecting her are viewed, and generalizations about the nature of the immune response dictate what information should be sought as relevant to making a diagnosis. Evidence from clinical trials, themselves based on inferences from theories, form a basis for decisions about therapy. A failure to understand the nature of scientific theories is also likely to stand in the way of making proper inferences from basic science to clinical situations.

As medicine continues its progress from a purely empirical, ad hoc enterprise to become a scientific discipline grounded on the principles of general theories, it is important to keep in mind the characteristics that it seeks to embody. To a considerable extent, medicine has already achieved a scientific character, although in some respects it still has far to go. As both an emerging discipline and an established discipline, medicine aims to be scientific. Accordingly, to focus on the nature of science, as we have in this chapter, is to characterize medicine as it is and to indicate what it can become. Furthermore, while it is clear that biomedical science provides clinical medicine with most of its theoretical superstructure, it also has theoretical concepts of its own. Central among them is the concept of disease, the topic of the next chapter.

Hypotheses, Laws, and Theories

RECOMMENDED READING

Philosophy of Science

Achinstein, P. The Nature of Explanation. New York: Oxford University Press, 1983. Earman, J., ed. Testing Scientific Theories. Minneapolis: University of Minnesota Press, 1983.

Einhorn, H., and R. Hogarth. "Judging Probable Cause." Psychological Bulletin 99 (1986): 3-19. Engaging discussion by two eminent psychologists.

Giere, R. Understanding Scientific Reasoning. New York: Holt, Rinehart, and Winston, 1979. A modern introduction with good examples.

Hempel, C. G. Aspects of Scientific Explanation. New York: Free Press, 1965. A collection of classic papers.

---.Philosophy of Natural Science. Englewood-Cliffs, N.J.: Prentice-Hall, 1966. An introductory text.

Kuhn, T. S. The Structure of Scientific Revolutions. 2d ed. Chicago: University of Chicago Press, 1970. The book most responsible for challenging and replacing the standard view.

Lakatos, I., and A. Musgrave, eds. Criticism and the Growth of Knowledge. New York: Cambridge University Press, 1970. A collection of papers on both Kuhn and the standard view.

Laudan, Larry. Progress and Its Problems. Berkeley: University of California Press, 1977. An alternative to both the standard view and Kuhn.

Munson, R. "Methodological Issues in Biology." In Man and Nature: Philosophical Issues in Biology, ed. Ronald Munson, 3-17. New York: Dell, 1971. A review of some of the issues that biology and medicine share.

---. "Why Medicine Can't Be a Science." Journal of Medicine and Philosophy 6 (1981): 183-208. Despite the fact that medicine is scientific, its aims and criteria of success keep it autonomous and distinct from science.

Nagel, E. The Structure of Science. New York: Harcourt, Brace and World, 1961. A wide-ranging, advanced text.

Newton-Smith, W. H. The Rationality of Science. Boston: Routledge and Kegan Paul, 1981. A challenge to Kuhn and a good review of all the issues.

Platt, J. R. "Strong Inference." Science 146 (1964): 347-53.

Popper, K. R.The Logic of Scientific Discovery. New York: Harper and Row, 1959. A view different from the standard one.

Rothman, K. J. Modern Epidemiology. Boston: Little, Brown, 1986. Chapter 2 discusses causal inference in epidemiology.

Salmon, W. C. Scientific Explanation and the Causal Structure of the World. Princeton, N .J.: Princeton University Press, 1984. Advanced text on causal inference.

Schaffner, K. F. "Theory Structure in the Biomedical Sciences. "Journal of Medicine and Philosophy 5 (1980): 57-97.

Scheffler, I. Anatomy of Inquiry. New York: Bobbs-Merrill, 1963. An intermediate text. Suppe, F., ed. Structure of Scientific Theories. 2d ed. Urbana: University of Illinois Press, 1977. A collection of papers critical of the standard view.

Susser, M. Causal Thinking in the Health Sciences. New York: Oxford University Press, 1973. An epidemiologic approach (somewhat dated).

Theories of Systemic Lupus Erythematosus

Golub, Edward S. The Cellular Basis of the Immune Response. 2d ed. Sunderland, Mass.: Sinauer Associates, 1981. A basic text in immunobiology containing a fine historical introduction.

Labita, R. G., ed. Systemic Lupus Erythematosus. New York: Wiley, 1987. A new text.

Ropes, M. W. Systemic Lupus Erythematosus. Cambridge, Mass.: Harvard University Press, 1976. The first chapter contains a useful historical survey.

Rose, N. R. "Autoimmune Disease." Scientific American 250, no. 2 (1981): 80-103.

                                  Disease: The Concept,
Classification, and Discovery

Clinical medicine aims to identify, diagnose, treat, and prevent disease. Indeed, a concern with disease, either directly or indirectly, is a fundamental feature of every medical enterprise. But what is disease? How are particular diseases already recognized to be characterized and classified into a rational classification scheme? Finally, just what does it mean to discover or identify a disease?

These are the three basic questions we are concerned with in this chapter. None of them is a straightforward question that can be given a direct and uncontroversial answer. Each is a thread leading into a labyrinth of subsidiary issues, but the passages also lead to interesting vistas.

WHY BOTHER WITH THE DISEASE CONCEPT?

At first it may seem that discussing the disease concept in medicine is a pointless or impractical undertaking. After all, physicians are already able to recognize and treat literally thousands of diseases so what is gained by focusing attention on the concept? Diseases are what they are; what we need is a better understanding of diseases, not the concept that includes them.

This point of view is understandable when it is held by people who are directly engaged in the pressing business of practicing clinical medicine. The medical enterprise requires action, and the situation in which medical care is delivered neither encourages nor rewards efforts made to analyze basic concepts. Thus we cannot expect a physician engaged in diagnosis and treatment to be concerned with the concept of disease any more than we could expect a runner to be concerned with oxygen exchange at membrane surfaces. Both are simply striving to achieve their respective goals.

However, medicine is also an intellectual activity; the network of concepts and theories that constitutes medicine's intellectual content shapes and directs clinical practice. Thus, from this point of view, there are serious theoretical and practical reasons for examining the nature and role of the disease concept. The following three reasons are just some of a number that might be offered to justify our inquiry. Yet these three are sufficiently important to make it unnecessary to cast about for others.

1. The disease concept is a central notion in medicine, and that, in itself, makes it worthy of attention. As we mentioned earlier, a concern with disease is a basic aspect of every enterprise that can legitimately be called medical. Accordingly, if we wish to acquire a better understanding of the intellectual basis of clinical medicine-if we wish to understand the paradigm or framework of ideas that guides medical practice-then we need to understand the concept of disease. This requires that we understand the meaning of the concept as it is actually employed in clinical medicine and pay attention to the role that the concept plays in directing and shaping medical practice.

In this same connection, an attempt to understand the concept of disease gives rise to other issues that are worth attention. For example, although we have spoken of the concept of disease, this is only a rhetorical convenience. It may well be that medicine does not employ a single or unified concept. Rather, there may be several concepts of disease that play a role in medicine. Whether or not this is so is something that inquiry and analysis might be expected to reveal. Furthermore, whether medicine ought to employ a single concept is a question that might legitimately be asked by someone concerned with both understanding and revising the intellectual basis of medicine and clinical practice.

2. What states or conditions considered to be diseases within medicine have implications that go beyond the practice of clinical medicine and affect other parts of society. This situation makes it crucially important to develop a critical understanding of the disease concept (or concepts) within medicine.

For example, consider the view that social values always play a role in determining what organic states or behavioral patterns are to count as diseases in the medical sense. Whether or not this view is correct, critics have pointed out that it contributes to the "medicalization" of social problems. When a problem is medicalized by recognizing it as a disease, then the way is open to attempt to control or eliminate the problem by some form of medical treatment. Thus, if excessive drinking, unruliness in children, or a tendency to act violently are diseases or symptoms of diseases, then medicine has an implicit mandate to eliminate them.

In such a case, there is the possibility that needed social reforms or social programs will not be introduced and medicine will be inappropriately called upon to solve problems that ought to be solved by social measures.

In a sense, then, the concept of disease is closely connected with the limits and scope of medicine. Thus, whether social values are necessary ingredients in determining what counts as a disease (and others like it) is more than a question of airy intellectual interest.

3. Diseases are discovered or identified, classified, and investigated in relation to other diseases and basic processes. Discovery and classification, in particular, are activities that can be conducted only in accordance with explicit or implicit assumptions about what a disease is. If the activities are to be rational and critical, if they are to be conducted in accordance with nonarbitrary principles, then we must make explicit the assumptions about the nature of disease (the criteria for counting something a disease) that are employed in those activities.

Disease is a concept like that of *species* in biology. It is possible to identify various diseases in the same way as it is possible to identify various species, to name them, and to classify them. But to take a step further and provide an account of the concept that makes sense out of the classification requires connecting the classification with additional ideas. In biology, for example, the species concept that we now accept is one that is based on genetics and evolutionary theory. The actual species identified before the rise of these theories are often unchanged. What has changed is the significance of the species as a category (taxon).

In medicine, the identification of particular diseases and their classification may remain virtually unchanged no matter what disease concept or concepts are offered as accounting for why conditions or processes are considered diseases within medicine. As in biology, the significance of the classification can be seen only in connection with more general theoretical considerations, and these considerations are expressed in the disease concept.

WHY NOT SIMPLY DEFINE DISEASE?

If we want to understand the concept of disease, it may seem only natural to attempt to do so merely by formulating a definition of *disease*. We could then say, "As the term is used in medicine, a disease is considered to be such and such." This approach would be analogous to attempting to understand, say, the way in which *even number* is used in mathematics.

The major difficulty with this approach is that, strictly construed, it assumes that *disease* is used in such a way in medicine that it is possible to present a set of characteristics that are necessary and sufficient for governing the use of the term. That is, the approach assumes we will be able to discover conditions such that all and only items or states called diseases in medicine will satisfy those conditions.

Such an assumption is often justified when dealing with formal concepts such as those found in logic or mathematics. (*Even number*, for example can be defined as "a number divisible by two without remainder." This is true of all and only even numbers.) Less often, the approach is sometimes justified in dealing with scientific concepts. (In population genetics, for example, *species* can be defined as "a population of organisms possessing mechanisms that reproductively isolate the population.") It is not at all obvious, however, that the assumption behind the approach is warranted in the case of the concept of disease.

It may well be possible to find criteria that are necessary and sufficient for forming a class of everything presently considered a disease in medicine. However, to get such criteria would mean facing up to such questions as whether a broken leg or agitation or fainting is a disease. Questions of this sort would have to be decided to get necessary and sufficient criteria, and the results would likely be ultimately unsatisfying. In the end, it would be quite doubtful whether the criteria actually captured the concept of disease as employed in medicine. Certainly the definition would closely resemble the way disease is used, but what, if anything, such a definition might achieve could be questioned. At best, it would seem that the definition rested on a series of doubtful resolutions of borderline cases in order that it might capture all the items listed as diseases in one of the standard statistical nosologies. As such, the definition would be hardly more than a kind of linguistic artifact produced by gerrymandering criteria to fit a preexisting classification scheme constructed for a variety of purposes (data collection, insurance payments, etc.).

Second, attempting to formulate a definition merely by focusing on what is or is not classified as a disease in medicine avoids the fundamental question about the disease concept: What is its status? That is, what sort of thing is a disease, any disease? This is a question that goes beyond merely analyzing a particular scheme of classification. The scheme is one that is, in effect, given for a particular society at a particular time. But the more important issue is whether there is not something fundamental about the concept of disease as it appears in contemporary clinical medicine.

To understand better the issue involved here, it is worthwhile considering some of the possibilities for constituting the disease concept that have been widely discussed and defended in recent times.

DISEASE: A CATALOG OF GENERAL CONCEPTS

In this section, we present briefly six general views or concepts about what types of conditions may be said to constitute a disease. We make no attempt to provide definitions of specific concepts of the sort "A disease is such and such." Rather, we present the general types or categories within which more detailed specifications of what it is to be a disease can be placed.

Not all of the concepts discussed here are mutually exclusive. Some are ones that might be further subdivided into "strong" and "weak" versions. Thus our discussion is, in a sense, a presentation of "ideal types." That is, a particular analysis by a certain author might not fit exactly into one of our categories, but the categories represent general positions. Though our catalog may not be complete, it includes the major views to be found in contemporary medicine and in writings about contemporary medicine.

Disease Nominalism

Disease nominalism can best be summarized by the statement "A disease is whatever physicians say is a disease." That is, a disease is a disease because it is called a disease by a certain group of people. Ordinarily, at least in our society, we would consider physicians to be the group that is appropriate to decide what is to count as a disease and what is not. Generally speaking, however, any group at all might make the decision.

From a sociological or anthropological perspective, this point of view can be quite useful. It permits someone to determine what is or is not *called* a disease by some identifiable social group. It is then possible to talk about the ways in which various states or conditions are classified by various groups. Medical sociologists, for example, sometimes provide an "operational definition" of disease for the purpose of conducting a research project. Furthermore, the criterion is one used for legal or financial purposes. Insurance companies, for example, are typically willing to pay claims only in those cases in which disease has been certified by physicians.

What the nominalist view does not permit, of course, is an understanding of disease. The obvious question to ask is why a particular group considers something a disease. The nominalist approach neither raises this question nor provides a means of answering it. Indeed, the approach forestalls inquiry, rather than furthering it.

Disease Relativism

As the term *disease relativism* suggests, what counts as a disease is relative to a given society or culture at a particular time. Furthermore, diseases are identified or labeled in accordance with explicit or implicit social norms and values.

For example, masturbation was considered a disease in part of the Western world during the nineteenth century. That it is no longer thought to be reflects a change in values. Similarly, in nineteenth-century Japan, armpit odor, which is greater in a small percentage of the Japanese population than in the rest, was considered a disease, and its treatment constituted a medical specialty. Also, various non-Western cultures in which there are high incidences of parasitic infection may consider the Jack of infection to be abnormal and so not regard those who are infected as suffering from a disease. Our culture, of course, would say that those infected are diseased.

In this view, there are no diseases in nature. There are only organisms undergoing change and displaying certain characteristics. The changes or the conditions become diseases only when they are labeled as such, and the labeling is done in accordance with social norms, values, attitudes, and so on.

Disease relativism gains its plausibility from cases of the sort mentioned above. It is a straightforward acknowledgment of the fact that the identification of diseases is something that shows historical and cultural variation. Like most relativistic theses, it seems to have common sense and a respect for the facts on its side. Furthermore, it suggests a kind of intellectual and cultural modesty.

After all, who are we to say that we know what a disease is and other times and cultures are in error?

The difficulty with disease relativism is that it assumes it is impossible to identify a condition as a disease in a value-free fashion. That we can point to cases in which cultural values do play a role is not adequate proof that a reference to cultural norms and values is necessary to the identification of disease. That cultural factors sometimes determine what is considered a disease does not prove that it is not possible to establish criteria for what is to count as a disease without relying upon norms and values.

After all, we know that there are cultures that count "one, two, three, many," but their lack of a numerical system does not show that it is impossible to develop an arithmetic. Nor need we say that their system of numeration is "just as good as" our system. It is not. There are reasons for saying that ours is demonstrably superior.

Various cultures have beliefs about the ways in which the world is constituted and organized, and we are all aware of the obvious fact that various historical periods in Western culture have had beliefs about the physical and biological parts of the world that are at variance with the beliefs we hold today. Yet if the reasons and evidence we rely upon in establishing scientific theories are to count for anything, then we are in a position to say that cultural and historical views that clash with those we now endorse are simply wrong.

It just is not true that the earth is at the center of the solar system or that all materials contain phlogiston. We are prepared to say this because of the well-supported and reliable theories we hold. Similarly, we have well-supported and effective theories of a biological kind that help us to understand the nature of disease. Consequently, any culture or society that believes that those with parasitic infections are not diseased are simply in error. And so it is with other diseases. A culture's tendency to classify a condition as a disease that, according to our theories, is not a disease is simply an error on the part of that culture.

The Sociocultural View

The sociocultural view resembles disease relativism in that it maintains that societies may possess a concept of disease that may differ from the concepts of other societies. However, and most important, the concept may also differ from that held by practitioners of medicine in the society itself.

Thus there can be a conflict in some cases between the sociocultural view and the medical view. For example, hypercholesterolemia is regarded as a disease condition in medicine but is not generally thought of as such in the society. As a result, medical treatment may be justified, but a person with hypercholesterolemia may not seek treatment, even when told of the condition. (The difference between the medical and the sociocultural view of what constitutes a disease is sometimes recognized by making a distinction between disease-the medical concept-and illness-the sociocultural concept.)

Of course, it is logically possible for the sociocultural concept and the medical concept to be identical. No doubt in recent decades our own society has moved far in the direction of establishing such an identity. Nevertheless, there still remains a large gap in many instances between people who are considered sick by society and healthy by medicine and vice versa. Obviously, in more traditional, less-developed societies the gap may be very large indeed.

In our society there are often pressures to get a particular condition recognized as a disease in medicine. The most obvious recent cases are alcoholism, compulsive gambling, and various forms of "mental illness." Once medical recognition is granted, two significant results follow. First, the condition becomes the object of scientific-medical inquiry. Its causes are sought, explanations are formulated, and treatments are devised. Those who are afflicted are offered hope that their suffering may be tractable.

Second, medical recognition influences sociocultural recognition and the condition that might have been regarded previously as an expression of evil or moral weakness may come to be seen as a (sociocultural) disease. If this occurs, then the "sick" person is no longer blamed for the condition and is treated with care and concern. Furthermore, he or she receives the benefits of the "sick role" in the society and is excused for a variety of kinds of behavior that would otherwise be condemned or punished.

Having said this, it is equally important to stress that the sociocultural concept of disease is not an appropriate one for medicine itself. The concept developed within medicine may be guided in part by the sociocultural perception of what constitutes a disease. What is missing, however, is an understanding of the biological conditions and mechanisms that are involved in any disease. At this point medicine must depart from the social concept and develop a concept that is more scientifically appropriate.

The Statistical Concept

According to the statistical view, a condition counts as a disease when it is abnormal, and a condition is abnormal when it deviates from the normal. The normal, in turn, is taken as a statistically defined notion. The normal (or "norm") may be construed as the median, the mode, the area within a standard deviation, or some more sophisticated statistical measurement. (A more complete discussion appears in chap. 4.)

Blood pressure measurements are a good example of the way in which statistics can be employed to define a condition as a disease. Someone with blood pressure of, say, 120/80 falls securely within the normal range, whereas someone with a measurement of 140/100 has a blood pressure that is abnormally high. Since high blood pressure readings have been associated with other physiological life-threatening conditions, blood pressure that is abnormally high is itself regarded as a disease condition.

The usefulness of statistics in clinical medicine is undoubted. Indeed, one of the great contributions of the late eighteenth and early nineteenth century to the development of a scientific medicine was the recognition of the importance of statistical measures in identifying diseases and evaluating treatments. Nevertheless, it has been clear to virtually every writer on the topic that there is no sensible way to rely on statistics alone to determine a disease concept. For one thing, a statistical concept does not make it possible to regard an entire population as having a disease. Thus, tooth decay, which is virtually universal in present-day humans, cannot be identified as an abnormal condition. Indeed, it is the person without tooth decay who is abnormal and hence, according to a strict statistical view, diseased. That is nonsense, of course.

Finally, the statistical concept, in itself, has no way of resolving the "line-drawing" problem. That is, given a range of measurements of some specific feature or function (blood pressure, visual acuity, cardiac output, lung capacity, etc.), exactly where does one draw the line that divides the normal from the abnormal? A choice point at the borderline (which may be wide) is rarely obvious and often seems arbitrary.

None of these criticisms is meant to suggest that the statistical approach is not useful. Notice that even in our example, however, the approach is not simply one of statistical distribution. The trait considered (blood pressure) is one that, to be considered abnormal, must be associated with other conditions that are life-threatening. A pure statistical concept of abnormality and, hence, of disease seems wholly inadequate both to the needs of clinical medicine and as an analysis of the actual use of the concept of disease within clinical medicine.

Disease Idealism

In the view we may call disease idealism, disease is the lack of health, and health is characterized as the optimum functioning of biological systems. As a matter of fact, every real system may fall short of the optimum in its actual functioning, yet by comparing large numbers of systems we can formulate standards that a particular system ought to satisfy to be the best of its kind. In this respect, then, health is a kind of Platonic ideal that real organisms approximate. The standards that specify the ideal of health are analogous to engineering specifications. Actual bridges are certain to show flaws and faults, for even when they are properly designed, construction materials and techniques are imperfect. We can evaluate a particular bridge by comparing it to the specifications that describe what it should be like, but of course the bridge will fail to meet the specifications in certain respects.

The implication of disease idealism is that everyone is less than a perfect physical specimen. We are all flawed to some extent in some ways. Hence, disease is a matter of degree. It is a more or less extreme variation from the normative ideal of perfect functioning. (This opens the way, clearly, to combine the normative view with the statistical view and to characterize disease as a statistical variation from the ideal.)

In favor of the normative view is the fact that disease is frequently (if not always) a matter of degree. For example, fundamental aspects of the immune response are the same in health as in disease, and the same is true for such matters as cardiac output and blood counts. Yet, even though this is so, the idealistic view suffers from the same significant difficulty that faces the statistical concept—the line-drawing problem. That is, at exactly what point does a measurable function qualify as characteristic of a disease? Since all biological systems fall short of the ideal, if we are not willing to say that everyone suffers from numerous diseases, then the problem of separating those who are really diseased from the rest become crucial.

Disease Realism

Disease realism is the view that diseases have a real, substantial existence quite independent of social norms and values. Furthermore, diseases exist independent of whether they are discovered, named, recognized, classified, or diagnosed. Thus, it is possible for someone in (say) the Maldive Islands to die of SLE, even though neither that person nor anyone else in the culture may have heard of the disease, recognize its symptoms, or know anything about the mechanisms of its operation.

From the point of view of disease realism, those in other societies or cultures who have labeled as diseases conditions that are not, in fact, diseases are simply mistaken .The nineteenth century was as wrong in thinking that masturbation is a disease as the sixteenth century was in believing that the rate of fall of a body is directly proportional to its weight.

Disease realism entails the notion that diseases are items that form the furniture of the world. It may be possible to identify them with the operations of biological systems (i.e., provide a reductionistic account of diseases in terms of system components and subprocesses, even down to the molecular level). Yet even if this is so, it does not alter the fundamental fact that diseases are not inventions and are not the product of arbitrarily or socially assigned names. Rather, diseases have a real existence, and that existence is as historically, socially, and culturally invariant as is the existence of Victoria Falls. The pharaohs of ancient Egypt suffered from bacterial infections and died of brain tumors, whether or not they or their medical advisers knew it.

The boldness of disease realism consists in the implicit claim that the scientific and medical theories we now hold are, if not true, at least the best guide to the truth that we have. Accordingly, when there is a conflict between our present beliefs and those of some other historical or cultural group, it is the latter ones that must give way. There is not sufficient space in the room of the world to accommodate the furniture of other groups, even though it is only imaginary. The most serious difficulty with disease realism is connected with just the aspect that makes it a bold, no-nonsense way of thinking about disease. According to philosophers of science like Kuhn (see chap. 6), what we say exists in the world is, in part, a function of the theories we hold. Thus, for example, it makes no sense at all to talk about "molecular diseases" apart from general theories about molecules and their structural and functional roles in biological systems.

Of course, our theories change over time, and virtually every scientific theory held even as recently as the last century has been either totally rejected or supplanted by a highly modified version of the original theory. If the identification of disease is connected with theories, then a change in theories may produce a change in what is considered to be a disease. Assuming that this is so, what justification do we now have for saying that we know what diseases are, whereas people in earlier times, with different theories, did not? Furthermore, are not our theories as likely to be as temporary as those of past times? And if they are, then why should we confidently assert that we alone know what counts as a disease? (Obviously, what we have said here about different times also might apply with only minor modifications to different cultures and their theories.)

The answer to this challenge to disease realism seems to require defending the view that the theories we presently hold are those most worthy of belief. Even if they should turn out to be false or inadequate, we have no way of knowing that at the present. Consequently, if we are to make decisions about what is to count as a disease, then we must rely on our present theories. Thus, it is not from a position of absolute certainty, something not obtainable by scientific theories, that we make our decisions about diseases. Rather, it is the comparison of our present theories with others that gives us confidence our theories are the most reliable. It is on this basis that we also consider our recognition of diseases to be the most reliable.

It seems reasonable to believe that each of the six types of disease concepts we have discussed is actually held by at least some people who engage in clinical reasoning and practice. This is not to say that each concept is explicitly recognized or that its use is accompanied by an understanding of its meaning and limitations. All of us, in all aspects of our lives, employ concepts that remain both unrecognized and unanalyzed. Nevertheless, such concepts may play a role in shaping our attitudes and behavior.

The point worth stressing in connection with our brief catalog has less to do with the particular kinds of concepts we have considered than it does with the fact that contemporary medicine employs a variety of concepts. Some are very strict (e.g., the statistical concept), while others are loose and vague to the point of arbitrariness (e.g., the sociocultural concept). It is very likely that the concept (implicitly or explicitly) employed by a clinician or researcher is to a great extent a reflection of the circumstances in which an enterprise is conducted and of the aims of the enterprise. A project in clinical research, for example, is very likely to make use of a statistical notion of what conditions constitute a disease, whereas a physician in practice is much more likely to rely upon a much less restrictive concept. Most physicians are almost certain to be disease realists, but those who work in non-Western societies or with ethnic populations are sure to recognize the existence of a sociocultural concept, even if they do not endorse it themselves. Furthermore, clinical researchers and epidemiologists may well accept disease idealism in their work, in addition to employing some specific version of the statistical concept of disease.

DISEASE AS A DEPARTURE FROM NORMAL FUNCTIONING: TOWARD A UNIFIED CONCEPT

In this section, we present a specific analysis of a disease concept. In particular, we recommend the adoption of the view that disease is best understood as a departure from normal functioning. We suggest that the concept, as defined and analyzed in this way, is one worthy of general acceptance within clinical medicine.

To an extent, this concept is already one that is employed in contemporary scientific medicine. Accordingly, our analysis should partially reflect actual medical usage. But of course, as we have already seen, there is not just a single disease concept in medicine. Because of this, our specific analysis must also be understood as a recommendation. We are suggesting, in effect, that the concept of disease as a departure from normal functioning is one that ought to be accepted. The concept is consonant with the aims of clinical medicine; it is also of potential usefulness in the pursuit of those aims. In this sense, then, our claim for the superiority of the normal-functioning concept is one that has a nonnative status. It is one that both reflects aspects of present practice and, if adopted, would also modify it.

When machines fail to function properly, we say that they are broken, defective, or just not working right. We do not say (except when we are being whimsical) that they are sick or have a disease. Yet it is by analogy with machines that we can perhaps best move toward an analysis of the concept of disease that is adequate for clinical medicine.

The machines that are of most use in providing help in the development of a disease concept are those like mechanical watches and clocks, automatic tracking devices (such as "smart bombs"), thermostats, and computers. Whatever may be the hardware from which such devices are constructed, they all share certain formal features. Specifically, such devices are all teleonomic systems, to use a term coined by the biologist C. S. Pittendrigh. That is, they are all, in various ways, goal-directed systems.

The goal may be simply to mark off equal intervals in a regular way (as in a clock), to maintain a variable within a certain range of values (as in a thermostat), to modify activities by a feedback mechanism to keep a target in sight, or any number of other possibilities. The inner mechanisms may be simple (as in a bimetallic thermostat) or complicated (as in a computer). The workings of the mechanisms may be part of the direct design of the hardware (as in a watch), or the workings may depend upon being supplied with a complicated external program of information (as in a computer).

Whether simple or complex, teleonomic devices require information for their operation. The information may be direct, as it is in the case of temperature change as sensed by a thermostat, or it may be indirect, as it is in computer programs. The fact that teleonomic systems are also programmed systems points the way to understanding disease as a departure from normal functioning. To lay out the background to make this claim plausible requires that we spend a moment examining the ways in which it makes sense to talk about organisms as programmed systems.

Organisms as Programmed Systems

Organisms and the cells that constitute them are complicated organized systems that display in their operations a variety of phenomena that can be regarded as the results of acting upon a program of information. As we mentioned above, this means that biological systems are physical systems of a very special kind. What makes them special is the presence of programs, acquired and developed during evolution, that control processes of the system. The programs that regulate occurrences within cells or in physiological or behavioral sequences are ones that impart a goal-directed character to the systems and subsystems of the organism.

Biological programs can be thought of as physical states of biological systems. Homeostatic phenomena, such as the maintenance of blood pressure and of sodium concentration within cells, can be viewed as produced by the operation of such programs. Similarly, the structural and chemical properties of certain complex molecules (DNA, RNA, for example) can be regarded as programs for carrying out particular sequences of operations upon appropriate materials. A clear and important case is the transcription of coded information from DNA into directions for protein synthesis. Another important example is the synthesis of appropriate antibodies in the presence of an antigen.

A major aim of biomedical research is to be able to write out the program of a process as an explicit set of instructions. Furthermore, as a part of this aim, the researcher wants to discover the manner in which the program is physically coded and the way in which it is uncoded and expressed in a characteristic end result. In some cases, such as in gene replication and protein synthesis, this goal has been almost wholly achieved. For other processes, the aim still seems quite distant.

Programmed processes are to be found at various levels of biological organization. Cells, tissues, organ systems, and behavioral complexes all exhibit phenomena that can be understood as being under the control of programs of information that become operative under specific, identifiable sets of conditions. Biological and medical research is directed at both the recognition of processes as programmed and also at the working out of their physical bases and operational sequences. Certain behavioral phenomena, for example, have only recently been identified as ones that have their basis in a genetically determined program. (A good example is the recognition of members of the same species by organisms reared in isolation and without prior experience.) There is reason to believe that as research progresses, more and more biological processes at all levels of organization will come to be understood as programmed processes.

The examples we have mentioned so far are all ones that constitute what Ernst Mayr calls "closed" genetic programs. That is, they are processes that are wholly the result of the decoding of information in the genome and its implementation through other intermediary elements such as the central nervous system, the cardiovascular system, and so on. Other biological phenomena, both physiological occurrences and behavior patterns, seem to require for their operation an interaction between the programmed system and the environment. Programming seems incomplete (hence, "open"), and more than the ordinary process of biological development (ontogenesis) is required to complete it. Some form of learning or conditioning is necessary.

To take an example from behavior, some birds develop species-specific songs without ever having heard them, while others do not but will acquire the songs of another species with which they are raised. A similar kind of open programming may well be present in the operation of the immune system, in which the production of appropriate antibodies is triggered by the presence of antigens.

Apparently, too, some programs that start out open become permanently closed after the conditions required to complete them are satisfied. Imprinting, for example, takes place during a certain phase of development and then afterward becomes impossible. It has been suggested (by Noam Chomsky and others) that language learning in human beings follows a similar pattern. If some language or other is not learned during a certain biologically determined period of development, then no language can ever be learned.

The development of sociobiology as a discipline can be understood, in part, as an attempt to identify and work out behavioral programs, both open and closed, that can be used to account for patterns of individual and social behavior. A fundamental claim of sociobiology is that such programs of behavior actually exist and that an attempt to understand behavior patterns by relying upon "empty organism" theories of learning is doomed to failure.

Evolution and Biological Programs

Any kind of program of information may be viewed from the standpoint of its construction or its operation. The construction of biological programs is an outcome of the evolutionary process. Natural selection, operating on the genetic variability of populations of organisms under environmental conditions, produces phyletic change. Whether the selection occurs at the molecular level, the level of the gene, or at the level of the phenotype (the organism and its traits), the outcome is the same, namely, the modification of genetic programs of information and the spread of those new programs differentially within the population.

Consequently, in any given time period a population of organisms will possess a characteristic genetic program. That program, in connection with external and internal environmental factors, will direct the development of individual organisms (ontogeny), and the developed organism will possess as part of its basic equipment programs of information that determine organic functioning at all levels of organization- molecular, organ system, physiological, cellular, behavioral, and so on.

Thus, programs are shaped and formed by evolution, but the programs themselves operate within organisms. It is the possession of evolutionary-shaped genetic programs that gives organisms their "historical" character and makes cells more than bags of biochemicals.

Normal Functioning

The view that organisms are biologically programmed systems offers a way of providing a notion of normal functioning that is independent of social norms and values. Put most straightforwardly, normal functioning consists in the operation of biologically programmed processes. This is to say, of course, that normal functioning is natural functioning. It is the operation of the programs of biologically stored information in the processes that take place within the various levels of biological organization. Because these processes are teleonomic ones, it is possible to characterize normal functioning by focusing on the *outcomes* of the processes, as well as on the informational programs that "direct" them.

Disease we can now characterize as a failure of normal functioning. Disease occurs (a disease condition is present) when something happens to frustrate or disrupt the operation of the biological programs of information.

The *evidence* that there has been a program failure and that, therefore, a disease condition is present can come from a variety of sources. In clinical medicine, the evidence most often available is the recognition that certain functions are not being carried out. Symptoms such as pain, fatigue, and headache, and signs such as temperature, color, swelling, and heart murmurs, may all be indicators of functional failure. The same is so of biological and biochemical assays of tissue, blood, bone marrow; and urine.

Of course, such evidence may be inconclusive or misleading. A particular measurement, for example, might indicate that a person is likely to suffer from a specific sort of functional failure, while there is no additional evidence to show this. That is, nothing indicates that there is a functional failure or that the biological program (or programs) has been disrupted or defeated. By contrast, a disease condition may well be present when no evidence of the failure of a particular biological program exists. For example, various compensating mechanisms associated with some other program or programs may have successfully maintained some expected functional outcome. Heart failure, for example, is compensated for by the accumulation of fluid to maintain tissue perfusion.

A clear-cut example of a disease that illustrates our analysis of disease as a failure of normal functioning resulting from the frustration or disruption of a biological program is alkaptonuria. Those who suffer from the disease excrete urine that contains homogentisic acid. Since this substance turns black upon exposure to air, urine color is a reliable diagnostic sign. In 1909 the British physician A. E. Garrod noticed that the level of homogentisic acid in the urine was increased when foods containing the substances phenylalanine or tyrosine were eaten in an increased quantity. This observation led him to suggest that the acid in the urine resulted from the absence of an enzyme required to metabolize it and that the lack of the enzyme was due to an "inborn error of metabolism."

In 1919 sufferers of the disease were shown to lack the enzyme homogentisic acid oxidase. Geneticists showed that the disease was inherited in a pattern consistent with its being the result of a homozygous recessive gene, a gene that presumably codes for the enzyme.

Diseases involving enzyme defects are persuasive examples for showing that disease involves a biological program failure. But other diseases at other levels of biological organization can also be understood in terms of the same concept.

Advantages of the Functional-Failure Concept

The concept of disease as a functional failure of a programmed biological process is offered here as one worthy of general acceptance. Although detailed arguments in favor of adopting the concept as adequate for clinical medicine have not been offered, a step (but only a step) in this direction can be taken by considering a few of the reasons for considering the concept worth accepting.

1. The functional-failure concept both entails and makes plausible the view that diseases have a real and substantial existence. That is, diseases exist quite apart from social norms and values and quite apart from the success of a society in identifying a condition as a disease. Granted that biological functions are the results of processes guided by inherent programs and that these functions, processes, and programs are real, then defects or frustrations of the programs that alter the processes and their functional outcomes are also real. (In principle, it is possible for someone to deny that biological processes are real. But this is not a matter we are concerned to argue. It is enough to say that, granted that biological processes are real, then diseases are real.)

Thus, the functional-failure concept makes sense out of saying (as we do) that physicians in the eighteenth century failed to identify SLE as a disease, although it existed then. Similarly, it makes sense of saying that physicians in the nineteenth century were wrong to identify masturbation as a disease: masturbation does not and never did involve any functional failure. Finally, the concept makes sense out of saying that societies that fail to recognize widespread parasitic infections as a disease condition are mistaken, for genetically programmed processes and their functional outcomes are disrupted.

2. The functional-failure concept helps explain the relevance and significance of basic research in medicine. Basic research aims at understanding the ways in which biological information is stored in programs, the ways in which programs operate to direct processes, and the ways in which processes are coordinated and combined to serve general biological functions. Since disease results in a failure or diminution of function at some level of organization, basic research is required to understand the mechanisms and sequences that may be involved in the failure.

In terms of our initial analogy, if a machine such as a clock does not work properly, then in order to understand its failure and to repair it in the most efficient and effective way, we must have knowledge of the mechanisms by which the clock operates. Obviously, it might be possible to get the clock to work properly by dropping it, kicking it, or hitting it with a hammer. The only knowledge or understanding involved here is the recognition that sometimes such actions produce the desired result.

This is just the sort of approach clinical medicine is forced to take when there is a lack of knowledge of basic programs and processes. "Empirical" modes of treatment are based on the clinical analogues of dropping, kicking, and hitting with a hammer. No one believes, of course, that such an approach forms the best foundation for therapy. The best foundation is that laid by basic research, the foundation that consists of understanding biological programs and their modes of operation.

3. The functional-failure concept makes clear the role of statistics in identifying diseases, while avoiding the difficulties that accompany the statistical concept of disease.

Measurements of particular somatic variables are associated, via statistical generalizations, with certain diseases with a certain degree of probability. In terms of the functional-failure concept, such probability measurements indicate the likelihood of one or more functional failures within programmed processes. As such, the measurements are evidence for functional failure and, hence, of disease. But the state of a particular variable does not in itself constitute a disease. It is possible (though perhaps rare) for an individual to be statistically unusual, in terms of measured somatic variables, while not having a disease. That is, the programmed processes may be operating properly and general functions may be served. In such an instance, it makes sense to talk about values that are statistically abnormal but are normal for the individual.

In summary, measurements may provide evidence for functional program failure, but the evidence of failure is not identical with failure. In practice, there may be no difference between the statistical and the functional-failure concepts of disease, but there is a significant epistemological difference between the two. Information viewed in terms of the statistical concept as constituting disease is viewed by the functional-failure concept as no more than evidence of a disease. As such, the latter concept comes closer to capturing the recognized facts about disease—that functional failure is not always properly captured by statistics—than does the statistical concept.

THE LOGIC OF DISEASE CLASSIFICATION

Diseases can be classified for a variety of reasons according to a variety of classification schemes. The scheme constructed and employed by the epidemiologist is not likely to serve the needs of the practicing clinician. Standard nosologies do exist in medicine, and they play a major role in helping to promote uniform diagnoses and data collection. Yet subspecialties frequently have their own special systems.

As useful as knowing how to use a particular classification is gaining an understanding of the principles and methods that may be employed in constructing any classification scheme. This makes it possible to invent coherent and useful schemes when necessary. Perhaps just as important, a knowledge of the principles of construction makes it possible to appreciate the strengths and limitations of schemes already in use. It will soon become clear that classification in medicine is not a matter of pure logic. As we mentioned earlier, the distinction between normal and diseased, in particular, is a matter that requires decisions that go beyond logic and statistics.

General Principles of Classification Systems

A classification system is a means of assigning a set of individual items to one or more groups or classes. The individuals may be patients, urine specimens, tissue samples, symptoms, or anything at all. The domain of a classification is the totality of individuals to which it can be applied. Thus clinical signs might be taken as a domain, or (much more narrowly) heart sounds might be a domain.

The tree structure is perhaps the most familiar type of classification system. In such a system, the domain is partitioned into subclasses, and these

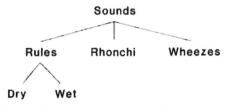

7.1.   Classification of adventitious sounds upon lung auscultation.

are divided into additional subclasses. The process can be continued until a level is reached at which it ceases to be useful or possible to make further distinctions. Such a classification system is easily illustrated by figure 7. 1.

We can describe such a system as a discrete tree structure. A degenerate case of such a structure is one that partitions the domain at one level but does not introduce further subdivisions. The division of baseball infielders into pitcher, catcher, shortstop, first, second, and third baseman is a discrete and degenerate tree structure.

Tree structures are frequently employed in medicine, but medicine also uses systems that not only partition the domain of classification, but also order it. Grouping patients by weight, height, temperature, or blood pressure produces a continuous ordering. Such an ordering can then be combined with a tree structure. For example, we might imagine a system for classifying cardiovascular disease in which a tree structure has a branch ending with systolic hypertension; under this heading is a continuous ordering by blood pressure readings.

In fact, medicine does not typically proceed in this way. Although systolic blood pressure arranges cases in a continuous ordering, many clinicians prefer to impose diagnostic ranges on the ordering. In this way, the cases can be classified as (say) mild, moderate, or severe hypertension.

If needed, classification schemes that are multidimensional can be constructed. For example, classifying patient by height and weight produces a two-dimensional scheme, and classifying them by height, weight, and age produces a three-dimensional scheme. We can think of a discrete, two-dimensional scheme as furnishing us with a surface divided into cells or squares like those on a sheet of graph paper. The cell in which an item belongs is then the intersection of the row and column appropriate to it. Discrete schemes of higher dimensions can be viewed as extensions of this representation. Continuous or discrete and continuous schemes of higher dimensions can be thought of as assigning each item of their domain to a point (pure continuous) or region (discrete and continuous) of n-dimensional space. In short, there are a variety of classificatory systems available to the clinician, and some allow us to use fairly sophisticated mathematical methods to represent and manipulate data.

Properties of Classification Systems

Exclusive and Exhaustive Divisions

From a logical point of view, a classification scheme of any type should employ divisions that are both mutually exclusive and exhaustive within each of its dimensions. This will lead to the assignment of items to one and only one cell, point, or region. Each dimension of a classification system consists of a collection of classes of members of the domain of the system. Thus, a one-dimensional system that classifies people by race consists of classes of people-one class for each race. Given that no person belongs to more than one race, we say that these classes (races) are mutually exclusive; given that everyone belongs to some race, the classes are exhaustive.

Simplicity

A logically impeccable classification system may still be useless. What makes a classification system useful? Generally that depends upon one's purpose in classifying. But there are several features that make any system more useful, no matter what the purpose may be. Simplicity is one. A scheme of classification should be as simply constructed as required for the job at hand. It should involve no unnecessary distinctions or dimensions. For example, if our purpose is to classify patients as possible candidates for heart surgery, then we have no need to segregate them with respect to eye color.

Ease of Application

Another virtue of a classification system is ease of application. It is easier for physicians in the United States to classify patients by weight measured in pounds than by weight in kilograms, since most scales in the United States are calibrated in pounds. As this example shows, ease of application is independent of simplicity. Indeed, a simple metric classification scheme might be harder for U.S. medical personnel to use than the more complicated conventional system. Generally, however, simplicity and ease of application go hand in hand. Conceptual complexities are usually reflected in the number and variety of observations needed to classify each item in the scheme's domain.

An Explicit Principle of Construction

Other things being equal, a classification system should have *a clear and explicitly formulated principle of construction*. For example, the classification scheme can be generated by this simple rule: Divide first according to gender, then according to stage of sexual development, and then according to substage, if any (fig. 7.2). A classifier who knows the sexes and developmental stages can memorize the one-line rule instead of the bulky tree.

The moral is that good classifications should not appear to evolve randomly, but rather they should be constructed according to a principle that can be recognized with reasonable ease.

Appropriateness

A classification system should be *appropriate to its domain and intended use.* For example, suppose we are designing a classification system for use at a medical screening clinic. We know that patients are given certain tests in a particular order. Furthermore, some tests are administered only if the patient satisfies specific criteria determined by the results of previous tests. Suppose our purpose is to classify the patients according to the information gathered from the screening procedure. Then our system will be appropriate to the extent that it is consonant with the procedures already in place. It will be inappropriate to the extent that it requires the administration of new tests or reordering or changing the candidacy requirements for the currently used tests. (To take a more homey example: Classifying horses according to mathematical aptitude would be inappropriate, but classifying them according to their ability to procreate would not be.)

Significant Divisions

Finally, a classification that makes theoretically significant divisions is generally more useful than one that does not. Classifying whales and porpoises as mammals, rather than as fish, proved to be far more useful to biologists and specialists in marine life, because biological theories are organized along reproductive and evolutionary lines. Similarly, medical theory makes it useful to segregate pulmonary tuberculosis from lung cancer although their clinical manifestations—coughing, radiographic abnormalities, and weight loss—are quite similar. Of course, such theoretical divisions cannot be an overriding

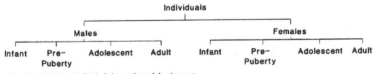

7.2.   Classification of individuals by gender and development.

factor in designing a classification. The clinician needs a classification of diseases according to clinical manifestations as well, even if this requires crossing theoretical divisions. After all, the first knowledge the clinician has is of the patients' clinical manifestations; these will be crucial to the subsequent diagnostic hypotheses and the decisions based upon them. Once the clinician determines a diagnosis or a reasonably small spectrum of diagnostic possibilities, then a theoretically oriented classification of the patient may prove quite helpful in suggesting treatment possibilities.

Classification Systems in Medicine

Classifying a patient by means of a diagnosis is a way of subsuming the patient under medical theory. But a more complicated interaction also occurs between classifying and theorizing. In the initial stages of a science, scientists typically classify in terms of features that are most obvious. For example, early botany placed trees and vines in different groups, and early medicine lumped all fevers together. Scientists then try to develop theories that address questions couched in terms of their initial classification systems. Thus early physicians and botanists asked, "What causes fevers?" and "Why do trees shed their leaves?" Their attempts led to revised types of classifications. For example, plants were divided into deciduous versus nondeciduous, and this, in turn, led to a different set of questions. This process has been a continuous one in history of medicine and biology, and the classification systems of both are always undergoing change.

In medicine, the realities of classification are far from any imagined ideal. No single, logically perfect, theoretically useful, and easily applicable system exists. Instead, medicine employs a motley of schemes inherited from earlier stages of its history, and even these are applied with less than full consistency. Early medicine classified in terms of clinical manifestations. The nineteenth century saw the rise of pathology and classification in terms of anatomical lesions. This, in turn, was superseded by classification in terms of physiologic dysfunctions and later in terms of the causal factors responsible for them. Yet none of these advances has been accompanied by a thorough purging of obsolescent classificatory ideas. (Partly this is because these ideas retain some usefulness.) For example, lupus is considered an autoimmune disease, a rheumatic disease, and a collagen-vascular disease.

The result is that today medicine classifies in terms of manifestations (angina), lesions (appendicitis), genetics (Down syndrome), infective agents (tuberculosis), and environmental factors (brown lung disease). This allows for flexibility, and it avoids forcing medicine prematurely under a single theoretical umbrella. However, it also creates problems for medical theory itself. The most important of these is its deleterious effect on the quality of medical data and statistics. For example, since cases of lung cancer and tuberculosis of the lung used to be counted as "consumption," much of the data acquired on the course and treatment of consumption cannot be used without further interpretation. In most instances, insufficient information is available for reclassifying the cases, and the data must simply be abandoned.

As particular diseases come to be better understood in terms of basic biological theories, it is likely that disease classification will become more uniform. Diseases will be identified in terms of the causal mechanisms responsible for the clinical manifestations, and other factors will be employed as evidence to establish that, in particular cases, specific mechanisms are at work.

Taxonomy versus Diagnosis

Strictly speaking, disease labels apply to cases, not to people. Jones has measles by having a case of them. Both the practicing physician and the medical taxonomist classify cases, but they do so with different ends in mind. The clinician classifies one case at a time. He or she determines whether the patient is diseased or normal (whether the patient has a case at all) and, if the patient is diseased, what the case is a case of. The clinician's purpose in so doing is to explain the patient's manifestations and to achieve the best possible disposition of the case. In so doing, the clinician makes use of a previously established classification system with no intention of modifying it.

By contrast, the taxonomist considers many cases at a time and has no concern at all with their disposition. (Many or all of the cases may have been resolved for years.) The taxonomist's aim is to group these cases in a manner that will promote medical knowledge and treatment. He or she may work with an extant disease concept, but may propose another conception of disease. The taxonomist may fit the collection of cases into current medical taxonomy and thereby enrich medical data. Or the taxonomist may argue that the current system must be modified to accommodate the cases. This could lead to the discovery of a new disease, or to a redrawing of old boundaries. But whatever is proposed, it should be judged by its usefulness for medical theory and practice.

DISEASE: INVENTION, DISCOVERY, AND INTERVENTION

Viewed from the perspective of history, diseases, like clothing fashions, seem to come and go. The scores of "fevers" so meticulously described in the medical texts of the middle of the last century are never referred to today. In the present century smallpox was wiped out of existence, and it may be that syphilis did not exist at all as a disease before the great scourges of the fifteenth and sixteenth centuries. Radiation sickness is a disease peculiar to modem times, and Legionnaires' disease and AIDS have only recently been discovered.

Yet to talk about diseases "coming and going" in this fashion is to trade on ambiguities and to ignore distinctions that ought to be made. Cases that are radically different cannot be treated as though they were the same without adding much confusion to the already confused talk about diseases.

The Origins of Disease

How diseases come into existence is, for the most part, a question that requires a biological answer. The spirochete that is the causal agent of syphilis may well have existed in some genetically similar form before the disease existed. The organism may have undergone one or more mutations that changed its character and made it into the causal agent of the disease.

The same may be true of various viruses and bacteria. The same sort of process of phyletic change that is accounted for by evolutionary theory may be expected, in principle, to account for the origins of various kinds of infectious diseases. The human body, after all, is the environment within which a great abundance of organisms flourish. A mutation that is successful within that environment may not benefit the host organism. Indeed, the mutation, as it spreads to successive generations of the parasite, may disrupt or destroy the programmed functions of the host. Hosts, of course, may acquire means of dealing with pathologic organisms through the same process of mutation, adaptation, and selection.

Nonbiological agents, such as chemical and radiologic materials, may never have existed before or may never have existed in the present combination or degree of concentration. Thus, the combination or concentration may induce changes in the programmed processes and become disease agents. Exactly how such a thing may happen requires a detailed biochemical and biological understanding of the mechanisms that are involved.

Particular diseases, like any other sort of natural phenomenon, may pass out of existence, as well as come into being. As we mentioned earlier, smallpox has been eliminated through the public health measures taken during the last century or so. Various genetic diseases may eventually cease to exist, if the technology of recombinant DNA becomes more developed. In principle, the sickness caused by radioactive poisoning could be eliminated by rigorous safety precautions.

The point is, diseases, like everything else in the world, have a natural history. Understanding that history requires the application and development of appropriate theories. Modifying that history, even to the point of eliminating specific diseases, may require particular kinds of intervention.

The Discovery of Disease

Are diseases discovered or invented? Are diseases, like the island of Tahiti, simply there whether anyone knows about them or not, just waiting for some medical explorer to come sailing into the harbor and declare them real?

Obviously, the way one answers this question determines whether (to use the terms we introduced earlier) one is a *disease nominalist* or a *disease realist*. A disease nominalist will say that diseases are social inventions. A society, or its representatives, simply decides in accordance with its own norms and values to characterize a phenomenon as a disease. By contrast, a disease realist will maintain that diseases are simply "out there" to be discovered. They will continue to be there, whether we know it or not and whether we discover them or name them.

Our analysis of the concept of disease as functional failure within a programmed process commits us to disease realism. However, the way in which the question was framed above assumes no middle ground exists between discovery and invention. There are good reasons for denying that this is so. If we think of discovering a disease as fundamentally the same as discovering an island, we will mislead ourselves about the nature of discovery in science and medicine.

Pasteur's famous dictum that "chance favors the prepared mind" is often taken to mean no more than that a researcher must be ready to follow up on anomalous findings. (After all, Rontgen was probably not the first person to discover that his x-ray plates had been fogged. He was perhaps just the first to attempt to discover the cause.) But in connection with discovery, the dictum cuts more deeply than this. The "prepared mind" is more than a psychological disposition to continue inquiry. A researcher's mind is "prepared" by the availability and acceptance of particular theories, methodological rules, and research techniques. Elements such as these constitute some of the conditions for inquiry and, consequently, of discovery.

No one is going to search for the agent responsible for producing an infectious disease, unless we already possess the concept of an infectious disease. That is, we must antecedently recognize that it is possible for organisms to be the carrier or cause of diseases. Similarly, no one is going to attempt to locate the missing factors that produce a deficiency disease, unless we already have the notion that faulty nutrition can result in disease.

We could obviously go on to list the many sorts of factors that contemporary clinical medicine recognizes as potentially involved in producing disease:

missing enzymes, physical blockage or damage, biochemical imbalances, neurotransmitter malfunctions, metabolic disturbances, faulty immune responses, and so on. The categories could be more specific or more general, but in either case, the point remains the same: the discovery of a disease is closely tied to the theories that we hold about the causal mechanisms responsible for producing outcomes that we identify as diseases.

A disease as a phenomenon is always "out there," manifested in the bodies of those who suffer from it. The disease is what it is, and what we say about it does not change it. Failing to recognize a condition as a disease does not change it. Similarly, explaining the disease only partially or improperly does not change it. Yet after all this has been said, it still remains true that the theoretical framework we have at a given time plays a major role both in the discovery of a disease and in the account we give of exactly what the disease is.

Let us consider as an example the disease we have been focusing on throughout these chapters-systemic lupus erythematosus. When was the disease first discovered? The question cannot be answered in any straightforward way, and any answer must be expressed in terms of "It all depends on what you mean by lupus."

This point is perhaps best illustrated by considering very briefly the history of the "discovery" of lupus. Lupus can probably be assumed to have existed from an indefinitely remote time. Certain infectious diseases, like malaria, or metabolic diseases, like diabetes, can be traced on the basis of their clinical descriptions to the writings of the ancient Egyptians and Greeks. Such is not the case with lupus. It loses its identity as a disease and disappears into the great mixture of diseases characterized by rashes. Chronic infections are almost surely among those diseases historically classified in the "wulf" or "lupus" category.

From our present perspective, we can now pick out some of the important steps in identifying elements that we now count as features of lupus. Here, in bare outline, are a few of them:

• Pierre Cazenave and Henri E. Schedel in 1851 described the skin lesions of lupus and observed that they usually appear as a rash on the faces of young adults. The lesions were characterized as involving induration, scarring, a butterfly distribution, and as sometimes affecting the exterior auditory canal. Casenave and Schedel introduced the term lupus erythemateux, which was later latinized.

• In 1872, Moritz Kaposi recognized the potentially fatal nature of the disease and its systemic manifestations. He associated lupus with fever, pleural and pulmonary involvement, and toxic manifestations, including encephalopathy. He recognized the "subacute remitting and relapsing course" of the disease and the correlations with skin and systemic changes.

• William Osler in 1904, without making a specific diagnosis, gave a detailed clinical account of two young women who died of renal failure within ten months of the appearance of a facial erythema. He distinguished the cutaneous from the systemic form of the disease and noted that patients with the systemic form might also show joint, gastrointestinal, cardiac, and renal involvement.

• In 1935, George Baehr and co-workers described the wire-loop pattern of glomerular lesions and pointed out the exacerbating effects of sun exposure.

• In 1940, Harry Keil called attention to the association of SLE and false positive serologic tests for syphilis.

• In 1948, M. H. Hargreaves discovered the LE cell phenomenon, which promised to permit a way of confirming clinical impressions. However, the test was rarely positive in patients with only the cutaneous form of the disease and not wholly accurate in identifying patients with the systemic form. Furthermore, some 20 percent of patients with rheumatoid arthritis were also found to have positive LE test results so the specificity of the SLE cell test was open to doubt.

To skip several important more recent steps, in 1970 the American Rheumatism Association (ARA), represented by a panel of its members, conducted a study to devise criteria that could be employed to diagnose SLE and to distinguish it from other connective-tissue disorders. The panel offered fourteen criteria. In the study, 90 percent of SLE patients met four or more of the criteria; in other studies, 94-96 percent met at least four.

In 1982, the ARA offered a revised set of criteria to incorporate new immunologic knowledge. The new criteria gained in sensitivity (96 percent) and specificity (96 percent). Although the number was reduced to eleven, a positive diagnosis still requires that at least four of the following criteria be satisfied:

1. Butterfly rash: fixed erythema, flat or raised, over the malar eminences, tending to spare the nasolabial folds.
2. Discoid lupus: erythematous raised patches with adherent keratotic

scaling and follicular plugging; atrophic scarring may occur in older lesions.

3. Photosensitivity: skin rash as a result of unusual reaction to sunlight, by patient history or physician observation.

4. Oral ulcers: oral or nasopharyngeal ulceration, usually painless, observed by a physician.

5. Arthritis: nonerosive arthritis involving two or more peripheral joints, characterized by tenderness, swelling, or effusion.

6. Serositis:

   a. pleuritis: convincing history of pleuritic pain or rub heard by a physician or evidence of pleural effusion; or

   b. pericarditis: documented by EKG or rub or evidence of pericardial effusion.

7. Renal disorder:

   a. persistent proteinuria greater than 0.5 g/day or greater than 3+ if quantitation not performed; or

   b. cellular casts: may be red cell, hemoglobin, granular, tubular, or mixed.

8. Neurologic disorder:

   a. seizures: in the absence of offending drugs or known metabolic derangements, for example, uremia, ketoacidosis, or electrolyte imbalance; or

   b. psychosis: in the absence of offending drugs or known metabolic derangements, for example, uremia, ketoacidosis, or electrolyte imbalance.

9. Hematologic disorder:

   a. hemolytic anemia: with reticulocytosis;

   b. Jeukopenia: Jess than 4,000/mm 3 total on two or more occasions;

   c. lymphopenia: Jess than J ,500/mm3 on two or more occasions; or

   d. thrombocytopenia: less than 100,000/mm3 in the absence of offend-ing drugs.

10. Immunologic disorder:

   a. positive LE cell preparation;

   b. presence of antibody to native DNA in abnormal titer;

   c. anti-Sm: presence of antibody to Sm nuclear antigen; or

   d. false positive STS known to be positive for at least six months and confirmed by TPI or FTA tests.

11. Antinuclear antibody: an abnormal titer of antinuclear antibody by immunofluorescence or an equivalent assay at any point in time and in the absence of drugs known to be associated with "drug-induced

lupus" syndrome.

Although the criteria are sometimes employed to make diagnoses in individual cases, they were formulated for the classification of groups of patients for research purposes. Furthermore, the ARA criteria themselves must be measured against an independent criterion. The expert opinion of experienced physicians must be the standard against which the criteria are tested. In the absence of such a standard, the criteria would constitute no more than an arbitrary definition of LE. The sensitivity and specificity of the criteria are determined by reference to the judgment of the experts. (See chap. 3 for a discussion of the validity of this approach.)

Even this summary review makes it obvious that we cannot provide a definitive answer to the question, "Who was the first to identify lupus?" Was it Cazenave and Schedel who coined the name we still use for the disease? Was it Kaposi who was the first to recognize its potentially fatal course and systemic manifestations? Was it Osler who provided the first detailed clinical account? Or was it Hargreaves's discovery of the LE cell phenomenon, the event that clearly pointed to an essential feature of the disease?

Our inability to answer the question is not due to a lack of detailed historical knowledge. Rather, the question itself is inappropriate. Since the way SLE is currently characterized identifies it as a so-called connective-tissue disease with a probable immunologic origin, in a sense it was only when these features were recognized that the disease was discovered.

Thus, the clinical signs of the disease, some of them probably recognized for centuries, do not really constitute the disease, and it is not until the causal mechanisms are clearly identified that we can say we have "really" discovered the disease. Indeed, in this strict sense, granted that so little is known of the essential nature of SLE, there is a sense in which the disease has not yet been discovered.

Yet this sense of discovery, knowing the underlying causal mechanisms, seems too strict. It seems more plausible to say that lupus has been recognized as a disease at least since the nineteenth century. However, if we say this, then we must also recognize that the concept of the disease has undergone changes over time. Cases once considered instances of the disease on the basis of incomplete or mistaken clinical signs are no longer considered to be such. Similarly, instances that were earlier unrecognized in terms of the criteria then employed are now considered to be instances on the basis of present understanding.

Lupus has been and continues to be an evolving concept. In effect, the theoretical understanding of the disease SLE is inseparable from the definition of the disease. Every theoretical advancement, every increase in understanding, is, in a sense, a discovery of the disease. The reason is quite simple, namely, each advancement is accompanied by a modification or reformation of the systemic lupus erythematosus category.

Thus, SLE has been discovered and rediscovered many times, and the process is far from being at an end. Yet, each time the disease is "rediscovered," it is characterized as a somewhat different disease. In this sense, then, SLE is not so much rediscovered as reinvented. The disease is what it is—our theories do not alter its independent nature-but at any given time, what we think it is, is what our theories and concepts tell us.

By contrast with the way in which diseases are discovered in this continuing process of advancing understanding and conceptual reformulation, consider the way in which an island is discovered. Tahiti was discovered by the Europeans only once. Even if they had forgotten about it, and the island had been rediscovered, it would have been the same island. The rediscovery would not have resulted from a conceptual revision, and the island itself would not be viewed in a different way than previously. Lyme disease, unlike Tahiti, has apparently been discovered many times. It was known in Europe for many years as the systemic manifestations associated with erythema annulare, its peculiar rash. Yet not until the sequence of events that occurred in Lyme, Connecticut, was the disease rediscovered and identified as a distinct entity. We are still learning about the extent and range of the disease's protein manifestations. In this sense, we are still in the process of rediscovery.

It is important not to end this discussion on a misleading note. The truth is, many diseases are discovered in ways that do not involve the conceptual revision of existing categories. Rather, what often happens is that practicing clinicians encounter patients with disorders that do not fit into existing disease categories and apparently cannot be explained in terms of known pathogenic agents, circumstances, or mechanisms. Repeated experience with such patients indicates that individual cases are not merely idiosyncratic or anomalous variations in a known disease process, and over time, a distinct clinical picture can be pieced together. The picture may eventually become clear enough to convince investigators that they are faced with a new disease.

When this happens, a concerted effort is made to identify new cases by means of the newly formulated diagnostic criteria. In the process, the criteria may become more refined and exact. At the same time, a search is initiated for the causal factors that might be responsible for the disease. The same sorts of methods employed in other empirical inquiries-statistical screening and correlation, the testing of causal hypotheses, and so on-are used to attempt to identify the cause of the disease. Roughly speaking, this is the sort of pattern that has been followed most recently in the discovery of Legionnaires' disease. It is the sort of pattern currently being followed in the investigation of acquired immune deficiency syndrome (AIDS).

Discoveries of a new disease introduce a new disease category, and in this respect they involve a conceptual revision in medicine. Over time, that category may be expected to undergo revision itself as we understand more and more about the disease. At this juncture, the points stressed earlier about lupus become applicable. The disease, once discovered, is continually rediscovered. That is, the category becomes altered and refined with increasing understanding of just what the disease involves. This process has been taking place with such great rapidity in the case of AIDS that it is difficult to remember that our understanding of most diseases has developed over centuries or decades.

The Identification of Disease

To identify a disease is to recognize a particular instance of the same kind. This is what we would ordinarily call diagnosis, but this is a term that is sometimes ambiguous between discovering a disease and classifying a specific set of clinical signs and symptoms as a disease.

Disease identification is an activity that takes place within an established framework of beliefs, categories, and procedures. Identification requires a thorough grasp of this framework and its elements, but it also requires experience and skill in employing them. Basically, it requires the ability to solicit information declared relevant by the framework and to fit a particular instance into the categories already established within the framework.

The clinician recognizes-identifies-a patient's illness as a case of a disease because the physician has memorized the elements that make up that pattern and through experience has gained a degree of expertise in recognizing the pattern when elements of the right kind are present in combination. There is, of course, more to the process of diagnosis than this. (See chap. 8 for a fuller discussion.) Nevertheless, this simple description is sufficient to distinguish diagnosis as discovery from diagnosis as recognition. The description acknowledges the fact that disease identification (recognition) is dependent upon the possession of disease categories (named diseases) and criteria for including particular disease manifestations within them.

It is quite possible for clinical medicine to employ a framework of disease categories, pattern, explanations, and methods of diagnosis that is wrong or incomplete in significant ways. For example, physicians in the early nineteenth century were trained to classify the various named "fevers" in ways that other physicians, in general, would also classify them. In this respect, then, they would all be identifying the same disease. At present, however, we consider the categories and criteria for the various fevers to be mistaken. What was actually being classified were clinical signs, not diseases.

The truth is, of course, that the framework of clinical medicine is always incomplete or faulty. Sometimes these defects are recognized and sometimes not. All the biochemical mechanisms involved in lupus are not yet known, and as they become elucidated, the general framework of clinical medicine will be altered to at least a minor extent. And of course various areas of ignorance exist in neoplastic and viral diseases.

Imperfect as the framework is at any moment in the recent history of clinical medicine, it is the only game in town, and it is in accordance with the rules of that game that diseases are identified. When the framework is altered and the rules change, then identification may change as well.

RECOMMENDED READING

Benedek, T. G. "A Century of American Rheumatology." Annals of Internal Medicine 106 (1987): 304-12.

Benedek, T. G., and G. P. Rodnan. "A Brief History of the Rheumatic Diseases."

Bulletin on the Rheumatic Diseases 32 (1982): 93-102.

Boorse, C. "On the Distinction between Disease and Illness." Philosophy and Public Affairs 5 (1975): 49-68.

Engelhardt, H. T., Jr. "The Disease of Masturbation." Bulletin of the History of Medicine 48 (1974): 234-48.

Feinstein, A. R. Clinical Judgment. 1967. Reprint. Melbourne, Fla.: Krieger, 1974. Disease as a category.

Fleck, Ludwik. Genesis and Development of a Scientific Fact. Translated by Fred Bradley and Thaddeus J. Trenn. Chicago: University of Chicago Press, 1979. In this 1935 book, Fleck traces the history of the concept of syphilis to illustrate a theory of science that influenced Thomas Kuhn's analysis.

Jarcho, S. "Notes on the Early Modem History of Lupus Erythematosus." Mount Sinai Hospital Journal 24 (1957): 939-44.

Labita, R. G., ed. Systemic Lupus Erythematosus. New York: Wiley, 1987.

Mayr, E. "Cause and Effect in Biology." In Man and Nature, ed. Ronald Munson, 101-16. New York: Dell, 1971.

Rose, N. R. "Autoimmune Disease." Scientific American 250, no. 2 (1981): 80-103. Schur, P. H., ed. The Clinical Management of Systemic Lupus Erythematosus. New York: Grune and Stratton, 1983. See Schur's "Historical Perspective and Changing

History," 1-8, for screening questions and a statement of the ARA criteria. Wallace, D. J., and E. L. Dubois. Lupus Erythematosus. 3d ed. Philadelphia: Lea and Febiger, 1987.

Wulff, H. Rational Diagnosis and Treatment. Oxford: Blackwell, 1976. See chap. 4, "The Concept of Disease."

CHAPTER 8   *Diagnosis*

Diagnosis is central to clinical medicine, and the need to establish a diagnostic decision places a demand on the physician's training, experience, and judgment. The physician must assemble and employ clinical data, call upon relevant medical and scientific theory, and use the powers of reason and the lessons of experience to integrate theory and data to arrive at a diagnosis.

Our aim in this chapter is to clarify the concept of diagnosis and to analyze the character of diagnostic reasoning. In previous chapters, we discussed the nature of clinical data, types of inferences, theories and predictions, the concept of disease, and the classification of diseases. In a sense, these previous discussions are brought to a focus in dealing with the topic of diagnosis, for diagnosis involves each of the matters discussed.

We begin with some general comments on diagnosis and diagnostic reasoning. Afterward, we turn to an examination of three stereotypes of diagnosis and show how their shortcomings make them unacceptable as models of the process. In the fourth section, we present a cyclical model of diagnosis that (we claim) correctly and accurately illuminates the basic features of the process. In the next section, we focus on the less formal and more practical aspects of diagnosis. Finally, we mention a few aspects of computers and their role in diagnosis and management.

DIAGNOSIS AS PRODUCT AND PROCESS

The term diagnosis has two distinct meanings within clinical medicine, and any effort to illuminate the nature of diagnosis must provide an analysis of both in order to be useful. First of all, diagnosis is the name for the process the clinician goes through to arrive at a conclusion about the state of health of a patient. Diagnosis, in this sense, is something the clinician does. It is an activity or action (making a diagnosis, or diagnosing). As such, it can be done well or poorly, hastily or carefully. The process is one that can be taught and learned, and it can be improved by practice. As common clinical experience indicates, some people have more of a talent for diagnosis than others. This is not particularly surprising. After all, to make a diagnosis is to exercise a skill, and although there are standard routines or procedures to be followed, they are not ones that can determine the quality of the outcome. In the same way that some people seem to be natural athletes or mathematicians, some seem to be natural diagnosticians. The process is one that has been studied psychologically, and a number of interesting findings about the influence of training, the maximum number of diagnostic possibilities considered by clinicians, and so on have been established.

Logically speaking, we can describe the diagnostic process as one in which the clinician is faced with the problem of selecting one or more diagnostic categories (named diseases or conditions) from the total range accepted by clinical medicine at the time of diagnosis. Of course, this is an idealization. First of all, no clinician is likely to know all the categories. Second, the presenting signs and symptoms are likely to narrow the range of possibilities at once. Furthermore, although new diseases are typically said to be diagnosed, we use the term *discovered* to describe the situation in which the number of diagnostic categories is increased. Accordingly, to diagnose a disease is to work within relatively fixed parameters.

Diagnosis in the second sense refers to the outcome of the diagnostic process. The clinician typically declares that the patient "has" such and such disease or diseases that the features displayed by the patient can be fit into one or more of the diagnostic categories. Such a declaration is often qualified by an accompanying estimate of how likely it is that the category identified is the correct one. The isolation of *Mycobacterium tuberculosis* from a patient makes it virtually certain that the patient has tuberculosis (given other typical signs and symptoms), whereas the features uncovered during the examination of Mrs. Halprin made it initially seem merely likely that she was having a drug reaction. Diagnosis in this second sense involves a labeling of the patient. The labeling has at least three important and distinct functions. First, it classifies the patient. In doing so, it facilitates communication with the patient and among those responsible for the patient's care. Furthermore, the classification provides a means of bringing to bear relevant medical information and theory, and in addition, data about the patient can then be used to extend the body of general information and confirm relevant theories.

Second, the diagnostic label is instrumental in providing an explanation of the symptoms, signs, and clinical data relevant to a particular patient. The body of medical information and theory can usually be counted on to provide a guide to the course of the patient's disease and its etiology. The diagnostic label, in effect, assimilates the patient's disorder into a known pattern and thus explains those features that are indicative of the disease.

Finally, the diagnosis aids the clinician in arriving at a prognosis for the patient. The recognition that the disease fits into a pattern, plus relevant theoretical information, permits the clinician to predict with some degree of certainty just what the course of the disease is likely to be and what the response to treatment is likely to be.

None of these three functions of diagnostic labeling can be performed without relying upon a system of disease classification and a body of medical information and theory. Most often, however, these simply lie in the background and are not made explicit unless some special circumstance (such as having to justify a diagnosis or prognosis) arises. Thus, at first view, it may seem that the diagnostic label alone is simultaneously a classification, an explanation, and a prognosis. In fact, the diagnostic label is no more than the tip of the diagnostic iceberg. Floating beneath the surface is the body of information and theory that give the label its meaning and significance.

SCIENTIFIC REASONING AND DIAGNOSTIC REASONING

Scientific hypotheses are typically tested by their predictive consequences. If hypothesis H predicts event E and E does not occur, the H may be rejected. H E occurs as predicted, this contributes some evidence toward establishing the correctness of H. (See chaps. 5 and 6 for a fuller discussion.) H may then be tested further by designing additional experiments. The continued success of H as part of a predictive base may eventually lead to the acceptance of H as correct.

Diagnostic reasoning follows this same logical pattern. Yet the testing of diagnostic hypotheses differs in a significant way from the testing of scientific hypotheses. The fact is, clinicians are not free to pursue the truth to the fullest possible extent. Instead, they must keep the interest and welfare of their patient at the forefront of their concerns. As a consequence, diagnostic inquiry operates under a constraint not present in scientific investigation. (Of course, some forms of scientific inquiry are also constrained in similar, as well as in other, ways. Experiments that may cause harm to subjects are not morally permissible. But this is the case with only some scientific inquiry, whereas it is the rule with all diagnostic inquiry.)

To illustrate this situation, consider the case of John Clark (as we will call him). Mr. Clark complains of severe abdominal pains localized in the lower right quadrant. Considering this and Mr. Clark's other clinical signs, his physician is fairly (but not fully) convinced that Mr. Clark has appendicitis. That is, to her that diagnostic hypothesis is a stronger contender than any other.

The most direct and persuasive way to test the hypothesis is to operate and examine Mr. Clark's appendix for signs of inflammation. But should she operate? If she decides that Mr. Clark is not a good surgical risk because of his age or physical condition, she may decide not to. Instead, she may carefully monitor his vital signs and white blood cell count, use antibiotics, and provide symptomatic relief. Suppose Mr. Clark recovers spontaneously, receiving no more treatment than this. Did he have appendicitis? His physician will never know. The hypothesis remains untested.

In a sense, Mr. Clark's physician did the right thing for him. After all, he recovered without the added risks of surgery. But did she do the most rational thing at the time? The answer to such a question hinges upon an appraisal of the features of the case. If Mr. Clark were young and in generally good health, he might be considered a good surgical candidate. If his physician did not recommend operating, many would question her decision. If Mr. Clark recovered anyway, this would only show that a poor decision can be rescued by good fortune. (Unfortunately, just the opposite may happen as well.)

Whatever decision Mr. Clark's physician made about operating, the grounds for the decision would have to involve consideration of Mr. Clark's welfare. It would not, legitimately, be open to her to decide to operate merely or even primarily to satisfy her own curiosity about the correctness of her diagnostic hypothesis. It is not legitimate within medicine to buy knowledge at the cost of health. Fortunately for Mrs. Halprin, the diagnosis of SLE was confirmed by a blood test and so involved little risk. This is not always the case.

Some theorists seem captivated by the scientific aim of diagnosis. This inclines them to describe the clinical situation as proceeding from data to diagnosis and then to treatment according to a two-step scheme: (1) from data, infer diagnosis; (2) from diagnosis, infer treatment. Inference (1) is a matter of arriving at a conclusion about a matter of fact, namely, what is wrong with the patient. It is a factual inference. By contrast, inference (2) is a matter of arriving at a conclusion about what to do. It is a practical inference. The two-step scheme recognizes that diagnostic reasoning involves a factual and a practical component, but it separates the two in its analysis.

As a picture of diagnostic reasoning, the scheme has much to be said for it. It is, at the very least, imprudent to treat someone without some idea of what is wrong. By representing treatment as following from diagnosis, the scheme recognizes this. Furthermore, once we have a diagnosis, we can then consult the body of medical information to determine the treatment of choice in such a case. Thus, having a diagnosis before instituting therapy seems to be the key to rational therapeutics.

In addition, the scheme is intellectually neat. Our understanding of the rules of scientific reasoning is not all we would like, but our understanding of the rules of practical reasoning is even more rudimentary and partial. The two-step scheme has the merit of decomposing the mixture and not forcing us to perform both tasks at once.

Yet despite everything favorable that can be said about the two-step scheme, in the end it is an unsatisfactory oversimplification of diagnostic reasoning. To be sure, there are cases in which good clinical procedure fits neatly into the two-step scheme. When a patient is not acutely ill and the diagnosis can be established at little cost or risk, then the scheme surely represents good medical practice.

However, establishing a diagnosis prior to any treatment is often a clinical luxury. The paradox in our case of Mr. Clark is that if he did have appendicitis, then treating it (by surgery) would be just what was necessary for directly confirming the diagnosis. Indeed, in countless instances, a patient's diagnosis can only be satisfactorily established by means of patient's response to treatment. If a disease fails to respond, it may mean (although not necessarily) that the diagnosis was incorrect. If the disease does respond to treatment, this is an indication that the diagnosis was correct.

In "A Cyclical Model of Diagnostic Reasoning" in this chapter, we present a general scheme of diagnostic reasoning that is more accurate and sophisticated than the process represented by the two-step scheme. We show that the two-step scheme is a special case, although not a generally correct portrayal. Before developing this scheme, we review briefly three other views about the forms and styles of diagnostic reasoning.

THREE STEREOTYPES OF DIAGNOSIS

The three views we discuss here are ones that are popular among clinicians. The views have some basis in fact and appeal to the imagination. This is reason enough to consider them carefully and to point out some of their limitations. But this exercise pays even more dividends, for it permits us to gain an appreciation of the features that a correct and accurate scheme of diagnostic reasoning must possess. Thus, we also pave the way for the presentation of such a scheme in the following section.

The Diagnostician as Detective

Readers of Agatha Christie are familiar with the final, crucial scene. The suspects are assembled in the same room .The detective then calmly reviews the evidence piece by piece, and as she does so, she rejects the hypotheses that particular people are guilty of the crime. ("I thought Lord Clarence was the one, until I learned that the great toe on his left foot was shot off during the war. Such a man would be incapable of balancing himself on a guy wire.") One by one the suspects are eliminated, until a single one remains. This must be the guilty one, but to clinch matters, evidence is presented to show that it could only be this person. Only he had the motive, means, and opportunity to commit the crime. The identity of the murderer has been established conclusively.

We are invited by some writers to imagine the diagnostician operating in a similar way. The crime is the manifestations of the disease-the symptoms, signs, and laboratory data. The suspects are the possible diseases. The job of the diagnostician is to sift through the evidence to eliminate as many suspects as possible and to establish the guilt of one (or more) of them -to identify the disease guilty of the "crime."

This is diagnostic reasoning at its most impressive-a real-life drama demonstrating the powers of "ratiocination." But let us now take a closer look at what such a process would have to involve for it to work as it is described.

Diagnostician-detectives are usually portrayed as reasoning from effects to causes. They observe a certain set of manifestations (such as joint pains, a rash, and a mild fever), then deduce one or more possible causes of these manifestations (for example, hepatitis or SLE). If they cannot deduce a single cause as the diagnosis, they then perform an experiment designed to eliminate conclusively at least one of the contending hypotheses. The information they acquire may lead them to infer new causes as well or it may suggest new experiments. Eventually, by repeating this process, they deduce the correct diagnosis.

The most important observation to make about this model is that it cannot be the complete picture. The reason is basic: causes cannot be deduced from effects. At least they cannot be without employing additional assumptions .The statement "This patient has joint pain" does not logically imply the statement "This patient has SLE." Joint pains are caused by SLE, but they are also caused by a variety of other factors.

Even the statement "This patient satisfies four of the eleven criteria for a diagnosis of SLE" does not logically imply that the patient has SLE. It is possible (even if unlikely) that the characteristics that satisfy the criteria may be produced by some other disease that we know nothing about.

Of course, it would be sensible and reasonable for the diagnostician to conclude that the patient has SLE. But this does nothing to alter the logical fact that manifestations alone do not imply a particular disease as their cause. In order to make the process work (in order to get the implication of causes from manifestations) it is necessary to assume that every disease manifestation can be explained by means of current medical information and theories. We call this the *explanatory completeness assumption.*

Given this assumption as a premise and given that a patient has certain manifestations only if he or she has some disease or other, we can deduce that the patient has one of the currently recognized diseases. Ordinarily, of course, we can go beyond this. The body of medical information contains generalizations to the effect that a certain manifestation is present if and only if a certain disease or diseases are present. For example, the Kayser-Fleischer ring is uniquely associated with hepatolenticular degeneration (Wilson's disease). Similarly, the body of medical information also contains generalizations to the effect that certain diseases are not present unless certain manifestations are present. For example, thalassemia (major) is not a diagnostic possibility unless hemolytic anemia is present. Thus, if the clinician can establish from clinical data that certain manifestations are absent, then certain diagnostic hypotheses can be eliminated.

Putting these observations together, we paint a fuller picture of diagnostcian-detectives. Clinicians begin by making observations of certain manifestations. Relying upon the explanatory completeness assumption, they then deductively conclude that the patient has the manifestations because he or she has one (or more) of the known diseases. They then infer that the patient cannot have some of the disease possibilities without certain manifestations. Clinicians may then be able to deduce that the patient does not have some of the diseases that are among those possible. But this is as far as they can go deductively. This may be far enough, for they may have eliminated all but one diagnosis. If not, they will have to make additional observations and acquire additional data in the hope of excluding more diagnoses.

The picture of the diagnostician-detective that emerges is quite a neat one. Unfortunately, it is not one that is representative of all good clinical reasoning. Three shortcomings are worth mentioning explicitly. First, the clinical data may be inadequate to eliminate many of the diagnostic possibilities. There is no guarantee that even additional data collection will reduce the possibilities to one certain one. Second, the data available may show that a diagnostic hypothesis under consideration is unlikely, while still failing to eliminate it completely. And since the world is the sort of place in which even the unlikely (statistically speaking) is sometimes true, this makes it impossible to arrive at a conclusive diagnosis. Finally, the decisive evidence may be obtainable only by autopsy or by performing a risky and possibly disabling or life-threatening procedure. It is quite possible to pay too high a price for a conclusive diagnosis. As these considerations show, in many instances the good clinician will be unable to act out the scenario of the diagnostician-detective and will find it necessary or advisable to enlist other strategies. This now puts us in a position to consider the next stereotype.

The Diagnostician as Gambler

At virtually every stage of diagnostic reasoning, the thoughtful clinician will have several diagnostic hypotheses under consideration. However, he or she will not usually consider them all equally likely, and as the evidence changes, the estimates of likelihood will also change. The likelihoods are ones that can be formally represented as the conditional probabilities of the diagnostic hypotheses given certain items of evidence. That is, for the ith diagnosis, the probability—Prob (d_i/e), where e stands for evidence. (See chaps. 4 and 9 for a discussion of conditional probabilities.)

Diagnostician-gamblers make use of the conditional probabilities to determine the most likely diagnosis, and this they declare to be "the" diagnosis. That is, "the" diagnosis is one for which Prob (d_i/e) is the greatest.

Having said this, we should go on to admit that few if any physicians function as gamblers in just this way. Typically, physicians opt for the most likely diagnosis only after they have made a thorough investigation of all likely possibilities; even then, they will name the most likely diagnosis only when they are in circumstances in which they must declare an opinion. (For example, pathologists serving as medical examiners are often forced to opt for the most probable cause of death.)

By contrast with physicians, however, a number of diagnostic computer programs are based on the gambler stereotype as we have described it. The patient is put through a screening process, the data obtained are fed into the computer, and a statistical or probabilistic algorithm is applied to yield a most likely diagnosis.

A storm of controversy surrounds the questions of what sort of computational algorithms are best and of whether automated diagnostic programs perform better than physicians. These are relevant questions in connection with the development and refinement of diagnostic programs. However, viewed in the context of understanding the process and practice of diagnosis, the questions are beside the point.

Unlike computers, physicians do not have stored in their memories the wealth of explicit, precise statistical and probabilistic information relevant to making decisions about, advising, and treating patients. The answers to such questions as "What are my chances of another heart attack?" and "How likely is it that this drug will do any good?" are ones that call for probabilistic inferences, and here the computer could be of value to the clinician.

Similarly, it is possible that the computer could assist a physician in determining the most likely diagnosis. However, the quality of the numerical data and other inputs from which the computer derives its probabilities is often inaccurate or incomplete. Furthermore, different computational algorithms may lead to different outcomes with the same input data. A computer program that uses regression equations will not always yield the same diagnostic judgment as one based on Bayes' theorem.

Despite the general usefulness of probabilistic reasoning, probabilistic approaches are not realistic models of the diagnostic process followed by good clinicians. Nor should such models be offered as a normative ideal to be followed by aspiring diagnosticians. Probabilistic reasoning has its place in diagnosis, but the model of the diagnostician-gambler does not properly represent it. First, it is wrong simply to gather a predetermined set of data, then at a predetermined time take a probabilistic leap to a diagnostic conclusion. The earlier in the investigation process the leap occurs, the more likely it is to produce unreliable results. The patient's initial complaint suggests some diagnostic hypotheses, and further examination rules out and replaces them with others. The process continues, with diagnostic candidates and their likelihoods constantly shifting as new data are acquired. A probabilistic leap threatens to end this process before it has produced at least some of the realistic diagnostic possibilities.

Second, a responsible clinician cannot base management decisions on probabilities alone. A conclusion of the form "The most probable diagnosis is X, therefore the most probable therapy that will be effective is Y" is simply a prescription for bad medicine. The probabilities have to be tempered with a variety of other considerations-considerations that are not part of the database employed to determine the probability assignments. The patient's age, general physical conditions, habits, life-style, allergies, current medications, and so on all must be taken into account.

Third, the diagnosis arrived at by probabilistic reasoning lacks explanatory and predictive power. Such a diagnosis is not based on causal laws but on statistical associations alone. The mechanisms of the disease process are, in effect, treated as though they are irrelevant to the diagnostic decision.

The Diagnostician as Artist

Diagnostician-artists figure prominently in the traditional lore of medicine. Like painters, potters, or blacksmiths, diagnosticians must have a special feel for the character of the materials and tools with which they work–the oils and canvas, clay and fire, steel and hammer, or human body and psyche. Like artists, diagnosticians must have a special talent for doing the right thing at the right time. They must make subtle observations, ask the right questions, pursue the proper lines of inquiry, and be open to new possibilities.

Clinicians who lack this talent, so the lore goes, may fail to be as effective with their patients. They will fail to notice the stare of the patient with Grave's disease or miss the peculiar foot drop that might indicate peroneal palsy.

This picture of diagnostician-artists represents an essential feature of clinical medicine. Clinicians remain the best diagnostic instrument. Some of the data they use to make a determination are not explicitly recognized by the taxonomic schemes employed to classify data. Furthermore, much of the data that are relevant must be interpreted by clinicians themselves for it to become useful. The rise of laboratory science and diagnostic technology should not be allowed to eclipse the fact that the clinician plays the crucial role in diagnosis as well as management. Ultrasound and thermography may now be employed to determine what was once determined by a stethoscope and a trained hand, but the use of such techniques has only supplemented the range of procedures. There is still an art to the practice of medicine, and there is still talent involved in diagnosis. Some clinicians will never be as good as others at diagnosis, in the same way that most actors will never be as good as Laurence Olivier.

To a considerable extent, diagnosis involves pattern recognition. The diagnostician perceives a pattern in the data, patient history, and clinical observations. While most people can be trained to recognize the same patterns, some few are better at it than others. These are, so to speak, the artists among diagnosticians. However, their skills and talents do not indicate that there is no rational scheme underlying diagnosis, that it involves nothing but creative imagination. It is the very existence of rational principles that makes it possible for new clinical students to learn to classify the diseases of their patients in just the way their teachers do. It is the existence of such principles that allow their teachers to instruct them in such classification, point out their errors, and improve their performance.

To the extent that diagnosis involves pattern recognition, we could employ computer programs to search for diagnostically significant patterns. However, although artificial intelligence researchers have developed pattern recognition models, so far the pattern dealt with have been restricted to such apparently simple cases as distinguishing a table from a chair, recognizing a discrete, physical edge, and so on. Even these cases have proved difficult, and so far pattern recognition models have not been developed for the complicated case of diagnostic reasoning.

A CYCLICAL MODEL OF DIAGNOSTIC REASONING

We have examined three schemes of diagnostic reasoning and pointed out some of the shortcomings that make each of them less than satisfactory. We now present a scheme that we believe correctly and accurately represents the basic aspects of the diagnostic process. We begin with a sketch of the scheme, then present some of the details.

The diagnostic process is best viewed as cyclical. Patient data prompt diagnostic hypotheses; diagnostic hypotheses prompt tests or treatments; tests and treatments yield new data; new data cause modifications of the diagnostic hypotheses, and so on. This is the process we see at work in the case history of Mrs. Halprin. Her initial complaint inclined Dr. Barton to consider certain diagnostic hypotheses, and these, in turn, guided her initial examination. Parts of the examination were routine, while others (such as questions about whether Mrs. Halprin had ever taken any sulfa drugs) were prompted by the hypotheses. The data garnered from this examination led to further diagnostic possibilities and these to additional tests. In the end, the diagnosis of SLE was confirmed. We tentatively represent the diagnostic cycle by figure 8.1. On an initial analysis, we find the clinician cycling through three phases: data generation or gathering (which produces data), diagnosis generation (which produces diagnostic hypotheses), and deliberation about testing or treatment (which produces a management plan for the patient). The mental and physical actions of the clinician are represented by the arrows, while their products are represented by the boxes. Even this simple picture shows us the sense in which the two-step scheme was on the right track-diagnosis generation precedes management in the diagnostic cycle.

The Generation of a Diagnosis

Let us begin by looking closely at the diagnosis generation portion of the cycle. Properly accounting for it will complicate our currently overly simple picture.

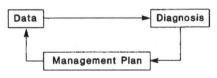

8.1.   A simplified diagnostic cycle.

Obviously, the clinician does not obtain diagnoses by making inferences from the data alone. Certainly a body of medical information is involved, especially the portion that contains the defining features, natural history, etiology, and prognoses for various diseases. (The current illness might be one not yet recognized, but we are ruling out this possibility by the explanatory-completeness assumption.) Yet the question remains: How could one deduce a set of diagnostic possibilities from such premises?

One way of explaining such inferences was central to the early diagnostic model developed by Ledley and Lusted. We start with their model and then refine it to obtain a more realistic account.

According to the model, medical theory (i.e., the body of medical information, generalizations, and scientific laws) associates certain clinical findings with each disease. The association may be between effect and cause (a malar rash is caused by SLE) or between cause and effect (smoking causes heart disease). It may be universal ("Every heart attack results in muscle enzyme release") or merely statistical ("Sixty percent of SLE cases demonstrate elevated DNA binding"). In any event, because certain findings are associated with each disease by medical theory, medical theory entails that each finding has certain diseases associated with it. More formally, each finding is associated with a class of diseases we call a *disease class*.

Now let us suppose we have established that a patient has certain signs and symptoms. That is, the data verify statements to the effect that the patient has certain findings. Each of the statements about findings, together with statements from medical theory of the form (S)-a patient has finding F only if the patient has disease belonging to disease class D_F-entails that the patient has one of the diseases in the disease class associated with that finding. The statements taken together imply that the patient has a disease or diseases belonging to one or more of the disease classes. The explanatory-completeness assumption is necessary to assert statements of the form (S). Unless the assumption is made, it is possible for a patient to exhibit a finding F without having a disease in D_F.

At this point, we have a large list of possibilities that will include at least some of the diseases our patient may have. We must say "some" because our patient may have diseases for which we have not yet observed any findings. The list is a long one because most findings have many diseases associated with them, and we (presumably) have several findings to contend with. Some of the possibilities may be eliminated at this stage, if they imply findings that are clearly absent. For example, if the finding of lassitude is present, then diabetes will be on our list of possibilities. But if urine and serum samples are normal, then that disease can be dropped from the list.

It seems reasonable to assume that our patient has no diseases other than those responsible for the current findings. This assumption will not rule out the recognition of asymptomatic subclinical diseases, provided that our findings contain evidence of them. It will rule out those diseases for which we currently have no evidence whatsoever. Also, the assumption will not prohibit the introduction of new disease possibilities as additional evidence arises. Each time we go through the diagnostic cycle, the assumption entails that all the diseases the patient currently has are present on the list derived from the disease classes. For future reference, we will call this the no-mere-possibilities assumption.

The list of possibilities can be narrowed considerably by assuming that the patient has just one disease. We can then restrict our attention to those diseases that belong to each disease class associated with current findings. That is, assuming the patient has just one disease permits us to exclude diseases not associated with all current findings. Of course, if no disease belongs to all disease classes under consideration, then we have immediate evidence against this assumption. We will call this the *one-disease assumption.*

As we construe this assumption, it must be applied to all current findings. However, this causes some difficulty. For example, recall that Mrs. Halprin displayed eosinophilia. It was difficult to explain this finding in terms of the diagnostic category to which Drs. Barton and Williams agreed the illness could best be assigned. Nevertheless, even though the finding did not fit, it was not used to exclude SLE as the most likely diagnosis. Yet if we make the one-disease assumption, we will be directed to search for a disease that makes sense of the eosinophilia. By doing so, we will have dismissed our best candidate for a diagnosis.

The rational thing to do here is obviously to ignore the data about eosinophilia. This does not mean ignoring the data altogether, but simply not attempting to account for it with a single diagnosis. We then proceed from the one-disease assumption to deduce the SLE diagnosis.

There are weaker diagnostic assumptions than the one-disease assumption, which clinicians might invoke when more than one disease is evident. These involve seeking the most comprehensive diagnoses. When a patient has more than one disease, it is safe to assume that some findings are associated with one disease, while others are associated with other diseases. If Mrs. Halprin's findings had included obesity and hypertension, as well as rash and joint pains, we would normally group the hypertension signs together and the autoimmune signs together. By considering the disease common to all disease classes in a grouping, rather than those common to all disease classes, we can conclude that our patient has more than one disease. This will also yield the most comprehensive diagnoses compatible with our groupings.

The explanatory-completeness assumption is characteristic of ordinary diagnosis. The no-mere-possibilities assumption is part of good scientific methodology. We certainly do not seek explanations for events unless we believe that they have occurred or will occur. However, neither the use of the one-disease assumption nor the grouping of findings is accepted unconditionally as good diagnostic practice. They are assumptions that are legitimate in some cases, but unwarranted in others. For example, the one-disease assumption might be more properly invoked to account for a generalized disorder of a twenty-year-old than to account for the same findings in a ninety-year-old. They are also assumptions that a good clinician is likely consciously to make or revise during the course of the diagnostic reasoning. For this reason, we segregate the explanatory-completeness and no-mere-possibilities assumptions from the others, putting the former under the heading of *background assumptions* (along with current medical theory) and placing the latter under the heading *simplifying assumptions.*

Additional simplifying assumptions can aid the clinician in narrowing the search for diseases to account for a patient's manifestations. Thus if a patient has chest pains, the clinician might assume that a cardiac disorder is responsible and omit consideration of such other causes as a tumor in the mediastinum. After additional investigation, the clinician may later assume that the problem is one concerning the coronary arteries and forego further investigations of the heart valves. Of course, at any point the clinician may reject come of these simplifying assumptions and consider again diagnoses or paths of investigations that were rejected earlier. We can think of medicine as organizing its diseases by means of a tree structure in which the branches closest to the trunk correspond to gross anatomical regions or functional systems. Then we can think of clinicians as working their way through this tree until they arrive at a twig containing a small number of diseases. As they choose a branch upon which to take their conceptual climb, they introduce a simplifying assumption. Taking back the assumption will send them down the tree some distance to a point where they can cross over to another branch. From a logical point of view, these assumptions function as further premises in the clinician's deduction of diagnostic hypotheses. They play a negative role by excluding those diagnostic possibilities corresponding to branches of the tree that have been passed over.

The background assumptions are justified by virtue of being part of the diagnostic methodology itself. The simplifying assumptions vary from case to case, and their adoption must be justified by the situation at hand. Since simplifying assumptions are factual (e.g., one patient has just one disease), at first sight one might think they should be justified in terms of the facts of the case in question. For instance, the one-disease assumption ought to be based upon the probability (given the available evidence) that the assumption is true, while the choice of a branch in the organizing system should be based upon the likelihood that it contains the correct diagnosis. If this view were correct, then the simplifying assumptions should be justified inductively in terms of the data available.

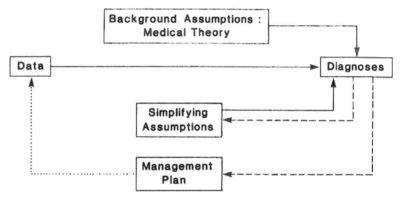

8.2.   A complete diagnostic cycle.

However, this view does not withstand a closer examination. Focusing on the most likely diagnosis may result in postponing the treatment of the true but rare disease while it is still curable. More often than not, good clinical practice mandates acting as if a poor diagnostic contender were indeed true. The reason is clear: pursuing an unlikely diagnosis is not based upon an inference to its truth but upon a decision that dealing with it now is crucial to the welfare of the patient. Simplifying assumptions are adopted in the context of diagnostic reasoning on the basis of decisions that it is optimal to do so. But here optimality is defined in terms of the patient's welfare, rather than in terms of the clinician's quest for the truth.

It is important not only to segregate the background and simplifying assumptions, but also to realize that the latter find their proper place in the deliberative phase of the diagnostic cycle. Only after a clinician has deduced a wide range of diagnostic possibilities from the current data and background assumptions will it make sense to consider introducing simplifying assumptions to further narrow the possibilities. With this in mind, we can revise figure 8.1 into figure 8.2.

In figure 8.2, the solid arrows represent results arrived at by deductive inference, the dashed arrows represent ones resulting from deliberate choices, and the dotted arrow represents interactions with the patient .Thus, the patient's initial presentation furnishes the clinician with a set of data to which is applied background assumptions and current medical theory to deduce an initial set of diagnostic possibilities. At this point, the clinician enters the deliberative phase and decides whether to follow a plan of tests or treatments (which might consist of merely continuing to observe the patient) or to introduce one or more simplifying assumptions. If the clinician chooses to employ tests or treatments, he or she will await further data before continuing with the diagnostic cycle, while if the clinician chooses to introduce assumptions, he or she will attempt to use them to narrow the range of diagnostic possibilities before proceeding to interactions with the patient.

Diagnostic Deliberation

During the course of diagnostic deliberation, the clinician chooses a plan for treating the patient or for the further determination of diagnosis. It is illuminating to distinguish two kinds of plans: thought plans and management plans. Thought plans involve the introduction of simplifying assumptions to aid the clinician in the search for the correct diagnosis. They are evaluated in terms of their ability to lead to genuine simplifications, their tendency not to lead the clinician seriously astray, and so on. In a sense, deciding on a thought plan is like deciding on a move in chess. The introduction of certain assumptions (such as, "it is a cardiac disorder") will rule out a number of diagnoses, which leads to the adoption of some management plans rather than others. This, in turn, could lead to failure to observe the very data that, if it were available, would refute the simplifying assumptions in question. Thus, it may be very difficult for the clinician to foresee the consequences of adopting certain assumptions. This, of course, could be a good reason in itself for rejecting such assumptions at the outset. On the other hand, the diagnostic process is potentially so enormously complex that the clinician usually must make some simplifications in order to proceed at all.

Management plans are patient oriented in ways that thought plans are not. They prescribe tests, treatment, or observation and are evaluated in terms of how appropriately they deal with what is perceived to be the patient's current situation. However, management plans also include such options as obtaining the opinion of a colleague, acting now rather than thinking further, or thinking now rather than acting. Although these are similar to thought plans, none feed directly back into the diagnosis-generation phase of the diagnostic cycle. These plans show us that our picture of the cycle must be further complicated, because a management plan that calls for further thought may throw the clinician directly back into the deliberative portion of the cycle. That could then lead to the adoption of a new management or thought plan.

The thoughtful clinician chooses plans—no matter what their type may be—by weighing them against the other available plans and comparing the potential outcomes of them all. The outcomes are determined, in part, by the plan implemented and, in part, by the true state of the patient's health. Since the clinician usually does not know the true state, he or she must weigh the likelihood of a number of hypotheses against the magnitude of the outcomes associated with a plan. For example, a plan calling for the administration of digitalis may be exactly the right action if the patient is in heart failure, but it might be fatal if the patient's manifestations are due to a pulmonary embolus. Deliberations such as these can be made much more exact by introducing numerical measures of likelihoods and outcome values. This casts diagnostic deliberations in the framework of modem mathematical decision theory. We discuss that subject and its applications in medicine in chapter 9.

The Acceptance of a Diagnosis

Often the clinicians can proceed without committing themselves to a specific diagnosis. So long as they can bring the range of possibilities within reason, they can implement a management plan that will cover all bases. For example, if the patient has an acute infection, clinicians may be well advised to administer a broad spectrum antibiotic immediately and quite independent of tests to determine the specific organism responsible. By contrast, there are also situations in which clinicians may be required to announce a diagnosis to which they are not fully committed. For example, while privately entertaining doubts, a clinician may declare a patient mentally stable or cured of alcoholism, because the consequences of pronouncing the patient unhealthy are undesirable in themselves. Such declarations are based upon personal and moral values as well as upon evidence and so are more properly represented in a decision- theoretic framework that incorporates such values.

It has been argued that good scientists should not accept hypotheses, for they are never in the position to establish one conclusively. The best they can do is accumulate more and more evidence in its favor and thereby increase its probability. Thus, scientists should restrict themselves to judgments about the relative probabilities of various hypotheses. In our view, this belies good scientific practice. Science progresses by taking some questions as settled. They become the facts by which further hypotheses are evaluated. Medicine proceeds in the same way. The acceptance of a diagnosis both explains a case and classifies it. The case becomes another statistic in the huge database with which medical science operates.

However, the acceptance of a hypothesis "as fact" does not preclude revising its status in the face of compelling evidence. Taking back a long accepted "fact" can lead to reverberations throughout science. For this reason, the standards for accepting a hypothesis should be high, and the evidence for retracting one previously accepted quite compelling. The very fact that we recognize that revision or retraction is sometimes necessary shows that just as scientists actually do accept hypotheses, clinicians accept diagnoses.

The question that needs answering is that of determining the standards clinicians ought use in accepting a diagnosis. When should clinicians accept a diagnosis and when should they suspend judgment and await further evidence? In science, hypothesis acceptance is usually based upon inductive inferences. Consequently, most hypotheses are never conclusively established, and acquiring more evidence bearing upon their truth or falsity is always possible. The situation with diagnosis is more promising. The diagnostic process is essentially an exercise in classification that presupposes that the general body of medical knowledge is held fixed. Thus there are natural points in which a case can be marked closed.

One such point is when evidence is found that medicine counts as pathognomic for the disease in question. Then, relative to the current medical classification scheme, the evidence entails the diagnosis deductively. Certainly the diagnosis should be accepted under those conditions. The natural histories of diseases provide another means of arriving at closure in diagnosis. The clinician can make use of them in two ways. First, when a disease has not run its full course and it is still doubtful whether the patient has it, then the clinician should suspend judgment. Second, when all the diseases under consideration have run their courses and the clinician is still in doubt as to the true diagnosis, then he or she should accept the most likely diagnosis, if any at all are accepted. When the disease has run its course and all the evidence is in, there is little point in the clinician's demurring on the grounds that more evidence is to be had. However, the quality of the evidence is relevant. If there is very little evidence and none of the competing diagnoses explains it well, then it is more appropriate for the clinician to acknowledge that rather than to accept any diagnosis.

Evaluating Models of Diagnosis

Diagrams of anatomical structures are frequently used in teaching and learning. Their usefulness would be severely compromised if the diagrams were so detailed as to reproduce literally every structure. No one would expect to find every capillary in a useful diagram of the circulatory system. We would expect to find the femoral artery, however, and any diagram that left it off would be clearly defective.

Similar considerations are relevant to judging models of diagnosis. A good model should contain all the elements that are to be found in cases of good clinical reasoning; furthermore, a good model should illuminate the structure of such reasoning (see chaps. 4 and 6). The model should help us understand and explain various features of diagnosis. A model that leaves out a crucial element or misrepresents a relationship is demonstratively defective. It becomes a candidate for correction, but if correction is not possible, then it should be rejected.

Before presenting the cyclical model of diagnostic reasoning, we examined three traditional models. We argued that each either omitted certain essential elements of diagnosis or presented a misleading picture of the process. We are now obligated to show that the cyclical model both escapes the faults of the previous three models and yet captures the features of diagnosis that each of them stresses.

The cyclical model clearly has a place for the deductions characteristic of the detective model. The deductions occur during the diagnosis-generation phase of the cyclical model. We criticized the detective model for attempting to solve all diagnostic problems via deduction and for placing the goal of finding the cause of the illness above the patient's welfare. In the cyclical model, the extra deductions (which the detective must make when the data and medical theory fail to entail a diagnosis) are based upon simplifying assumptions. These are adopted only as a result of deliberations in which the patient's welfare and other nonscientific values are weighed against the likelihood of various contending diagnoses.

The gambler model we criticized as requiring the acceptance of diagnoses on the basis of probabilities, without considering whether the acceptance would be appropriate to the diagnostic context. In the cyclical model, probabilities are tempered with values in the context of diagnostic deliberation, and no diagnosis is accepted as true until all available and relevant evidence has been considered within the constraints of the situation.

We objected to the artist model on the grounds that it conveyed the impression that there are no principles of inference in good diagnostic practice. The cyclical model allows the clinician-artist to enter the picture in several ways. First, in interacting with the patient, the clinician must see the most effective means of soliciting information about the patient's health and concerns. History taking is no more a mechanical and impersonal enterprise than portraiture. The clinician-artist will be much more able to make informed decisions during the process of diagnostic deliberation than will the clinician-mechanic. Second, in developing management plans and thought plans, the clinician must use creativity. The cyclical model does not assume the availability of a fixed list of plans. Third, in evolving plans to further the patient's welfare, the clinician must display the sort of understanding of people and their needs and wants that apparently cannot be captured by any formal theory. What is wrong with the artist model is not its insistence on these features of clinical practice, but its assumption that the entire process of diagnosis is essentially intuitive and nonrational.

REAL-LIFE DIAGNOSIS

In the last section, we developed a formal model of diagnostic reasoning. The main purpose in doing so was to achieve a better understanding of the logical structure of that form of reasoning. The focus on structure required that we deliberately suppress the richness of content in favor of abstraction and idealization. In this section, we hope to restore the balance to some extent by giving an account of what diagnosis can be like in the hands of human clinicians with human concerns and limitations.

Clinicians usually have little or no information about a patient until they meet. The clinician generally opens a discussion with a patient by asking an open-ended question such as "How are you?" or "What can I do for you?" The question is intended to prompt the patient to tell about the problem in his or her own words—to present the "chief complaint." The patient's account may indicate both the symptom the patient considers most important and also the way it is affecting him or her. For example, someone might say, "I've got this cough, and it's keeping me awake at night" or "I'm getting quite worried about it." Information about the relevance of the illness for the patient is very important, because of its usefulness in planning for management.

At the early stage of the history-taking process, conversation is kept fairly general and undirected to encourage the patient to supply a personal account of the illness. From the clinician's perspective, the overt objective of history taking is to establish a chronological account of the illness. But two other objectives should also be pursued: The first, as we mentioned earlier, is to assess the effect of the disorder on the patient. The second is to begin generating diagnostic hypotheses that will later be considered in greater detail. Failure to achieve any of these three goals marks a serious deficiency in the clinical encounter.

The most problematic of the three objectives is the generation of diagnostic hypotheses. In terms of our model, the chief complaint suggests a class of disorders that are then whittled down to a reasonable number by available data. Our patient's cough would define a class of diagnoses (disease class) that includes bronchitis, pneumonia, lung cancer, and so on. At this point the clinician would characterize the cough further: Is it productive? Is the expectoration blood-streaked? What time of day is it worse? The clinician is likely, at this stage, in an informal way, to assign probability ranges ("one in ten," "about 50-50," "very likely") to some of the diagnoses that occur to him or her. Additional features of the patient's history, physical examination, and laboratory studies may then narrow the choices.

Clinicians, because they are mere humans, do not have the full compendium of currently recognized diagnoses at their fingertips. They primarily rely on associations produced by their knowledge and experience to yield the diagnostic hypotheses that they actually entertain. The number of hypotheses they consider is thus limited by their associative capacity, knowledge, and experience. Studies generally show that clinicians are limited to fewer than seven variables they can deal with at one time.

This limitation is rarely a source of problems, for it is unusual to face a situation requiring serious consideration of more than four diagnostic hypotheses. When there is great diagnostic uncertainty, physicians tend to think in broader categories of disease than individual diagnoses—Is it infectious, neoplastic, immunologic, and soon? The crucial limiting factor at this phase of the diagnostic process is not psychological capacity but ignorance. If a clinician does not know that a disease exists or that it has certain manifestations, then obviously it is impossible to consider the disease a diagnostic possibility. This is, in part, why a large knowledge base is necessary for clinicians.

After permitting the patient to give an initial description in his or her own words, the clinician enters the next stage of this history-taking process—the directed portion of the history—in which the patient is asked specific questions. In terms of our model, these questions are tests to acquire more data about the patient, and their selection is governed by a management plan. Thus, the clinician who proceeds to the directed history can be said to have passed through the deliberative phase of the diagnostic cycle. This explains why clinicians feel uncomfortable directing a history until they have at least one diagnostic hypothesis under consideration. In the absence of a hypothesis, more circumstantial evidence may be sought in hopes of uncovering something useful or suggestive.

What do clinicians do if diagnostic possibilities worth pursuing fail to occur to them? They have two choices. First, they can go to the library or to a colleague and try to obtain more knowledge about the problem in the hope of generating new diagnostic hypotheses. Second, they can proceed with the interview and subsequent examinations by employing a prescribed routine that they have been taught or that has evolved from experience in handling such dilemmas. Beginning clinicians and medical students often find themselves in this position, and usually opt for completing the routine portions of the examination (the database) before reading about the problem.

The second phase of the interview is marked by more directed questioning of the patient in order to complete the original three goals-a complete chronological account of the illness, a maximum set of diagnostic hypotheses, and a clear notion about the effects of the illness on the individual. However, there is now also a fourth objective-to acquire data supporting or refuting the various hypotheses being considered. If lung cancer is a possibility, then the questions will likely be ones about weight loss, fatigue, bloody sputum, and a smoking history, if the answers have not already been obtained.

One might argue that all of these questions are relevant to a patient with a cough. That is true if cough is the only thing that is known about the individual. But during the course of the initial history, the patient will divulge information that limits the possibilities, often to a reasonable number and occasionally to only one possibility. It is usually the case that the individual's chief complaint, the primary symptom, is a common manifestation of a large number of diseases. The number is usually so large, in fact, that clinicians rarely consider a specific list of possibilities until well into the patient's account of the problem, until after the patient has narrowed the range of possibilities to a number that can easily be dealt with. An eighteen-year-old woman with a week's history of low fevers, cough, and runny nose is not giving a history consistent with lung cancer, just as the sixty-year-old two-pack-a-day smoker with a hacking cough of six months' duration and a ten-pound weight loss is not indicating he has strep throat.

Once the clinician has started this more directed phase of the interview, the door to new-hypotheses generation is at least partially closed. There are no specific rules on how long the first phase of the interview should be or when to start specific questioning. If the account is complex or if the patient continues to provide useful information, the first phase of the interview will continue. If not, the clinician should proceed to the second phase. It may be a mistake to let a patient ramble on about a problem, but a more commonplace and more serious mistake is to terminate the first phase before the patient has had an opportunity to communicate all the relevant information. It is vastly more efficient to narrow the diagnostic possibilities via the patient's account than by the clinician's questioning. If we had to enumerate all the possible causes of a cough and all their different manifestations and ask the patients about each one, we would be in for a very long night indeed. Simply letting the patient recount the problem usually provides sufficient information to narrow the field immensely in a short time.

The past medical history, family history, review of systems, and the social history constitute a set of information called the *database*. The information is relevant and necessary, but it rarely causes revision in the initial set of diagnostic hypotheses. However, it often adds other possible diagnoses that are not related to the present illness. (A common example is the presence of an allergy or a history that includes a previous operation.) Occasionally, an entirely separate present illness may be suggested by a response during this portion of the history taking. Our patient with a cough might describe varicose veins on specific questioning about the extremities during the review of systems. If this occurs, then the same procedure that was carried out with the primary history should be applied—a chronological account generating specific hypotheses, followed by specific questioning about those hypotheses.

The physical examination and the initial laboratory studies complete the database. In both areas, a routine series of procedures are performed similar to the questions in the review of systems. The choice of what to include in these routine examinations is controversial. The kinds of data commonly sought are those that indicate the presence or absence of a broad spectrum of possible disorders and do so in a relatively uniform and sensitive fashion. That is, the data are often present or positive when the (or a) disease is present. A good example of this is the sedimentation rate of red blood cells when left standing in a tube. The more rapid the rate, the more likely the patient is ill from a wide range of possible disorders.

Another desirable feature of these routine screening tests is a high predictive value. Recall from our earlier discussions that this means that the presence of the feature predicts the presence or absence of the disease in question. Recall also that this feature depends on the prevalence of the disease in the population (or more precisely the prior probability of the disease in the individual) and so cannot be uniformally determined for large numbers of patients. At least part of the controversy surrounding the use of screening tests involves the variation in predictive value of these tests in different populations. Screening for lead exposure should include questions concerning lead paint ingestion in the North and moonshine drinking in the South. The controversy also arises from the different orientation of clinicians. Clinicians who believe in prevention and early intervention tend to screen more, whereas more conservative and skeptical clinicians screen less.

In addition to this screening function, the physical examination and laboratory tests allow the clinician to investigate diagnostic hypotheses by acquiring more data on each possibility. In this sense, they are analogous to the specific questions at the end of the history.

This entire process is by no means uniform in different clinicial circumstances. (A comatose patient will not give a detailed history.) However, as we discussed in chapter 3, it is more uniform than one might expect. For example, in the case of a comatose patient, history may be obtained from those who brought the individual to the hospital, from family, and from friends. This history might suggest possible diagnoses that could be examined for in the physical examination and in the laboratory. The patient's lifestyle might suggest drug overdose as a cause of coma. Needle puncture sites and other signs of drug abuse could be examined for, and a toxicology screen could be performed by the chemistry lab. Alternatively, a history of diabetes suggests the possibility of hypoglycemia so various determinations by physical and laboratory examination become relevant.

At the end of the examination, the various diagnostic hypotheses that remain as possible explanations for the present illness are weighed against each other. This process leads to a more or less precise ordering of likelihoods for the possibilities. At least an ordinal ranking should be generated. The two major considerations that operate this ordering are, first, the posterior probability of the diagnostic hypothesis after all the information has been assessed and, second, the explanatory power of the hypothesis. Thus, the diagnostic process utilizes both inductive and hypothetico-deductive reasoning.

Two warnings are worth stressing. First, the ranking of diagnostic possibilities is not necessarily the order of importance in the generation of a management plan. A plan necessitates other considerations such as urgency, availability of effective therapy, and so forth. Second, data that were inadequately explained by the diagnostic possibilities need to be addressed. Their importance may be discounted in light of the evidence supporting the existing diagnostic hypotheses. Alternatively, some attempt to explain the data within the confines of the existing hypotheses may be undertaken. As we pointed out earlier, this may lead to reading about the diagnostic possibility or by asking colleagues about their experiences in similar circumstances. These kinds of discussions are commonplace and usually begin with "Have you ever seen...?"

Data may be explained in a nonempirical fashion by analogy to a known mechanism or model of disease. For example, the observation that gout attacks occur primarily in the early morning hours has been explained by an appeal to certain principles and laws of fluid physiology. Specifically, at night when legs are elevated in a recumbent position, there is less hydrostatic pressure in the blood vessels of the leg. Fluid in the joint spaces of the foot tends to return to the blood vessels, leaving the joint fluid more concentrated. If the uric acid (actually, sodium urate) concentration is high to begin with, the added concentration can make it precipitate in the joint and start the inflammatory response called a gout attack.

Data that cannot be explained either empirically or theoretically must be either discounted or explained by new diagnostic possibilities. Usually this requires expanding the clinician's knowledge base since, if the clinician knew how to explain the data in the first place he or she would not be having difficulty at this point. Again, this requires discussions or reading about the problem. Those cases with manifestations that cannot be either ignored or easily explained are among the most troublesome. If the features noted are truly novel and the disorder is proven, then it may be the subject of report in the medical literature to alert other clinicians of its occurrence.

COMPUTERIZED DIAGNOSIS

During the past two decades there have been a number of impressive applications of computers to diagnosis. Computers have a tremendous capacity for swiftly and accurately executing complex computations and for instantly recalling vast amounts of information stored in their memories. Scientists and engineers have used them to perform tasks that even teams of unassisted humans could barely begin to accomplish in a lifetime. The use of computers in medicine promises to revolutionize our approach to patient care. Unfortunately, short of presenting a course in computer science, we can offer only a brief glimpse of computerized diagnosis.

Computers can only do what they are programmed to do, and to write a program to do a task requires analyzing the task into its most simple and basic components. Thus, writing and testing programs for such complex processes as diagnostic inference and decision making may take years. Furthermore, even when such programs are developed, the number of separate computations involved in their operation may be so huge that they not only compare miserably to humans, but also are uneconomical to run.

To take just one example from the field of computer diagnosis, it is quite easy to write a program for computing probabilities using Bayes' theorem or the inverse probability law. Thus, it is not particularly difficult to develop simple diagnostic programs that assign probabilities to various diagnoses and revise them as new data become available. However, if one applies such programs to an area such as internal medicine, where the number of diagnostic possibilities and items of information are large, then the number of calculations these programs must execute reaches astronomical levels. Consequently, computer scientists must be concerned not only with what is mathematically correct, but also with what is feasible now or in the foreseeable future. This must be borne in mind when assessing the current batch of programs for computerized diagnosis.

There are three major approaches to computerized diagnosis: physician-substitute programs, interactive programs, and simulation models. So far, the physician substitutes are at their best in tasks involving routine gathering and processing of patient information. For example, instead of having a clinician or a nurse conduct an initial screening interview, patients can sit at a computer terminal and answer simple yes-or-no questions, much as they would deal with an automatic bank teller. The computer can be programmed to refer the patients for further interviewing or laboratory tests. As long as the interview can be organized into a series of set questions, each requiring one of a definite number of set responses, and so long as each set of possible responses has a definite action associated with it, there is little difficulty in writing a computer program for carrying out the interview. The computer merely follows algorithms similar to those already widely used by the lay staff of screening clinics as a means to free the clinical staff for tasks in which their knowledge and training is genuinely required.

Of course, computer interviews pass over data that may be crucially important to a clinician. Patients may not perceive that they are depressed or slightly jaundiced, but it will be readily apparent to any trained clinician who takes a careful look. Thus, there are clearly circumstances in which it is not advisable to rely upon a physician substitute alone. In such instances, an interactive program might be very useful. Programs of this sort allow the computer and the clinician to pool their talents. The clinician plans strategies, exercises clinical judgment, and gleans subtle information eluding quantitative characterization and measurement; the computer searches through large data banks and performs computations. An internist, for instance, to be sure of considering all the disease associated with a cough and fever, could use an interactive program to generate a list of the relevant diseases. The list could even be ordered in terms of seriousness or rarity. Similarly, given a diagnosis or set of diagnoses one could quickly retrieve lists of therapies or management plans from the computer; the same program could calculate dosages appropriate to the patient's age, weight, known allergies, and other relevant factors. Of course, the clinician could obtain the same information through traditional sources, but nowhere near as quickly.

Artificial intelligence (AI) is a branch of computer science concerned with the computer simulation of intelligent behavior. Programs that attempt to duplicate the results of human reasoning have certain characteristics in common: they are goal or task oriented; they involve processes that are guided by rules or heuristics; they usually specify a hierarchy of procedures; finally, they are never simply computational. AI researchers have developed programs for proving theorems in logic and mathematics, recognizing patterns, playing chess, translating languages, and carrying out diagnostic reasoning. Spectacular successes have been achieved with simple tasks drawn from each of these applications. However, they have been accompanied by almost as dramatic evidence demonstrating that the same programs are not adequate to deal with the more complicated tasks they were intended to handle, despite the fact that humans perform their tasks with relative ease. In logic, for example, there are algorithms that, yield proofs of every logical theorem, something that can be demonstrated as a mathematical certainty. The early theorem-proving programs implemented these algorithms and managed to prove the totality of theorems of a freshman logic text in seconds. Yet the same programs bogged down hopelessly when applied to more demanding theorems that were still within the range of, say, an above-average undergraduate mathematics major. In theory, the computer could have found proofs, but its search for them would have demanded an unreasonable amount of computer time. The cyclical model of diagnostic reasoning that we presented earlier in this chapter suffers from the same problem. It is possible to design a computer program to implement it, but the program's efficiency would be limited to very simple diagnostic problems and to restricted areas of medicine.

To cope with this situation, experts in artificial intelligence have sought algorithms that, though not entirely satisfactory from a theoretical point of view, work reliably for the domain of their intended application. For example, a programmer who knows that a program will never need to calculate interest on a loan that extends more than thirty years may find it easier to write a program for scheduling loan payments than if there were no upper bound on the number of years the loan extends.

Another useful device is to design programs that mimic what from a mathematical viewpoint are human frailties. For instance, humans hold only a small number of ideas in their active consciousness at one time. In other words, their short-term memory is limited. However, when properly prompted humans can recall information that they acquired quite some time ago. Their long-term memory is at least as impressive as that of most computers. Association seems to play a large role in recalling information from long-term memory into short- term memory. Some diagnostic programs make use of this limitation as a device to restrict the number of diagnostic hypotheses that are actively considered. The program might generate a large set of diagnostic possibilities (much as our model does) by inferring disease classes from information stored in long-term memory. Then, thresholds, defined in terms of likelihoods or seriousness, can be set in order to narrow the diagnostic possibilities and to avoid the computational explosion attendant upon large sets of them. Diagnostic contenders falling below the thresholds can be stored in long-term memory and recalled when the appropriate associative cues appear.

Another approach replaces probabilities with certainty levels or ranges of probabilities. This reflects the fact that humans are poor at judging exact probabilities. Some programs combine several of these features. At present, those working in artificial intelligence often borrow from psychology, but their own efforts may lead not only to programs useful for practicing clinicians, but also to ones that will improve our understanding of the human mind.

For illustrative purposes, we discuss three of these programs: the Internist program of Harry Pople and Jack Myers, the Mycin program of E. H. Shortliffe and others, and the Casnet program of S. M. Weiss and others. These programs are major undertakings requiring years of effort and illustrate the spectrum of conceptual tools investigated to date.

Internist

Internist is a massive attempt to catalog all the diagnostic situations encountered in internal medicine. The program is apparently well on its way to completion.

Conceptually, Internist employs a predominantly Bayesian scheme. Each disorder is associated with a set of manifestations, and each manifestation has two conditional probabilities associated with it-the probability of the disease given the manifestation $P(D/M)$ and its inverse, the probability of the manifestation given the disease $P(M/D)$. However, these are scored only roughly on a scale of 0 to 5, and there is no explicit prior probability of the disorders for the population, $P(D)$.

This program must deal with the problem of common manifestations invoking large numbers of diagnostic possibilities, which in turn require computations of even larger numbers of manifestations. This consequence of unbridled probabilistic schemes is called combinatorial explosion and must be controlled. Internist does this by relating specific diagnoses to more general disease categories, unless evidence is present that sufficiently specifies an individual disease. This corresponds to the physician's awareness that a patient has heart disease and, further, that the patient has valvular heart disease, without knowing which valve is dysfunctional. In a sense, the program is a form of chain reasoning leading to smaller and smaller subsets of disorders. Scoring diagnoses involves incrementing the probability of the disorder, given the manifestation $P(D/M)$ for each one of the patient's manifestations, adding points for causally confirmed diagnoses, then subtracting the probability of manifestations given disease $P(M/D)$ for each manifestation not found and subtracting a certain score for each manifestation not accounted for. The total score for each diagnostic contender is generated, but Internist does not stop there. It then pursues competing diagnoses with a questioning strategy to confirm a single diagnosis, if possible. Confirmation is achieved by exceeding some arbitrary numerical threshold.

Mycin

Mycin is a therapeutically oriented consultation program to aid physicians in the treatment of patients with infectious diseases. In many ways, the Mycin system is the opposite of Internist. The fundamental scheme is entirely deductive (but not causal), rather than probabilistic. It is based on a series of production rules that derive from empirical observations and are formulated in an "if... then..." format. Probabilistic influences are inserted as a "certainty factor" (between 0 and 1) for each rule and as measures of belief and disbelief for data. Additional positive data tend to lessen disbelief and, in a probabilistic but not Bayesian fashion, increase belief. Belief and disbelief are combined to give a certainty factor for each fact. The overall strategy provides the user with diagnostic possibilities arranged in certainty order and with therapeutic recommendations. The system has explanatory capabilities based on its rules and can even acquire new knowledge.

Casnet

Casnet is a deductive, causally modeled system for the management of glaucoma. The central feature of glaucoma is increased pressure within the eye globe. Both the antecedents and the consequents of this feature are causally related, though it is quite a complex area. Probabilistic elements enter when the likelihood of an individual pathophysiological state is estimated. The likelihood is estimated from causal associations that give it weight and, separately, by the strength of association with other confirmed or disconfirmed states. Both states are confirmed by testing, which requires exceeding an arbitrary threshold value. Thus, weights are used to define a test strategy-high-weight states are likely to be confirmed by testing, and low-weight states are likely to be disconfirmed. A pathway that contains no denied state (node) and ends in a confirmed state is confirmed and defines the disorder. The disorder network defines preference values for therapeutic options, but it can be modified by subsequent observations on the patient. On the whole, the program performs much like an experienced ophthalmologist.

These models are quite instructive. They suggest that a mixed set of formalisms are necessary to capture diagnostic and management reasoning. The initial set of diagnostic hypotheses is generated from the starting information on the patient. A set-theoretical approach seems most consistent with physicians' reasoning at this stage. An initial set of manifestations defines a set of diagnostic hypotheses. However, many disorders can be generated from a small set of manifestations. In fact, additional symptoms narrow diagnostic possibilities, since they require that the diagnostic hypothesis explain more information. Thus, some sort of flexible mechanism of initial data acquisition is necessary to define a limited number of disorders.

For the most part, the diagnostic set must be pursued by the acquisition of new data to focus on a very small set of highly likely possibilities. This focusing mechanism must order the possibilities and must pursue them by acquiring new information that bears on their presence or absence. This new information might be acquired in a strictly rote fashion (e.g., "When x is a possibility, do test y"), or it may be acquired by appeal to a more general rule. These rules may be based on general classification schemes, such as "If x is a possibility and x is a member of z class of diseases, do tests T_z." Rules also may be causal, such as "If x is a possibility and x often causes y, then test for y." However, strict causality is unlikely to be successful, because disease biology is simply too complex and too poorly defined to accommodate that degree of formalism. Nevertheless, a causal system has far greater explanatory power than either a classificatory or an empirical-rule-based system. In general, the explanatory power of these latter two systems is augmented, because they usually are higher-order rules. That is, both of them are based on a foundation of scientific data. In Mycin, for example, a rule might state that certain bacteria will be sensitive to a certain drug. This may be an empirical observation. However, a large collection of data about the molecular biology of the organism, the drug's mechanism of action, and its pharmacology may be subsumed under this rule.

If necessary, these data could be brought forth to establish a causal explanation. Associative reasoning clearly plays a role in diagnostic reasoning. Physicians tend to seek additional supporting data that, while not strictly related to the patient's disorders in a biological sense, may lend support. For example, if an inherited disorder is a possibility, a physician might look for evidence of consanguinity in the family. Computer analysts conceptualize this in terms of inference networks.

The acquisition of new evidence may lend support to a hypothesis. However, this is unlikely to be appropriately modeled by a strict Bayesian system. The notion of data independence is too restrictive, and the enormous numbers of calculations necessary to assess possibilities is unrealistic. Furthermore, the classificatory scheme is nebulous enough to prevent mutually exclusive possibilities from being generated.

The artificial intelligence models are obviously quite sophisticated. Yet certain aspects of diagnosis are not clearly addressed. One is the time-dependent nature of diagnosis. Physicians often choose to wait, to do nothing except observe, usually because the acquisition of new data is not warranted at that time. Another aspect is the question of when to expand and when to contract the set of diagnostic hypotheses. Another is why physicians often request more information than is necessary to achieve a given level of certainty.

In a pragmatic sense, these models may be very prophetic. One set of formalisms may be useful for one domain of medical knowledge, while another area might necessitate other formalisms. If this is so, then the future of computer diagnosis may consist of taking only small nibbles at the medical apple. The hope is that eventually the entire domain will be understood, bit by bit.

Value judgments must enter the scheme at various stages. Is it worthwhile to do the test? To pursue a diagnostic possibility? To pursue a treatment plan? The only model proposed for this aspect is decision analysis, and it is to this topic we now turn.

RECOMMENDED READING

Mathematical and Conceptual Models of Diagnosis

Card, W. I. "Mathematical Methods in Diagnosis." Journal of the Royal College of Physicians of London 9 (1975): 193-96. Statistical treatment.

Cohen, L. J. "Bayesianism versus Baconianism in the Evaluation of Medical Diagnoses." British Journal for the Philosophy of Science 31 (1980):45-62. This paper reviews the philosophical and practical objections to the approach to diagnosis based on Bayes' theorem (i.e., the approach taken in this chapter) and proposes an alternative.

Einhorn, H. J. "Diagnosis and Causality in Clinical and Statistical Prediction." In D. C. Turk and P. Salovey, eds., Reasoning, Inference and Judgment in Clinical Psychology. New York: Free Press, 1987.

Einhorn, H. J., and R. M. Hogarth. "Prediction, Diagnosis, and Causal Thinking in Forecasting." Journal of Forecasting 1 (1982): 23-36.

Feinstein, A. R. Clinical Judgment. 1967. Reprint. Melbourne, Fla.: Krieger, 1974. This classic attempt to use rigorous methods in medicine contains a number of discus- sions of diagnostic reasoning.

---. "An Analysis of Diagnostic Reasoning." YaleJournal of Biology and Medicine 46 (1973): 212-32, 264-83; I (1974): 5-32. This article proposes a non-Bayesian and nonprobabilistic model of diagnostic reasoning.

Ledley, R. R ., and L. B. Lusted, "Reasoning Foundations of Medical Diagnosis."

Science 130 (1959): 9-21. The first formal model of diagnostic reasoning.

Miller, M. Clayton, Ill, M. C. Westphal, Jr., and J. R. Reigart, II .Mathematica/ Models in Medical Diagnosis. New York: Praeger, 1981. A discussion of multivariate approaches.

Murphy, E. A. The Logic of M edicine. Baltimore: Johns Hopkins University Press, 1976. A critical-thinking approach to medicine written by an eminent biostatistician, this book contains a discussion of diagnostic reasoning.

Price, R. B., and Z. R. Vlahcevic. "Logical Principles in Differential Diagnosis."

Annals of Internal Medicine 15 (1971): 89-95. An early attempt.

Wulff, H. Rational Diagnosis and Treatment. Oxford: Blackwell, 1976. This clear and accessible discussion of critical thinking in medicine contains a discussion of diagnostic reasoning.

Artificial Intelligence Models of Diagnosis

Clancy, W. J., and E. A. Shortliffe. Readings in Medical Artificial Intelligence. Reading, Mass.: Addison-Wesley, 1986. A collection of important papers.

Croft, D. J. "Is Computerized Diagnosis Possible?" Computers and Biomedical Research 5 (1972): 351-76.

Jacques, J. A., ed. Computer Diagnosis and Diagnostic Methods: Proceedings of a Conference on the Diagnostic Process, University of Michigan. Springfield, Ill.: Charles C. Thomas, 1972.

Psychological and Sociological Studies Bearing on Clinical Judgment and Diagnosis

Eddy, D. M., and C. H. Clanton. "The Art of Diagnosis: Solving the Clinicopathological Exercise." New England Journal of Medicine 306 (1982): 1263- 68.

Elstein, A. S., L. S. Shulman, and S. A. Sprafka. Medical Problem Solving: An Analysis of Clinical Reasoning. Cambridge, Mass.: Harvard University Press, 1978. Kassirer, J. P., and G. A. Gorry. "Clinical Problem Solving: A Behavioral Analysis."

Annals of Internal Medicine 89 (1978): 245-55.

Pauker, S. G., G. A. Gorry, J. P. Kassirer, and W. B. Schwartz. "Towards the Simulation of Clinical Cognition: Talcing a Present Illness by Computer." American Journal of Medicine 60 (1976): 981-96.

Wolf, F. M., L. D. Gruppen, and J. E. Billi. "Differential Diagnosis and the Competing- Hypothesis Heuristic." Journal of the American Medical Association 253 (1985): 2858-62.

Hypothesis Acceptance

Klemke, E. D., R. Hollinger, and A. D. Kline, eds. Introductory Readings in the Philosophy of Science. Buffalo: Prometheus Books, 1980. Essays 14-17 in this volume are useful introductions to hypothesis acceptance and the role values play therein.

CHAPTER 9   Decision Making and Patient
            Management

Even when a diagnosis has been conclusively established, physicians must make innumerable decisions in caring for patients. The decisions are often routine and uncomplicated, but they are occasionally agonizingly difficult. An unexpected consequence of a course of action can be a brutal reminder to both physician and patient that we live in a world of uncertainty.

The skill to deal effectively with complex and uncertain situations is precisely what constitutes clinical judgment. Physicians with outstanding clinical judgment are marked by their keen analyses of clinical situations, the knowledge of relevant options, their careful evaluations of competing concerns, and their capacity to integrate information from a variety of sources. In the practice of medicine, decisions concerning the use of dangerous or costly tests or marginally beneficial or dangerous therapies are likely to require just those skills. The question in our case study of whether to perform a renal biopsy on Mrs. Halprin is an example of such a decision. On the one hand, the biopsy could help predict the course of her disease and the effectiveness of various therapies, and, consequently, it might dictate a change in therapy; on the other hand, it involves a definite risk of morbidity and mortality. Because decision making of this sort plays a crucial role in medical thinking, it requires careful analysis. What we need is a logically sound and mathematically rigorous means for assessing the consequences of medical decisions.

During the past forty years, economists, mathematicians, and philosophers have developed a methodological framework for dealing with decisions in a rigorous and quantitative manner. Although decision theory, as the approach is called, was developed in a highly theoretical setting, it has been extensively applied by analysts assisting business and governmental decision makers. More recently, physicians have incorporated its tools and insights in developing methods for making clinical decisions. In this chapter, we present and discuss the general decision-theoretic framework and examine the question of applying decision theory in medicine.

INDIVIDUAL DECISION MAKING: THE BASIC
FRAMEWORK

In discussing the value of biopsying Mrs. Halprin's kidney, Dr. Williams

228

presented a clear example of clinical reasoning and decision analysis:

Sometimes, the usefulness of a biopsy in helping achieve the best patient outcome is something that can be evaluated by decision analysis. Basically, what we want to know is whether the results will redirect our strategy to a more effective therapy.

For that to happen, it is necessary for there to be different and effective treatments for different biopsy results. What's more, we have to be unable to predict the biopsy results beforehand by using other data. Finally, the test cannot have an excessive rate of mortality or morbidity.

Let us try for a more exact understanding of Dr. Williams's reasoning. He was stating conditions that warrant a decision to biopsy. Presumably, Dr. Williams believes we should be sure that the following three conditions hold before biopsying:

1. If the biopsy results will not affect the choice of treatment, then it is pointless to biopsy.

2. If we can predict the biopsy's results using other more easily obtainable data, then it is pointless to biopsy.

3. If risk of the biopsy exceeds its expected benefit, then it would not be reasonable to biopsy.

Although all three of these points are a matter of "common sense," the last involves an explicit reference to balancing risks against potential gains. Clearly, we need a mathematical approach to make such a comparison.

Let us begin by reviewing the considerations that Dr. Williams brought to the biopsy decision. First, he stated two choices or acts or options-to biopsy or not to biopsy. (We will ignore for the moment the option to wait.) Each of these options could result in one or more outcomes. If he performs the biopsy, then, depending upon the state of Mrs. Halprin's renal disease, several things may happen. First, he will learn that her disease is severe, moderate, or mild. Second, it is possible, though unlikely, that she will die from biopsy. Assuming this does not happen, Dr. Williams will make a choice of therapy based on the biopsy results. The therapy may or may not succeed. (We are simplifying matters considerably. There are plainly different kinds of success and failure and many different ways the biopsy could lead to Mrs. Halprin's death.)

If Mrs. Halprin does not have the biopsy, then the choice of treatment will have to be made without this information. Keep in mind that the choice of whether to biopsy is separate from the question of success or failure of any treatment, since it depends on the severity of the disease. (Whether we get to our destination depends on whether we take the proper route. Having a map may help, but it does not ensure success.) This analysis is represented by the decision tree in figure 9.1. Boxes (decision nodes) are used in decision trees to represent choices for actions open to the decision maker. Circles (chance nodes) are used to represent factors that determine the outcome of the decision. At the time the biopsy decision was made, we did not know whether Mrs. Halprin would survive the operation or whether she had mild, moderate, or severe renal disease. Thus the biopsy line is followed by a circle with those possibilities branching from it. The tips of the tree are called outcome or terminal nodes. In analyzing a decision it is essential that the states be chosen so that they are mutually exclusive and exhaustive. In terms of decision trees, this means that the branches emanating from a chance node should represent all the relevant possibilities and that it should be impossible for two different branches to apply at once. One might wonder, for example, whether Dr. William had already failed to use an exhaustive set of states by not including the possibility that Mrs. Halprin's kidneys were perfectly healthy. But given the severity of her disease, he could safely exclude that possibility (a process called "pruning the tree").

When the branches of the chance nodes can be assigned definite probabilities, then the decision is called a decision under risk. By contrast, if the situation is less clear and probabilities cannot be assigned, the decision is called one under ignorance or ambiguity. In the other extreme, when one knows exactly what will happen, the decision is one under certainty. Medical decisions are almost always under risk.

To determine the best option in decisions under risk, we need to calculate their expected values, which are sums of the products of the probabilities of the states with the values of the outcomes. We should then choose the outcome with the highest expected value. The explanation that follows makes this clear.

DECISIONS UNDER RISK

Let us invent some numbers and suppose that the probability of mild, moderate, and severe disease is each one-third and that of biopsy-related mortality is .01. Then the probability Mrs. Halprin will survive the biopsy *and* that Dr. Williams will learn that her kidney disease is mild (or moderate or severe) is not exactly one-third but rather .33. Thus, the total .33 + .33 + .33 plus the probability of .01 that she dies equals 1.

Now that we have the probability assignments fixed, we can consider the values or utilities of therapy. The effect of therapy is to improve Mrs. Halprin's

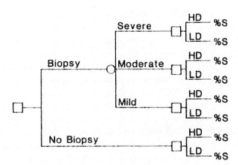

9.1.   A decision tree. Should a kidney biopsy be performed on a patient with systemic lupus erythematosus? Will the biopsy results influence the choice of high-dose (HD) or low-dose (LD) coricosteroids and result in improved survival (%S)?

chance of survival. For simplicity, we will represent survival as 1 and death as 0. Let us suppose that the probability of survival using high-dose therapy is .9 when the disease is mild, .5 when it is moderate, and .15 when it is severe. By contrast, with low-dose therapy the probabilities are .95 when the disease is mild, .4 when it is moderate, and .1 when it is severe. These assignments are represented in figure 9.2.

If for each terminal node, the high-dose therapy resulted in a chance of survival better than or equal to the chance of survival with low-dose therapy, then Dr. Williams should treat Mrs. Halprin with high-dose therapy and not biopsy. In this case, the high-dose therapy is said to dominate the low-dose therapy. Information that might be acquired by biopsy is irrelevant. (This is just a restatement of Dr. Williams's condition (1) for biopsying.)

However, in our example neither high-dose nor low-dose therapy dominates. If Mrs. Halprin's kidneys are only mildly damaged, the high-dose

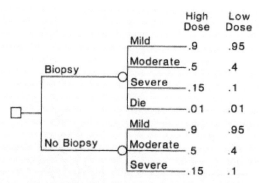

9.2. A decision tree for a biopsy problem, indicating the outcome with high-dose and low-dose therapy.

therapy results in a lower survival rate (90 percent) than low-dose therapy (95 percent). However, if the disease is moderate or severe, the high-dose therapy results in greater survival: .5 versus .4 for moderate and .15 versus .1 for severe.

Let us now calculate the expected value for not biopsying and treating with low- or high-dose steroids versus biopsying and treating with the therapy best for the biopsy result. If we treat with high-dose therapy without biopsying, the probability of survival is

.9 x 1/3 (mild disease), plus
.5 x 1/3 (moderate disease), plus
.15 x 1/3 (severe disease), which equals .5167.

Similarly, the probability of survival for low-dose therapy without biopsying is

.95 x 1/3 (mild)
.4 x 1/3 (moderate)
.10 x 1/3 (severe), which equals .483.

However, if we biopsy and treat accordingly, the result is

.95 x .33 (mild, low dose)
.5 x .33 (moderate, high dose)
.15 x .33 (severe, high dose)-total of .99 not 1.00—which equals .528.

Thus it is clear, given these numbers, that the preferred course of action is to biopsy and treat accordingly.

Where do the numbers used as values come from? How can we justify physicians making life and death decisions on their basis? Answering these questions occupy us for most of this chapter. We need to consider how probabilities can be estimated and how they can be revised in light of new information. We also need to consider how to represent outcomes. And, finally, we need to examine the validity of using decision theory in clinical medicine.

PROBABILITIES FOR DECISIONS

Estimating Probabilities

How can physicians derive the probabilities they need for decision analyses? Those who define probability in terms of relative frequency (see chap. 4) will go with the available statistics. When there are none, they will forego probabilistic approaches to decision making. Our view is that physicians cannot avoid using personal or subjective probabilities. Even when physicians are familiar with good statistical studies, they must tailor them to the case at hand. Thus, suppose that the published figures state that 3 percent of patients die as a result of a kidney biopsy and that there are no specific figures for females in their thirties being biopsied at Dr. Williams's hospital. Since Dr. Williams would surely consider all these factors as relevant, he might be justified in using a number smaller than .03-for instance, the .01 we used above. If he had to perform the procedure under primitive circumstances in a third world country, then he would probably be justified in revising his probability upward.

We cannot condone uninformed or wild probability assignments, even when they satisfy the subjectivist criterion of coherence (see chap. 4). Physicians should seek statistical information to use as a first approximation to the probabilities they assign. Where no statistics are available, they should attempt to arrive at informed judgments by reasoning analogically from statistics concerning similar cases and by drawing upon their experience and that of their colleagues.

Revising Probability Assignments

During the course of diagnosing or treating a patient, clinicians may find good reasons for revising their probability assignments. Consider the case of Mrs. Wu. She has just learned that her breast biopsy is positive for cancer. When she presses her physician about her chances, he tells her that right now she falls within a statistical group whose five-year survival rate is 60 percent. Later, when her lymph node biopsies prove negative, he reassures her by pointing out that she has now moved into the 85 percent survival category.

As we saw in the last chapter, diagnosis and management are cyclical processes that constantly generate new information, leading the clinician to revise probability assignments. How should we model the process of probability revision? The rule most commonly used is conditionalization. It states that when one acquires new evidence E, then one should use Prob (S/E) (the probability of S, given E) rather than Prob (S). More formally,

$$\text{Prob}_n(S) = \text{Prob}_o(S/E),$$

where the subscripts n and o are used to indicate the "new" and "old" probability assignments. These are usually called the posterior and prior probabilities, respectively. We can use the inverse probability law (see chap. 4) to expand the right side of the equation:

$$\text{Prob}_n(S) = \text{Prob}_o(S/E),$$

(In other words, the posterior probability of the state is its prior probability times the probability of the evidence given the state, all divided by the probability of the evidence.) When the probability of the evidence is not known, we can replace the denominator $\text{Prob}_o(E)$ by $(\text{Prob}_o(S) \times \text{Prob}_o(E/S)) + (\text{Prob}_o(\text{not}S) \times \text{Prob}_o(E/\text{not}S))$, which yields the equation

$$\text{Prob}_n(S) = \frac{\text{Prob}_o(S) \times \text{Prob}_o(E/S)}{(\text{Prob}_o(S) \times \text{Prob}_o(E/S)) + (\text{Prob}_o(\text{not}S) \times \text{Prob}_o(E/\text{not}S))},$$

a form of Bayes' theorem.

Consider the situation of a physician who has observed a spot on a chest x-ray. The physician knows the probability of observing such spots, given that the patient has TB; the physician also knows the prevalence of TB and the frequency of spots on chest x-rays. By applying the inverse probability law our physician can calculate the probability that the patient has TB given that there is a spot on the chest x-ray. This is

$$\text{Prob}(TB/S) = [\text{Prob}(TB) \times \text{Prob}(S/TB)]/\text{Prob}(S).$$

Having observed the spot on the chest x-ray, the physician should use the Prob(*TB/S*) as the probability that the patient has TB and should base decisions on it.

Posterior probabilities can also be used as "new priors" in further applications of the inverse probability law. For example, if the physician now tests the patient with a TB skin test and obtains a positive reading, the physician can apply the formula again and use the previously calculated Prob(*TB/S*) as a new prior.

The use of the inverse probability law has been criticized on the grounds that the probabilities used in the denominator are often more difficult to obtain than the probabilities calculated by means of them. Clinicians can be expected to know prior probabilities of diseases (prevalence) or of findings given diseases, since these are often given in textbooks or in published studies. However, statistics on symptoms and other clinical findings per se (e.g., statistics on the prevalence of coughs or fevers) are virtually nonexistent. However, using the "odds-likelihood" form of Bayes' theorem (see Weinstein and Feinberg 1980, 105-8), clinicians can base their deliberations on two kinds of probabilities: (1) the prior probabilities of the diagnoses under consideration, and (2) the probability of the evidence relative to each diagnosis. While these may be quite difficult to ascertain, they represent knowledge that a good physician can be expected to have. The first represents the prevalence of disease in the physician's practice; the second is a measure of the ability of each diagnosis to explain current evidence.

Calculating the Value of Additional Information

It is a commonplace that having more facts on which to base a decision can make a radical difference to our choices. But how can we determine how much those facts are worth? By using Bayes' theorem or the inverse probability law, we can calculate how our probabilities and decisions would change if we had an additional piece of information. We can then determine how much our expected values would change. The change in expected values is the upper bound on the value of that information.

We have already seen a simplified version of this idea at work in our biopsy example. If Dr. William s performs the biopsy, then he will know for certain whether Mrs. Halprin's kidney disease is mild, moderate, or severe. Provided she survives the operation, he will then treat her appropriately. If he does not do the biopsy, then he will proceed with the high-dose therapy, whose expected value is .516. We saw that even when the possibility of operative mortality is included in the reckoning, the expected value of the biopsying is .528. Thus, the value of the information obtained from biopsying is positive (.012).

A convenient way of representing the value of additional information was suggested by S. Pauker and J. Kassirer. They depicted the prior probability of a disorder as a continuum from 0 percent to 100 percent. A test would function at intermediate prior probabilities to confirm the diagnosis if positive or reject it if negative. At the low end of prior probability below the test-no test threshold there is no reason to test because even a positive result would not confirm the diagnosis. Similarly, at the high end of the spectrum—the "test treat" threshold—there is no reason to test since a negative result would not reject the diagnosis.

The basic formula for a threshold is $T = \dfrac{1}{1 + B/C}$, where B is the benefit and C is the cost. For the test threshold this expands to

$$\frac{(P_{pos/nd}) \times R_{rx} + R}{(P_{pos/nd}) \times (R_{rx}) + (P_{pos/d}) \times (B_{rx})},$$

whereas the treatment threshold is

$$\frac{(P_{neg/nd}) \times (R_{rx}) - R_t}{(P_{neg/nd}) \times (R_{rx}) + (P_{neg/d}) \times (B_{rx})}, \text{ where}$$

P = probability;
pos, neg are positive and negative test results;
d, nd are disease and no disease;
B = benefit of treatment or test;
R = risk of treatment or test;
rx = treatment;
t = test.

To illustrate how this works let us reconsider the biopsy question. We confine the question to the dichotomous decision between biopsy with appropriate treatment and low-dose steroids. The risk of high-dose steroids pertains to mild disease, .90 - .95 = -.05; but for moderate and severe disease there is benefit .5 versus .4 and .15 versus .10. Since all three patterns are equally likely, the net benefit is -.05 + .1 + .05 or a total of .1. However, for the threshold equation we keep them separate, that is, the benefit of therapy is .15, whereas the risk of therapy is .05. The risk of the test is .01. The test accuracy we will assume to be 100 percent.

$$\text{Test threshold} = \frac{(0 \times .05) + .01}{(0) \times (.05) + (1.0 \times .15)} \text{ or } \frac{.01}{.15} = 6.67\%.$$

$$\text{Treatment threshold} \frac{(1.0 \times .05) - .01}{(1.0 \times .05) + (0 \times .15)} = \frac{.05 - .01}{.05} = 80\%.$$

Thus if Dr. Williams thinks Clara Halprin's chance of having moderate or severe disease on renal biopsy is between 6.67 percent and 80 percent he should recommend the biopsy. If below that, he should recommend treatment with low-dose steroids and above that treatment with high-dose steroids.

This means of representing the decision to test or treat is convenient and focuses on the value and quality of the information gained by the test as well as on specific benefits and risks.

Dr. Williams could also analyze the decision to perform the lung scan for a possible pulmonary embolus. It is, however, important to realize that the benefits and risks cannot be uniformly applied to all patients. For example, Mrs. Halprin had pericarditis. If indeed she had had a pulmonary embolus on lung scan, her risk of therapy was higher than most people's since she had a greater chance of bleeding into the pericardia] sac, a rare but serious consequence. Specifically, her R_{rx} was higher than many other patients. This would have to be taken into account in the threshold equation.

UTILITY THEORY

There is just one rule for making decisions under risk: choose an act whose expected value is maximal. However, for this rule to make sense, we must be able to assign numerical values to outcomes. So far we have glossed over this problem by representing outcomes in terms of chances of a cure for the patient. But clearly this approach will not work in general.

First of all, in many clinical decisions, getting a cure is not in question at all. Whether or not a postoperative patient is given aspirin or morphine for pain, the chances of healing remain virtually the same. It would make more sense in this case to represent outcomes in terms of measures of the duration or intensity of the patient's pain. Second, it is not clear that quantitative means are always available to clinicians. How should cosmetic surgeons proceed? The intangibility of the outcomes with which they deal (e.g., refined noses, beautiful breasts) would seem to defy numerical representation (although people do pay for them). Third, actions lead to definite outcomes. A patient with SLE such as Mrs. Halprin will either live or die. Thus how can we be justified in making decisions by appealing to expected values or chances of success?

All of these difficulties are addressed by utility theory. This theory explains not only how to measure the value of nonquantitative outcomes, but also how to justify making one-time choices on the basis of expected values. However, the theory comes with a built-in restriction. The theory requires that outcomes be represented on a special type of scale known as a *subjective utility scale.* Before we plunge into the deep waters of this theory, let us take a look at scales in general.

Types of Scales

Scales are simply devices for representing information by means of numbers. There are several different types of scales. The simplest are nominal scales, which merely use numbers as substitute names. Any distinct numbers in any order will suffice, for a nominal scale encodes only the information that there are distinct outcomes. Obviously, nominal scales will not serve as bases for calculating expected values.

An ordinal scale reflects rankings by assigning higher numbers to items that are valued more. Using an ordinal scale in a decision analysis presupposes that we can rank each outcome as "better than," "indifferent to," or "worse than" any other outcome. In our biopsy example, it is clear that a successful treatment would count as the best outcome since it portends the best health for Mrs. Halprin. By contrast, dying as the result to the biopsy is probably the worst outcome. Previously, we have counted a treatment failure as equally bad, but it is probably more realistic to rank this above a postprocedure death and below a successful treatment. Henceforth, let us use this ranking in place of the one used in the section "Individual Decision Making." Then we can

Death	Failure	Success
0	25	100

represent the three outcomes on this ordinal scale.

Since ordinal scales encode only rankings, any change that preserves the order of this scale could serve equally well. For instance:

Death	Failure	Success
−10	250	251

For this reason, ordinal scales are not appropriate for assigning values to outcomes for decisions under risk. Like nominal scales, they encode so little information that an information—preserving change of scale can lead to radically different decisions.

By contrast, *interval scales* do suffice for the purpose of calculating expected values and making decisions under risk. They not only represent rankings, they also represent the relative distance (or intervals) between the items ranked. The Fahrenheit and Celsius temperature scales are interval scales; the relative distances between two pairs of temperatures remain the same in both cases. For example, if 122°F is replaced by 50°C, the temperature remains one-half the distance between the boiling and freezing points of water.

Interval scales may be transformed by means of *positive linear transformations* without destroying the information they represent. A transformation of a scale s to a scale s' is a positive linear transformation, just in case s and s' are related by an equation of the form

$$s' = as + b.$$

where a and b are real numbers and $a > 0$.

It can be shown that the relative ordering of expected values remains constant when a scale used is subjected to a positive linear transformation. Thus interval scales are appropriate for making decisions under risk.

For completeness, we should mention ratio scales. These represent the ratio a given quantity bears to a given unit of that quantity. Our familiar scales for measuring lengths (feet, meters), weights (pounds, grams), and speeds (MPH, KPH) are ratio scales. Ratio scales permit transformations that satisfy equations of the form

$$s' = as,$$

where a is a positive real number.

The four types of scales mentioned have been given in order of increasing precision. Moreover, every ratio scale is also an interval scale, and every interval scale is also an ordinal scale. Obviously, the converse relationships do not hold.

Interval Utility Scales: Some First Approximations

Many applications of decision theory in medicine and business use some generally recognized values to approximate interval scales for representing outcomes. We have already used cure rates. Survival rates are a popular variant on this system for assigning values, but monetary values are used just as frequently. In this case one chooses an act that maximizes expected monetary values (EMVs) instead of maximizing cure rates. For example, in deciding whether to administer a vaccine to the general populace of a country, government health officials might assign values to possible epidemics by estimating their effect upon the nation's GNP. This, together with the costs of administering the vaccine, could be used to calculate EMVs for the various options. Cost-benefit analysis, in which one evaluates options by subtracting expected costs from expected benefits, is a variant on the EMV approach.

The practical advantages of EMVs and cure or survival rates are that they are familiar and relatively easy to measure or estimate. However, it is plain that in most decisions, money or a cure is not the only factor at stake. Studies have shown that patients are concerned not only with their chances for surviving, but also with the quality of life they can be expected to lead. They are also concerned with the shape of the survival curve: one that remains high for five years and then drops will usually be preferred to one that drops precipitously at first and then levels off, even if the five-year survival rates are the same for both curves. Furthermore, as we have already mentioned, many medical decisions (such as performing some cosmetic surgery or prescribing a drug for a bad cold) should not be evaluated in terms of cure or survival rates. The same holds for EMVs, since it is difficult, if not impossible, to assign monetary values to such outcomes as restored sight, years of crippling pain, or a disfiguring postoperative scar.

Of course, the courts often do assign monetary values to some of these outcomes, and economists and management scientists have attempted to develop other indexes for valuing "intangible" factors. Thus, in place of survival rates we could use expected "quality-adjusted life years," an index in which the length of a life is inflated or discounted by its quality. To deal with quickly dropping survival curves, we can use a discounting factor that assigns a greater weight to the earlier years of the survival period than to the later ones. Willingness to pay and expected lifetime earnings are sometimes used in legal and insurance situations.

But there are obvious problems with these devices. How do we measure the quality of a life? What discount factor should we use? Should we use a different one for young patients than for old ones? Furthermore, the scope of these devices is limited. If a patient is concerned with having a knee injury repaired so that he or she can run a marathon next month, then using quality-adjusted life years or discounting to evaluate the outcomes may be beside the point.

Von Neumann-Morgenstern Utility Theory

The version of subjective utility theory that we present is due to the mathematician J. von Neumann and the economist 0. Morgenstern. They had two fundamental insights. The first was that choosing an act in a decision under risk is in effect choosing to gamble. The second was that the value persons place on a given item will be reflected in the risks (gambles) they are willing to take to obtain it. Using these two insights von Neumann and Morgenstern showed how to evaluate both outcomes and options in terms of gambles.

A humdrum example illustrates how the idea works. Suppose we prefer going to a football game to going to the movies to staying at home. This orders our preferences for these three outcomes from best to worst; they can be represented on an ordinal scale. We rank going to the movies somewhere between going to the football game and staying at home. But exactly where? Do we like the movies almost as much as the football game? Or just a little more than staying at home? Well, suppose we had a ticket in hand for the movies, and someone offered to exchange it for a bunch of tickets in a lottery (to be paid off immediately), which would permit us to go to the football game if we won but would require us to stay at home if we lost. What must the chance of winning be for us to be willing to trade the ticket to the movies for the lottery tickets? If we say 75 percent then the movie ranks at the three-quarter point in the "interval" between staying at home and going to the game. If we say 50 percent then it ranks at the midpoint, and so on. This is where the bet in the lottery ranks too, since we are indifferent between it and going to the movies.

Let us suppose that we rank the movies and the bet at the three-quarter point. Then if, using a popular convention, we assign the value Ito our best option and the value 0 to our worst, then the movies and the bet should both be assigned the value 3/4. By considering further bets, we can even find the midpoint, the one-quarter point, and the seven-eighths point on our scale. These correspond to bets that give us, respectively, a 50, 25, and an 87.5 percent chance of going to the football game and a 50, 75, and 12.5 percent chance of being forced to remain at home. Other points on the scale can be associated with gambles in this way too. If a new item comes under consideration, say, going to a play, we can measure it on the scale by comparing it with various gambles until we find one for which we would trade the new item. (This assumes that the introduction of the new item does not affect the preferences by which we have generated the scale.) The scale thus established is a *subjective utility scale* for the items scaled. It is an interval scale and the information it represents—the order and the intensity of our preferences—will remain unaffected by positive linear transformations of our scale.

Let us use this idea in the case of the biopsy decision. First, we must identify the options with gambles. Bypassing the biopsy and using the high dose is one possibility, a gamble that consists in certain chances (.516) of the successful treatment of Mrs. Halprin and certain chances of failing (1.0 - .516 or .484). These are determined by the chances that her kidney disease is mild, moderate or severe. Bypassing the biopsy and using the low dose is a similar gamble associated with different chances of success (.483) and failure (.517). However, the biopsy option turns out to be the simple gamble that gives the physician a .01 chance of having the patient die, a .528 of a success and a .472 chance of failure.

Once Dr. Williams recasts all the relevant outcomes in terms of gambles, he can use these to assess his options and finally to choose the one he has ranked highest. In so doing he maximizes his (subjective) expected utility. We have already assumed that he prefers a successful treatment to an unsuccessful one and that in turn to a surgical fatality. Let us set the first outcome at 1 and the last at 0. Let us further suppose that we are indifferent between having the treatment fail for certain and a gamble that gives it a 10 percent chance at success and a 90 percent chance of Mrs. Halprin's dying from the surgery. Then the utilities for the three outcomes are 1, .1, and 0, and the expected utilities for the three options are

Biopsy, then treat: $.01(0) + .528(1) + .472(.1) = .5752$.
High dose without biopsy: $.516(1) + .484(.1) = .5644$.
Low dose without biopsy: $.483(1) + .517(.1) = .5347$.

Thus, given these preferences, we should biopsy.

However, suppose that Dr. Williams regards the potential surgical loss as a relatively bad outcome-so bad that he is indifferent between a treatment failure and a gamble that gives him a 90 percent chance of success and only a 10 percent chance at a surgical loss. In other words, success and failure are both close to the top of his utility scale and the surgical loss is at the bottom .Then the expected utilities are

Biopsy, then treat: $.01(0) + .528(1) = .472(.9) = .9528$.
High dose without biopsy: $.561(1) + .484(.9) = .9966$.
Low Dose without biopsy: $.483(1) + .517(.9) = .9483$.

In this case Dr. Williams should forego the biopsy and use the high-dose therapy.

We turned to utility theory because it promised to solve two major problems that confronted more familiar measures of value. It promised to be universally applicable and to explain how one can be justified in making one-time decisions. You should now begin to understand why, at least in principle, utility theory can be applied to any set of outcomes. To calibrate the outcomes on a subjective utility scale, a decision maker need only follow the procedure we illustrated above and *ordinally rank* both the outcomes in question and gambles among them. The surprising thing is that an ordinal ranking of this kind produces an interval scale.

Explaining why utility solves the second problem is more complicated. Given his first set of hypothetical preferences, why should Dr. Williams do the biopsy? It has a higher expected utility than the other options. But why should that matter?

There is a tempting answer that will not work. One might point out that if Dr. Williams performed a biopsy on many patients like Mrs. Halprin, he would, on the average, have better results than he would were he not to biopsy. This point would be relevant if Dr. Williams had been trying to develop a general policy for dealing with SLE patients-one that he expected to apply to many patients. But Dr. Williams may well have made a one-time decision here, and certainly many clinical decisions are one time or relatively rarely made. So the answer in terms of average results will not do; there may be too few cases to average.

The answer is found in recalling that we have identified Dr. Williams's options with gambles, and they are gambles whose "payoffs" are the various outcomes associated with his decision. Dr. Williams's utility scale is so constructed that one item is given a higher utility number than another if and only if Dr. Williams prefers the former to the latter. In short, Dr. Williams should biopsy because that is what he prefers to do. More generally, in maximizing expected utilities, a decision maker is only doing what he or she prefers to do. For all this to work, Dr. Williams must be able to rank all the outcomes and gambles associated with them. If he did not satisfy this *ordering condition*, the process of constructing a utility scale for him would soon break down. Furthermore, he also must subject his ranking to certain other conditions. He must be indifferent between a compound gamble and one that is probabilistically equivalent to it. This constraint, called the *reduction of compound gambles condition*, was used when we reduced the biopsy option to a simple gamble. Without it the expected utility of a gamble need not equal its utility. Also given any three outcomes or gambles A. B, and C, which Dr. Williams ranks in that order, he must be indifferent between B and some gamble with A and C as payoffs. This *continuity* condition played a crucial (but implicit) role in generating Dr. Williams's utility scale. Additionally, if Dr. Williams prefers some outcome or gamble A to another one B, then he must prefer a gamble with just A and B as outcomes to another one if and only if the first gamble gives him a better chance at A. Without this *better chances* condition his preferences need not match the risks he is willing to take. For the same reason, Dr. Williams must abide by a final condition, the *better prizes* condition. This states that if there are two gambles, the first of which gives Dr. Williams a certain chance at A and C, while the second gives him the same chance at B and C, then he must prefer the first to the second if and only if he prefers A to B.

Von Neumann and Morgenstern proved that, provided an agent satisfies these five conditions, preferences for outcomes and gambles can be represented on an interval scale. On this scale the utility of a gamble will equal its expected utility. Finally, any other utility scale constructed from the same data will be a positive linear transformation of the first. The von Neumann-Morgenstern expected utility theorem, as it is called, thus provided the theoretical underpinnings for the use of subjective utility scales in decision theory.

Some Common Misconceptions about Subjective Utility Scales

Suppose an agent assigns a utility of 2 to having a dish of ice cream. Can we conclude that the agent will assign a utility of 4 to having two dishes? No, utility is not an additive quantity; that is, there is no general way of combining prizes, with the result that the utility of the combination equals the sum of the utilities of the components. As a result, it does not make sense to add, subtract, multiply, or divide utilities. In particular, we have no license to conclude that two dishes of ice cream will be worth twice the utility of one to our agent. If eating the second dish would violate the agent's diet, then having two dishes might be worth even less than having one.

It would also be fallacious to conclude, for example, that something assigned a utility of 2 on a given scale is twice as preferable to something assigned 1 on the same scale. For suppose that the original scale is a 1-to-10 scale. If we transform it to a 1-to-91 scale by the permissible transformation of multiplying every number by 10 and then subtracting 9, then the item originally assigned I will continue to be assigned 1 but the one assigned 2 will be assigned 11. Thus its being assigned twice the utility on the first scale is simply an artifact of the scale and not a scale-invariant property of the agent's preferences.

Finally, remember that we are dealing with *subjective* utility scales and not with some intersubjective measure of value. Dr. Williams and Mrs. Halprin had conflicting preferences concerning dialysis. He was prepared to put her on it, she wanted no part of it. Thus on his scale it ranked higher than her death; on her scale the ranking was reversed. So we cannot conclude that she assigned it a utility greater than zero just because Dr. Williams did. Furthermore, even when two people have the same ordinal rankings for outcomes, it does not follow that they assign each the same utility. Mrs. Halprin could have preferred dialysis just a bit more than dying, while Dr. Williams preferred to put her on dialysis quite a bit more than having her die. Finally, even when two people assign the same numbers to the same items, it does not follow that their preference intensities are identical. Although the most preferred thing for one may be the most preferred for the other, one may have a very wide range of preference and the other a very narrow range. The problem of interpersonal comparisons of utility scales is one of the major difficulties confronting the use of utility theory in the analysis of group decisions.

Can We Make Utility Theory Work?

Decision theory is beset with practical difficulties that raise questions about its usefulness for clinical purposes. Let us take a look at some of them and at how decision analysts are attempting to cope with them.

In a complicated decision, such as the choice of therapies for a serious illness, decision makers may be unsure of what some of their preferences are. They may know the best outcome, but may be unable to rank some of the middle or worse ones. In short, they may not even be able to set up an ordinal ranking. If so, they cannot even begin to construct a utility scale. Furthermore, people often resist the idea of trading gambles involving extreme payoffs for the certainty of an intermediate one. This is likely to happen when a patient whose condition is currently stable is faced with the choice of a procedure that carries a risk of death. This is why most patients resist kidney biopsy. Similarly, because there is a chance of dying under a general anesthesia, a patient with a reducible hernia may be unable to fix the exact chances of a successful repair that is needed to make him indifferent between having the procedure and living with his current condition. Yet utility theory requires the patient to do so.

One thing a decision analyst can do for a patient who is having difficulty refining personal preferences enough for utility theory to apply is to obtain as many definite preferences as possible and construct the rest of the preference structure by extrapolation and curve fitting. By questioning the patient, a decision analyst can decide whether this structure is appropriate for the decision at hand or needs further modification. After some interchange, the analyst may have arrived at an approximation that is good enough for the decision at hand. (Sensitivity analysis may be useful here. See "The Role of Decision Analysis" below.)

Another technique open to the decision analyst is to turn to multidimensional utility scales. Instead of assigning a single number to each outcome, these scales assign lists of numbers to each outcome, where each number on the list is a value on a more easily applicable scale. For instance, in deciding whether to have dialysis or a kidney transplant, a patient has many factors to consider: the risk of death, the time lost during hospitalization and treatment, the discomfort of vascular access, the risk of complications, the nature of the complications, and so on. Because of this, patients may be unable to fix their preferences with enough accuracy to support an ordinary utility scale. By contrast, the decision analyst may find that patients are able to rank each factor associated with an outcome against the corresponding factors associated with other outcomes. Other things being equal, the patient prefers more life to less, less pain to more, less time in the hospital to more, fewer complications to more, more mobility to less, and so on. In this way the decision analyst may be able to construct one utility scale for measuring risks of death, another for measuring risks of pain, another for measuring the inconvenience of hospitalization, and so on. Using these separate scales the decision analyst can assign a vector (list) of utility numbers to each outcome and then attempt to order outcomes in terms of the vectors.

If so, the decision analyst's problem is how to order the vectors, that is, how to combine the values on the various dimensions in order to arrive at an overall ranking of the options. Suppose, for instance, that on a two-dimensional scale of risk of death and pain, a patient associates having coronary artery bypass surgery with the vector (5,10) and not having it with (10,5). Then we know that the patient prefers less risk to more and less pain to more, but how can we decide between the two treatments?

Sometimes the decision is easy. If the vectors had been (5,10) and (5,5), respectively, then we could confidently choose the bypass surgery. For the patient is indifferent between the two actions on the first dimension and prefers the bypass on the second. This illustrates a more general principle: if one act is at least as good as another on all dimensions and better on some, then it should be preferred to the other. (This is a variation on the dominance theme.)

Furthermore, if the decision analyst can get the decision maker to establish a priority ranking of the dimensions, then the acts can be easily ordered in terms of their vectors: acts are first ordered by the value assigned to the most important dimension of their utilities on the dimension given the highest priority; ties are broken by going to the dimension given next highest priority, remaining ties by going to the dimension next in priority, and so on. Suppose, for example, that the dimensions used are (in order of priority) risk of death, pain, and cost, and that the patient prefers to minimize each. Then less risky options are preferred to more risky ones, no matter what the pain or cost; of two equally risky options, the less painful is preferred; of two equally risky and painful options, the least costly is preferred.

Some studies show that once the options have been analyzed into a number of factors, patients try to use the lexical approach to ordering illustrated in the last paragraph. But there are certainly many situations in which decision makers are willing to concede on one dimension in order to gain on another for example, to chance death in order to gain relief from pain. Thus, the lexical approach is not always the solution. Currently, there is no consensus concerning how to proceed in such cases.

DECISIONS UNDER IGNORANCE

Physicians are used to estimating probabilities—such as the chances of a favorable outcome or of a positive test result—and they are uncomfortable with situations where they cannot estimate them. Yet there are circumstances where they simply must make a choice and they find that they cannot justify introducing even a range of probabilities. On the night that Mrs. Halprin was first admitted to the hospital Dr. Barton had only vague hunches concerning the nature of her illness-lupus had not even occurred to her as a hypothesis, and she certainly could not confidently assign probabilities to the various diagnostic hypotheses she entertained. Decision theorists have proposed a theory of decision making under ignorance for dealing with predicaments like hers.

An agent's decision is made under ignorance (or ambiguity) when the agent is not warranted to assign probabilities to each of the states. Several methods have been proposed for handling such decisions, and they vary according to the demands they place upon the agent's ability to rank the outcomes involved as the decision. At the very least, however, they all require the agent to generate an ordinal value scale. That means that each outcome must be ranked as better, indifferent, or worse than any other outcome. We have already observed that even this may be a difficult task for some patients or physicians.

The Maximin Rule

There is a simple and intuitively appealing rule for making decisions under ignorance for which an ordinal scale suffices. Applying this rule will avoid many of the difficulties we discussed in connection with interval utility scales. The rule is called the *maximin* rule because it enjoins us to pick an act whose minimum outcome value is maximal among the minimums. More precisely, to apply the rule, we list the minimum values for each act and then pick an act having the greatest value on the list. The rule embodies the assumption that the worst will happen, no matter what the true state, and that the decision maker should pick the least of the evils.

If Dr. Williams does the biopsy then the worst outcome possible is that Mrs. Halprin dies, whereas if he bypasses the biopsy and uses either the high- or low- dose treatments then the worst outcome is that his treatment fails. We have already stipulated that Dr. Williams ranks the latter two outcomes above the first; so if he used the maximin rule to make the biopsy decision, he would be free to flip a coin to choose either treatment.

The maximin rule is clearly not very useful in dealing with Dr. Williams's biopsy decision since probabilities can be estimated. However, it can be useful in dealing with medical decisions in which the paramount concern of the physician is bypassing a serious illness. Earlier in Mrs. Halprin's case Drs. Barton and Williams considered a number of diagnostic possibilities—some quite rare—and ordered a number of tests with a high degree of specificity in order to rule out those possibilities. But to take a more readily formalized example, suppose a physician suspects that a patient has an uncomplicated cough but admits tuberculosis as a diagnostic possibility. The physician's decision to order a skin test for TB can be analyzed as a simple two-act, two-state decision in which the worst that can happen if the test is ordered is that the patient may be unnecessarily alarmed and inconvenienced by a false positive, whereas if the physician does not order the test then the worst that can happen is that the patient is actually seriously ill with TB. The maximin rule supports the conservative decision to order the test.

Using the maximin rule clearly violates the assumption of maximizing expected utility, which is the defining principle of rational decision making. The same decision, cast in terms of risk, can lead to a different conclusion. Does this mean that we have more than one form of decision making? We do, in the sense that we should use the rule that best suits the situation, but we do not, in the sense that the rules do not necessarily conflict. If Dr. Williams has a good idea about the probabilities of the outcomes, he should use the rule of maximizing expected utility. If he does not, he should use a rule of decision making under ignorance. In an analogous case, he would be foolish to use expected utility as a basis for decision making if he were omniscient and knew the outcome of his actions ahead of time. There is a hierarchy of decision making from certainty to ignorance, and the decision maker is obliged to use the rule appropriate to his or her state of knowledge about the chances of the outcomes.

There are other rules under ignorance, and there are many arguments and counterarguments attacking and defending each rule. It seems to us that different rules are appropriate for different circumstances. We already mentioned that the maximin rule seems appropriate when a physician is very concerned about missing a serious illness. We think there is too much controversy surrounding these rules and too little known about their clinical applicability to recommend any of them at this time.

VALIDATING A DECISION ANALYSIS

The past few sections have focused on difficulties that arise in applying decision theory and some proposals for dealing with them. These difficulties make the question of how we can validate a decision analysis all the more pressing. This section attempts to begin to answer that question.

Right Decisions versus Rational Decisions

Let us call a decision *right* if the outcome it produces is one that the decision maker prefers to the other possibilities. Furthermore, let us call a decision *rational* if it was the best decision the decision maker could make using the values and information available at that time. Poorly made, nonrational decisions can turn out to be right, for good luck can intervene. By the same token, well-made, rational decisions can fail to be right. Bad luck can wreck the most careful plans.

There is no way we can guarantee that every rational decision will be right. However, it could be argued that, on the average, rational decisions are right, while nonrational ones are not. This is a plausible consequence of the rule of maximizing expected utility. But rather than delve into the deep philosophical question of whether it is better to be rational, let us assume that it is. The question that now arises is: How can we be sure that our decisions are rational? Answering it calls for another distinction.

Soundness versus Validity

In logic a valid deduction from premises that are true is called a sound argument. The argument establishes categorically that its conclusion is true. Every sound deduction is valid, but not every valid deduction is sound. Some valid arguments are based upon one or more false premises. Consequently, they establish their conclusions only hypothetically. They show that if all the premises were true, then so would be the conclusion. (See chap. 5.)

By analogy with deduction, we can usefully distinguish decisions that are merely valid from those that are sound as well. Let us call a decision *valid* if it results from correctly applying one of the rules of decision theory. (For the purposes of this discussion we will assume that there are no disputes about what these rules ought to be.) Let us call a decision *sound* if it is valid and based upon an appropriate set of actions, states, probabilities, and utilities. Finally, let us identify rational decisions with sound ones.

Assuming that we have not made some arithmetical error, Dr. Williams's decision to biopsy was a valid one. It resulted from correctly applying the rule of maximizing expected utility to the decision problem we have formulated. To check the decision for validity, we need only verify that our calculations are correct and that biopsying is an act whose expected utility is maximal. This is the sort of task that can be left to a computer and for which computer programs currently exist.

Checking for Soundness

Checking to see whether a valid decision is also sound is quite another matter. There are many ways in which a valid decision can fail to be sound: it might use the wrong probabilities or utilities, it might be based upon some irrelevant states (such as using the state of the weather in a biopsy decision), or it might omit a critical state, it might consider some inappropriate options, or it might omit an important one. All of these errors can and do arise in clinical practice.

How then can we determine whether the inputs for the calculations are appropriate? Since these are determined to a large degree by the terms in which the decision is cast—that is, by the acts, states, and outcomes used—this is where we must start. Consider the biopsy decision again. Dr. Williams might have gone astray by limiting himself to just three options. Perhaps Mrs. Halprin would do better if she were given the high dose for one week, the low dose the next, and the high dose the week after. But Dr. Williams never considered this option. Nor did he consider the option of not treating Mrs. Halprin at all. Furthermore, in our analysis we have not distinguished a failed low-dose therapy from a failed high-dose therapy. Possibly this is a dangerous oversimplification. For if the low-dose therapy fails, then Dr. Williams can follow it with the high-dose therapy, but if the high-dose therapy fails he has no alternate treatment. Moreover, our choice of states might be inappropriate. Perhaps there is another possibility. For instance, instead of dying from the biopsy Mrs. Halprin might develop a condition for which the two therapies are contraindicated (such as an infection).

There is no way we can prove that Dr. Williams considered exactly the right acts, states and outcomes. (It is not even clear whether such talk can be given any precise sense.) But we could check our set of acts, states, and outcomes against a previously drawn checklist (if there were one) in order to see whether we had omitted something crucial or included something inappropriate.

To be sure, this check would be no better than the checklist. However, checklists can be composed at one's leisure and amended as new alternatives are discovered. They can also be computerized when they can no longer be conveniently committed to memory or to one's pocket notebook. Finally, it would be possible for groups of experts in the various areas of clinical medicine to compose checklists for a variety of clinical decision making contexts.

Turning next to the probabilities that go into a decision analysis, clinical decision makers can check these by consulting other physicians and medical statisticians. They can also check whatever computations they used in calculating probabilities from other probabilities or statistical data basis. But again there can be no guarantee that a given decision is based upon an appropriate set of probabilities.

The same holds for the utilities, for it is always possible that the decision analyst has misrepresented the preferences of the decision maker—even when the decision maker and the analyst are one and the same person. In the first place, the clinical decision maker, typically the attending physician, may be trying to make the decision on the basis of the patient's preferences. For instance, although Dr. Williams did not find the prospect of dialysis as terrible as Mrs. Halprin did, he might have felt obliged to respect her preferences by assigning dialysis a utility that was very low in comparison to those given to other outcomes. Furthermore, even when decision makers are not attempting to incorporate someone else's values, they may fail to know their true preferences. Even then a decision analysis can be a useful tool in revealing a decision maker's true preferences. If a valid decision and otherwise sound analysis leads to a choice that is unacceptable to a decision maker, then there must be something wrong with the preference ordering on which it is based. The repugnant choice is a signal for the decision maker to reconsider his or her preferences. There are many sources of error in preference assessment. Some of the better-known problems include different preferences depending on the questions asked—framing effects—or preference reversals by individuals, but there are also deeper issues than these. Some individuals do not seem to have a coherent preference structure for a given set of alternatives. If this is the case or if the result of an analysis seems to be genuinely counterintuitive, there are no fully accepted methods of resolving the problems.

Sensitivity Analysis

Often decision analysts cannot fix exact probabilities or utilities, or be certain that a given state can be excluded or that two outcomes can be safely collapsed into one. This is where sensitivity analysis can prove useful. It is most easily explained in terms of probabilities or utilities, but it applies to the other elements of a decision analysis as well. To illustrate the technique, let us suppose that in our role as decision analysts we are confident that the probability of Mrs. Halprin's dying from the biopsy is somewhere between 0 and .01, but we cannot fix an exact number. Then we can run the calculations for the biopsy decision using these two extreme values and see whether there is any difference in our recommendation. We have already done the calculations using the value of .01, and they resulted in recommending the biopsy. If we use the value 0 in place of .01, then instead of assigning .33 to the possibility of Dr. Williams's learning that Mrs. Halprin's kidney disease is mild we assign 1/3 (and similarly for the other two possibilities.) As one might expect, this raises the expected utility of biopsying (from .5752 to .5796). Thus the decision to biopsy is not sensitive to changes in the probability assigned to Mrs. Halprin's dying so long as they are within the range cited.

We can actually do better than this. Using algebra we could determine how high the probability of Mrs. Halprin's dying can get before biopsying is no longer recommended. If we found that we are not confident that the true probability falls within this range, then we could postpone the decision until we have a firmer grasp of the true probability. Or if we thought that the decision is too sensitive to inaccuracies in our data, we could recommend that Dr. Williams consider an entirely different set of management plans. Sensitivity analysis of utilities proceeds similarly, and we saw in the section "Utility Theory" that if Dr. Williams assigns a utility of .9 to a treatment failure, the biopsy is not recommended. Thus, the decision to biopsy is sensitive to changing the utility in question from .1 to .9. Again, we can locate the range within which it remains insensitive and decide whether we are confident that the true utility falls within that range.

To see whether a decision may be sensitive to different sets of options, states, or outcomes, we must construct alternative analyses of the decision-from the decision tree on up-and then see whether the same act is recommended by each analysis. Suppose, for instance, that we decide that we need to include (as an additional state) the possibility that Mrs. Halprin does not die from the biopsy but develops an infection for which the steroid therapies are both contraindicated .We would need to put a new branch in the decision tree, emanating from the circle in the biopsy branch, to represent the new state. Ife assign this outcome a very low probability and a utility of 0, then the utility of biopsying will still remain higher than not doing so. Under these assumptions, the decision to biopsy is not sensitive to the addition of the extra state.

Some of the tasks of sensitivity analysis are simply a matter of finding break-even points and thus can be relegated to a computer. However, many, such as recasting the analysis from the ground up, demand imagination, patience, and time. Of course, even the initial decision analysis demands these too. This once again raises the question of the role decision analysis can actually play in medicine—our next topic.

THE ROLE OF DECISION ANALYSIS

Our discussion of the application of decision theory in medicine has revealed a number of serious obstacles. Decision theorists have long been familiar with these and several others. One of these is that experiments have repeatedly shown that, in their day-to-day decision making, people do not reason according to the models of decision theory. Apparently, people do not estimate probabilities well. They tend to crowd them into the middle, deflating high numbers and inflating low ones. Furthermore, they fail to keep their estimates fixed from one time to the next, and do not keep their probability assignments independent of their preferences. (For instance, they assign unrealistically high or low probabilities to outcomes that they desire or fear.) Cognitive psychologists have identified numerous biases that affect peoples' ability to estimate probability. The most well-known of these is framing bias where the context may determine the probability estimate given. Usually individuals will inflate desirable event probabilities and deflate objectionable ones. Treatments that save two-thirds of patients are preferred to alternative therapies that lead to one-third mortality. However, there are other biases and there is no doubt that people are not entirely rational when estimating probabilities.

On the utility side, people often pick an option that is good enough without bothering to develop even an ordinal ranking of the prospects open to them. In Herbert Simon's terms, they satisfice rather than maximize. If the applicability of decision theory is limited and it fails as a realistic description of how people actually make choices, then what role can it play?

Some decision theorists have answered this question by proposing modified versions of decision theory that purport to be more realistic. However, this does not address the problem of applications. The majority of decision theorists have taken an opposite position. They claim that the theory is best viewed as prescriptive. The theory is not supposed to tell us how decisions are actually made, rather it is supposed to tell us how they should be made or how an ideally rational agent would make them. On this view, decision analysis is a mathematically precise tool with rigorous foundation, whose use will undoubtedly improve the quality of our decisions. The major drawback to this proposal is that, since computational complexities or poor probability or utility estimates often prevent us from applying decision theory, it appears to be offering us an ideal that is impossible to realize.

This drawback leads to the more moderate view that we should try to emulate decision theory where it is practicable. Most people do not hold a totally consistent set of beliefs, but that does not mean we should refrain from calling inconsistent beliefs to a person's attention. Indeed, by doing so we help people improve the quality of their thought. Similarly, even trying to use decision theory usually illuminates a decision problem. Being forced to come to grips with the components of an important decision requires us to address its critical aspects. Just enumerating options is often revealing, and particularly helpful if done as a group project. (In Mrs. Halprin's case it might have led her doctors to treat the infection that eventually killed her.) Identifying the important aspects of outcomes is further enlightening, and trying to assign probabilities to states often reveals a striking lack of data to support one's contentions. Thus learning that we are not in a position to apply the theory can be useful in and of itself. At the very least, decision analysis forces us to consider issues and options we might easily overlook or ignore. It keeps us honest and makes us perspicuous.

In our opinion, each approach embodies part of the truth. There is no denying that trying to apply decision analysis is a good thing. Furthermore, it can function as a useful tool for teaching novice decision makers. But we are willing to go further than that. Decision theory, in our view, is an appropriate nonnative ideal. It states the degree of perfection that we ought to strive for when perfection is both required and possible. Finally, there are situations that may be usefully described by decision-theoretic models. Such descriptions will be idealized, but this may be just what gives them their explanatory power, just as the gas laws gain their power from idealization.

GROUP DECISION MAKING

As in Mrs. Halprin's case, many people have a say in an important clinical decision. Not only the patient and the family, whose stake is obvious, and the attending physician, who must carry out and assume responsibility for the decision, but also hospital personnel and administrators, whose policies or politics may be affected by the decision, may participate in making a major clinical decision. Emergency situations in which clinicians find themselves isolated and forced to decide then and there are relatively rare. Thus we must address the question of how a number of interested parties with possible conflicting values and professional judgments can arrive at a rational and equitable plan for the management of a patient.

There is little consensus among experts on group decision making about the proper analytic framework to use in group decision making or the proper rule to use within a given framework. Thus, our approach breaks new ground. We propose a framework for formulating group decisions in medical contexts and suggest how a group choice might be achieved.

The Goal: The Amalgamation of Differing Points of View

Let us place ourselves in the context of the decision to dialyze Mrs. Halprin at the time she was semicomatose. When fully conscious, she was vehemently opposed to the procedure, but her family strongly favored it after she became semicomatose. Her physicians were not certain whether her coma was due to uremia alone or to central nervous system lupus. If the coma was due to uremia alone, the dialysis would restore her to consciousness; if not, she might well remain in the coma indefinitely. This decision cannot be given a simple analysis in terms of expected utility, because no single person's values or probability judgments can be used in the analysis, while excluding those of the other parties to the decision. At the very least, the values of Mrs. Halprin and members of her family must be incorporated, and the conflicting probability judgments of her physicians must be balanced against each other. Even if a single individual is ultimately responsible for the decision, this decision maker will try to amalgamate the inputs from the others and is obviously obliged to try to do so. Thus, we take the amalgamation problem to be the fundamental problem of clinical group decisions.

The problem could be approached as one of combining individual decisions into a single decision. If we used majority rule, for example, then we would decide to dialyze Mrs. Halprin, since more parties to the decision favor it than oppose it. However, the use of majority rule is objectionable, because the outcomes do not affect a large group and involve Mrs. Halprin quite specifically and personally. But any method of combining decisions after they have been made on an individual basis is inadvisable. These bypass the utilities and probabilities that went into the separate decisions. We lose information. The patient's values, in most instances, should count for more than those of the physicians, and the opposite should hold for probability judgments. Thus, to retain this information we shall split the amalgamation problem into two sub-problems: (1) the problem of combining the values of the parties, and (2) the problem of combining their probability judgments.

Firms or Republics?

In approaching problems of social choice, two pictures of decision-making groups are prominent in the literature. One of these is appropriate to groups such as baseball teams, university departments, corporations, and armies, in which the group has an overarching interest that it promotes and to which interests of its members may be sacrificed. For example, a professional baseball club has winning teams as its goal. To achieve that goal, it may release individual players, however distasteful that may be to the players discarded or to their friends on the team. It may be that, from a purely personal point of view, no one wants to see a teammate go, but all the same everyone readily acknowledges that their friend is a poor ballplayer. With firms, the main problem is arriving at decisions that are rational in terms of the firm's overarching interest. The other picture of decision-making groups is more appropriate to groups acting politically, such as a town meeting to decide on zoning regulations, a professional association meeting to decide whether to take a side on a political issue, or a labor union meeting to decide how to set the wage scale for the various categories of membership. These groups are concerned either with adjudicating or resolving the possible conflicting interests of their members or with distributing a scarce resource among their members. We will call such groups republics. Group decision methods such as voting, bargaining, and arbitration by a disinterested party have been proposed as suitable for decision making by republics. Here the main problem is that of arriving at fair, just, or equitable decisions.

Most group decisions in medicine involve determining the best thing to do for the health or well-being of a patient or a class of patients. This is certainly true of clinical decisions generally and of the dialysis decision for Mrs. Halprin in particular. Thus, groups concerned with clinical decisions function as firms. Furthermore, decisions by firms may be appropriately treated as a kind of individual decision. Just as individuals choose so as to promote their interests, a firm chooses the option it believes maximizes its interests. Of course, this presupposes that the members of the firm have an understanding of what the firm's interests are and how they are best maximized. In terms of individual decision theory, this means that both a utility scale and a probability measure for the firm must be determined. Because republics have no overarching interests, this would be inappropriate for groups functioning as republics, but it is neither unrealistic nor irrational for firms.

The problem of group decision making in the clinical context thus reduces to amalgamating the probabilities and utilities of its members into group probability and utility assignments.

A Proposal for Amalgamation

Each participant in a clinical decision has his or her own area of authority. Physicians are authorities concerning diagnosis, prognosis, and the effectiveness of various treatments. In most instances, the patient's knowledge of this area is minimal. Patients, by contrast, are authorities concerning their personal tastes and values, their ability to tolerate given treatments, and their willingness to accept certain outcomes. In deciding whether to treat a cancerous breast by radiation or surgery, the patient must certainly be given a large say.

These considerations suggest the following initial approach to group clinical decision making: In a simple two-person (one-physician, one-patient) case, the patient supplies the utility function and the physician supplies the probabilities. The decision is then made by calculating the resulting expected utilities.

If several physicians are involved and their probability estimates do not agree, then the following approach seems reasonable. First, carry out decision analyses using the different probabilities; if all lead to the same decision the matter is settled. This is another application of sensitivity analysis. Second, if and only if the sensitivity analysis does not endorse one decision, then average the probabilities, assigning greater weights to the more experienced and expert physicians in the group, and use the resulting probabilities to calculate expected utilities.

The same approach can be applied when there are several parties to the decision whose values are relevant and possibly conflicting. Mrs. Halprin's case is a good example. She was opposed to dialysis, but her family, which had some voice in the decision, wanted it. Parents of children furnish numerous examples. If, for instance, a child shows signs of seizure activity, one parent may favor aggressive treatment with drugs (and be willing to risk the side effects), the other may be willing to wait and see whether the signs go away on their own (and risk the child being injured as a result of seizing). Using weights can give each parent a say. Indeed by assigning each party some positive weight, one could permit every party to the decision to have some say concerning both probabilities and utilities.

The averaging model we are proposing is rudimentary and leaves many questions unresolved. It could be refined by using a multidimensional analysis that would not only permit a more detailed analysis of the decision itself, but would also permit one to vary over different dimensions the weights given to the opinions and values of the various parties. The patient's utilities could be given the bulk of the weight on such dimensions as pain and disfigurement, while the utilities of the family members could be accorded some weight on the dimension of cost. Finally, even the physicians' utilities could count heavily on some dimensions. If a given treatment is unfashionable or relatively untried, the physicians' preferences against it could be permitted to override a patient's desire for it.

We have no proposal concerning how specific weights can be assigned to the various parties to the decision. This is clearly a serious practical problem. It is a deep theoretical one too, since assigning weights can be seen as a way of making interpersonal comparisons of utilities. Nor do we have any firm evidence concerning how realistic our analysis is. The best we can say is that when clinical groups make decisions the exchange of ideas and information that occurs tends to bring about a convergence toward a single option or ranking of options. An averaging approach is a reasonable mathematical approximation to this. Finally, there is the question of rationality. In what sense does our approach represent the rational approach? Is there any rational approach? A unique one? Is an individual member of the group being rational in acquiescing to the group decision when it conflicts with a personal choice? These questions open up an entire field of research. We wish we had answers to them, but as matters now stand, we do not.

DIAGNOSIS, MANAGEMENT, AND DECISION ANALYSIS

Now that we have examined decision theory as a general framework and examined its chief elements, we can bring our discussions together by considering how the theory can be applied clinically. Keep in mind that there are still many open questions concerning probability and utility and their use in medical contexts. Nevertheless, clinicians frequently consider probabilities and weigh costs, benefits, and other values. It is fitting, therefore, to consider how these deliberations could be represented within a theoretical framework. Decision theory, as currently conceived, is the only viable option. Furthermore, as we argued in the preceding section, its acknowledged problems have by no means destroyed its usefulness.

We focus on diagnosis because virtually every clinical decision is made against a diagnostic background. Even the clinician who appears to be involved in a simple management decision (for instance, whether to decrease a certain patient's medication) does sounder a diagnostic hypothesis, which the clinician would be prepared to question if the prescriptions led to unexpected consequences. Because diagnosis is central to clinical decision making, to represent decision making we must combine our analysis of diagnosis from the last chapter with the decision-theoretic framework we have developed in this chapter.

Recall that our model of diagnosis is cyclical. Data concerning the patient lead the physician to diagnostic hypotheses, which in turn lead the physician to plans, one of which is chosen and implemented by testing or treating the patient. This produces more data, and the cycle is repeated until the clinical problem resolves itself. Clearly, decision theory enters this picture primarily at the point where we try to model the physician's rational choice of a plan for moving on to the test/treatment phase of the cycle.

A decision problem is specified by enumerating the acts, states, and outcomes relevant to the decision and then representing these systematically by means of a decision tree or some other scheme. In a diagnostic decision the acts are obviously the plans currently under consideration, the states are the diagnostic possibilities currently entertained, and the outcomes are the various events the physician believes might result from a given action under a given diagnostic state. For instance, early in the diagnosis of Mrs. Halprin's condition her physicians discussed a variety of clinical options. Some called for giving her this or that medication, while others called for giving her this or that diagnostic test. At that time they entertained a number of diagnostic hypotheses (states), such as hepatitis, a venereal disease, or a rheumatic disease, and believed that the actions they were considering would lead to many different outcomes, which varied according to the states. They believed, for instance, that if she had hepatitis then not obtaining liver function tests could lead to a confusion; if she had a rheumatic disease, the indomethecin might provide some immediate relief, and so on.

According to our model of diagnosis, the diagnostic states considered by physicians are determined by the information on the patient currently available and the physicians' background knowledge concerning correlations between diseases and findings. If the physicians' memory or training is faulty then they may omit a relevant diagnostic hypothesis. This would mean first that they would incorrectly assume that the states used would exhaust all the possibilities. Furthermore, unless the diagnoses omitted were very unlikely, the physicians' probability assignments would be wrong. For by failing to assign any probability to the omitted diagnosis they would overstate the ones they did consider. Obviously, this could adversely affect subsequent decisions. There is no way to guarantee that one has omitted a relevant diagnosis, short of having an absolutely complete list of the diagnostic possibilities currently recognized by medicine. (Recall that we treated diagnosis as a process that fits patients into currently recognized categories, not as one that creates new categories.) Computers and algorithms could help physicians by making sure that they have not overlooked a diagnostic possibility. Discussing the case with colleagues is also a valuable check, one that has always been popular. Finally, physicians will often intentionally exclude diagnostic possibilities from consideration, on the grounds that they do not fit well with the current data on the patient. Again, there is no way to guarantee against mistakenly excluding a diagnostic possibility. Excluding a relevant diagnosis will obviously affect the quality of any decision in which it figures.

We have no place in our model that corresponds to plan generation. We distinguished two sorts of plans—management plans, which call for test or treatments, and thought plans, which call for the physician to change diagnostic strategy, for instance, by reconsidering a diagnosis or treatment options previously excluded or by giving up an assumption concerning the general nature or number of diseases the patient has. Physicians derive most of their plans from the same sources from which they derive the diagnoses they consider. Whether it is from texts, lectures, colleagues, or personal experience, information concerning the signs and the course of various diseases tends to be clumped with information concerning how to deal with them. Thus, we can expect a good physician to have "stored" mentally a wide variety of plans for dealing with various diagnostic possibilities, together with information concerning how effective and appropriate they are in various circumstances. Of course, just as physicians may fail to consider the true diagnosis, so too they may fail to consider the most effective treatment. In this connection, computers could prove to be as valuable as colleagues currently are.

It can be difficult to evaluate management plans. More often than not, even when considered under a fixed diagnostic state, they do not lead to unique outcomes, but rather to a spectrum of possibilities associated with different probabilities. Thus even when Dr. Williams was virtually certain that Mrs. Halprin had SLE, he could not be sure that either therapy he considered would produce a favorable outcome. This happened because his analysis used diagnostic states that were too crude. If, instead of analyzing Mrs. Halprin's case in terms of the broad state description "SLE," Dr. Williams had used (as he eventually did) the descriptions "SLE with mild kidney damage," "SLE with moderate kidney damage," and "SLE with severe kidney damage," then he would have had a firmer idea of his chances for a successful treatment under a fixed state.

By repeatedly refining his analysis, theoretically it would have been possible for Dr. Williams to be certain of the outcome associated with a fixed state. The price would be in the complexity of his analysis. Thus, in practice we simply refine our analyses to the point where the probability that our actions will lead, under a fixed state, to specific outcomes is high enough for us to have a firm enough evaluation of our options to justify implementing one of them.

If a physician is operating under the assumption that the patient has just one disease, then each state will correspond to a single disease. If a thought plan calls for the physician to drop the one-disease assumption and assume that the patient's condition is the result of multiple causes, then it will also call for the physician to reanalyze any further decisions so that he or she can use conjunctions of several diagnostic possibilities as new states. The problems with evaluating management plans become even more pressing in evaluating thought plans, because they are yet another step away from outcomes.

Furthermore, thought plans give rise to their own problems. Let us suppose that Dr. Williams decided, at least momentarily, to reconsider his working hypothesis that Mrs. Halprin's deterioration was due to the action of just SLE and not to some other cause either by itself or working together with SLE. At the very moment that he wondered whether he should reconsider his hypothesis, it is unlikely that he would have anything but vague ideas of which new diagnoses should be entertained or which new management plans should be considered. He would know only that if he gave up his current assumption that just one disease was operating in Mrs. Halprin, then his subsequent management of her case could lead to a vast number of new possibilities. Unless something or someone came along to remove this indefiniteness, it would be virtually impossible for him to evaluate this thought plan. Thus, prudence would urge him to stop such useless speculation, to put his doubts aside, and to press on with the plan that, to the best of his knowledge, he had already considered carefully and rationally.

Put in this light, Dr. Williams's failure to treat Mrs. Halprin for infection would seem like less of a mistake than it was. (Unfortunately, it was a serious mistake. Although Dr. Williams should not be faulted for assuming that SLE was the primary cause of Mrs. Halprin's illness, a reasonable management plan for this single disease would call for guarding against secondary infections.) The moral is that because thought plans are usually quite difficult to evaluate, physicians need fairly dramatic reasons for deciding to consider giving up one overall approach to a case and trying another. Unfortunately, such dramatic events are common enough. Patients do take sudden and unexpected turns for the worse, which will cause the good physician to rethink the approach to the case. Patients occasionally present with signs and symptoms that do not fit any simple or familiar pattern, and this will prompt a good physician to consider interacting diseases and even the possibility of a brand new disease.

The remaining ingredients that go into a decision analysis are probabilities and utilities. Since we have already discussed these at length, we can be brief now. Obviously, ascertaining utilities is a serious problem that can be excruciatingly difficult in cases involving high risks of mortality or morbidity. Also there may be hard questions concerning whether the patient's preferences, the physician's, or some combination of both should determine the utilities on which a decision is based. Hospital or governmental policy or the law may be a relevant factor, too. Specialists in medical ethics have much of value to say about these issues, but their work goes beyond the scope of this book.

Probabilities enter the diagnostic picture in a special way because many of them are revised as new evidence is acquired. As we mentioned earlier, there is as much debate about the proper methods for revising probability assignments as there is about the meaning of probability. Earlier we used the rule of conditionalization supplemented by the inverse probability law (or Bayes' theorem) to represent probability revision. That is how we also propose to model probability revision as it occurs during the diagnostic process.

This completes our model of diagnostic reasoning and clinical decision making. As we have conceded all along, there are serious questions concerning various components of the model and many places where our model is sketchy and incomplete. Despite this, we offer our model as an attempt to shed light on the type of deliberation and reasoning that leads, in actual as well as in ideal circumstances, to diagnostic conclusions and clinical choices. We hope it will help researchers of clinical inference, as well as students trying to become thoughtful clinicians. We also hope it will prompt further attempts to achieve a fuller understanding of diagnosis and patient management.

RECOMMENDED READING

Clancy, W. J., and E. H. Shortliffe. Readings in Medical Artificial Intelligence. Reading, Mass.: Addison-Wesley, 1984. Collection of important papers.

Eraker, S. A., and P. Politser. "How Decisions Are Reached: Physician and Patient." Annals of Internal Medicine 97 (1982): 262-68.

Kassirer, J. P., A. J. Moskowitz, J. P. Lau, and S. G. Pauker. "Decision Analysis: A Progress Report." Annals of Internal Medicine 106 (1987):275-91; with accompanying editorial, "Decision Analysis: What's the Prognosis?" by A. S. Detsky, 321-22.

Keeney, R.L., and H. Raiffa. Decisions with Multiple Objectives: Preferences and Value Tradeoffs. New York: Wiley, 1976. Advanced text on multiattribute utility theory.

Lusted, L. B. Introduction to Medical Decision Making. Springfield, Ill.: Charles C. Thomas, 1968. Early attempt to apply decision theory to medicine.

Pauker, S. G., and J. P. Kassirer. "Decision Analysis." New England Journal of Medicine 316 (1987): 250-58; with accompanying editorial, "Decision Analysis: A Basic Clinical Skill?" by H. C. Sox, Jr., 271-72.

Raiffa, H. Decision Analysis: Introduction Lectures on Choices under Uncertainty. Reading, Mass.: Addison-Wesley, 1970. A business approach.

Rapoport, A. Two-Person Game Theory. Ann Arbor: University of Michigan Press, 1966. Elementary game theory.

Rawls, J. A Theory of Justice. Cambridge, Mass.: Harvard University Press, 1971. Decision-theoretic-influenced philosophy of justice.

Resnik, M. Choices. Minneapolis: University of Minnesota Press, 1987. Philosophical approach to decision theory.

von Neumann, J., and 0. Morgenstern. Theory of Games and Economic Behavior. Princeton, N.J.: Princeton University Press, 1944. Original description of decision theory.

Weinstein, M. C., and H. V. Feinberg. Clinical Decision Analysis. Philadelphia: W. B. Saunders, 1980. Excellent text.

We have traveled a long road to reach this point. After presenting the case of Mrs. Halprin, we discussed the characteristics of clinical data, then considered the nature of both inductive-probabilistic and deductive inferences. We explored aspects of scientific theories and the place they occupy in the background of clinical medicine. We offered a new analysis of the concept of disease and presented a new model of diagnostic reasoning. We ended by considering the nature of decision analysis and the role it can play in diagnostic and management decisions.

We are now in a position to take a brief look at Mrs. Halprin's medical history and reinterpret it from the new perspective we have acquired. For lack of a better term, we can call this new perspective a philosophic viewpoint. It can be regarded as supplementing the ordinary pathophysiological view, in much the same fashion as anthropological or psychosocial evaluations supplement it. As we review Mrs. Halprin's case, our goal is to elucidate the theoretical presuppositions that clinicians characteristically employ. To be more exact, we want to demonstrate how her physicians utilized the available information and the tools of reason to generate hypotheses about her disorder and to make claims about prognosis and treatment. We also want to examine how they reached the conclusions they reached, consider whether the conclusions were justified, and make explicit the assumptions that led them to their conclusions. It does not seem too much to hope that the broadened perspective on clinical medicine that we have presented in the earlier chapters will pay off in terms of better patient care. The recapitulation of the case of Mrs. Halprin will help show how this might be so.

Mrs. Halprin made the initial determination of her illness. She mentioned to her husband that she felt ill, and she eventually consulted Dr. Kline. In turning to Dr. Kline, Mrs. Halprin was following a characteristic pattern. People seek medical care as a result of their own interpretation of their health. (Obligatory screening, such as tests for syphilis or AIDS, constitutes an important exception to this rule.) Two important consequences follow from the fact of the self-determination of illness.

First, it blurs the distinction between illness and disease. Our analysis of the concept of disease as involving a failure in programmed biologic function makes clear how a physician may legitimately claim that an individual does not have a disease. The physician need only show that the person does not possess the characteristics required to satisfy the criteria for any given disease. More precisely, the physician is unable to find evidence to support the presence of a functional failure that constitutes a recognized disease.

By contrast, it is difficult to imagine how a physician could support the claim that someone who has sought medical care for real or imagined symptoms is not ill. Indeed, the very notion of "imagined symptoms" makes no sense, unless we are speaking of someone with a thought disorder. There can be no distinction between "imagined pain" and "real pain," and someone who honestly reports "I have a stomachache" necessarily has a stomachache. In general, if patients think they are ill, they are ill until they think they are not. (Of course, this is not to say the patient has a disease.) Unfortunately, all too often patients leave the physician's office complaining that the doctor said there was nothing wrong with them or that it was all in their head. Furthermore, it is difficult to believe that even the most skillful and knowledgeable physician can be even reasonably confident that a patient who is ill is not also diseased.

Second, the self-determination of illness means that patients' symptoms are biased. They are perceived in a distorted fashion by persons who are burdened by a fear that they have a disease. This is undoubtedly true, but instead of denigrating the quality of the information, physicians are accustomed to evaluating the importance of the findings in conjunction with the source of the information. For example, the complaint of headache means something different coming from a healthy, twenty-year-old male college student than from his female counterpart, let alone from a depressed middle-aged person or a young child. In a sense, the bias is the same sort that one encounters in trying to extrapolate from the results of a clinical study of a group of patients to one's own patient.

Toward the end of summer, Mrs. Halprin first thought she was ill. Whether this was when the first symptoms of her illness appeared is difficult to ascertain. In chronic illness, it is often hard to establish an exact starting date. Lupus erythematosus is notorious in this regard, because individual episodes may appear to be related only in retrospect, after the disease has been diagnosed .It is not uncommon to string together unexplained problems, such as a childhood seizure disorder and vague joint pains or a periodic rash occurring over several years, into a pattern of disease in a patient with lupus. Furthermore, lupus is not alone in this respect. Other types of arthritis and many neurological diseases, such as multiple sclerosis, share this feature. Thus, there is a great deal of uncertainty about the actual date Mrs. Halprin acquired lupus.

When Mrs. Halprin did feel ill, she did what most individuals do and attributed the problem to a common disorder—a cold. If her symptoms had been gastrointestinal, she probably would have attributed them either to a stomach virus or to something she ate. The effect of this reasoning is multifold.

First, she was invoking some notion of the probability of common disorders. If a common disorder is a sufficient explanation, then it is a useful tentative causal hypothesis. (Incidentally, this is exactly what a physician would do, albeit with a more sophisticated notion of prior probabilities and of whether the hypothesis was an adequate explanation.) Second, she was invoking some form of Ockham's razor. (If a single explanation is sufficient, then there is no reason to postulate a second.) In effect, she was relying on the single-disease hypothesis. Third, she was buying time. Many disorders attributed to viruses, food, and so on never get explained, but they are transient and require little or no intervention. Fourth, she was providing a very useful screening procedure by allowing transient (often called intercurrent) illnesses to run their course before seeking the advice of a physician. This last aspect varies among individuals. One end of the spectrum is occupied by stoics and people who fear doctors and the other end by hypochondriacs who imagine every sensation to be the manifestation of a dread disease.

After a week, Mrs. Halprin decided to see her doctor, because she was feeling no better. She had not altered her hypothesis about what was wrong with her, even though it was toward the end of a normal duration for a cold. However, she was fatigued and wanted some relief from her nagging cough. Dr. Kline listened to the history, performed a brief physical examination, established a tentative diagnosis, and made certain diagnostic and therapeutic decisions. We did not delve into the details of this encounter, but presumably Dr. Kline listened to her story of a coldlike illness, then asked her several questions to establish a possible source for the presumed virus and to make certain she was not dehydrated or developing pneumonia. He probably included several maneuvers in his physical examination to explore these possibilities further. It is unclear why he did a throat culture. Mrs. Halprin's illness was not characteristic of a streptococcal sore throat. Either he saw some finding suggestive of this diagnosis on physical examination, or he did it to appease her (unlikely), or perhaps he was just wrong. His conclusion that she had an upper respiratory infection was, in all probability, based on the compatibility of the findings and the prevalence of the disease. That is, his prior probability assignment was high, given the frequency of URI in the population, and the posterior probability assignment was higher still, given Mrs. Halprin's history and physical examination. Furthermore, the diagnosis of URI had substantial explanatory and predictive power. It accounted for Mrs. Halprin's symptoms and formed the basis for specific projections about the course of her disease and the likely outcome of various therapeutic maneuvers.

It is doubtful that the possibility of lupus entered Dr. Kline's mind. It really should not have, because lupus is not a common cause of an apparent intercurrent illness and Mrs. Halprin's complaints would be an unusual presentation. In fact, this illness may not have been the start of her lupus. There are a host of diagnostic procedures that he could have ordered and did not, including cultures and serological tests for viral conditions, certain bacterial diseases, and other infections, such as mycoplasma pneumonia. In this situation, he adopted the posture that the disorder was most likely transient, that he had no specific signs to lead him toward another problem, and that if he was wrong, it would become evident in time, and that time lost would not result in any irreversible catastrophe. This is probably a legitimate argument, although some physicians might have ordered a chest x-ray.

Dr. Kline's decision to give Mrs. Halprin an antibiotic and specifically Septra is more questionable. However, he made the decision based on the possibility of a bacterial infection (such as purulent bronchitis or sinusitis), the efficacy of a broad spectrum antibiotic like Septra, and its low rate of side effects. With this treatment, Mrs. Halprin apparently improved for several days. Whether this was spontaneous and coincidental or due to the medication is unclear, but when she relapsed, one possibility was that this was due to the medication. While this possibility always exists, and perhaps up to 25 percent of patients have some sort of reaction to medication, it is not a common cause of a disease relapse. However, Dr. Kline acted appropriately in stopping her medication. What seems to have been a relapse might well have been a drug reaction, since the fever and joint pain are compatible with this, even though Mrs. Halprin had taken sulfa eight years earlier for a urinary tract infection and showed no reaction at that time. Also, and most important, we may assume that Dr. Kline did not want to take the chance of doing something to make Mrs. Halprin worse, something for which he would bear the brunt of responsibility. Furthermore, he probably did not believe that she actually needed the drug. Four days would probably be enough for the drug to begin to control purulent bronchitis or sinusitis. Obviously, there are a large number of considerations in Dr. Kline's decisions to prescribe an antibiotic and then to withdraw it. They are not ones easily modeled in a decision-theoretic framework.

In any case, the new symptoms were probably not a drug reaction, since they continued to accumulate after the drug was stopped (although this is not entirely impossible). Dr. Kline's decision to have Mrs. Halprin admitted to the hospital was based more on what he did not understand about her problem than a specific disease or diseases that he identified as possible explanations. Many of the decisions that antedate a confirmed diagnosis suggest decision making under ignorance (no probability assignments available), rather than decision making under risk. We may suppose Dr. Kline started the antibiotic to minimize the maximum risk and then discontinued it for the same reason. In the beginning, he feared failing to treat a bacterial infection that, left untreated, would have serious consequences. Afterward, he feared that continuing the antibiotic would extend the drug reaction, which would also have serious consequences. Admission to a community hospital might be plausible in a case like Mrs. Halprin's, although it would be very unusual for her to be admitted to a medical center like Boston Central without some specific plan.

As is commonplace in teaching institutions, several individuals formed the team responsible for Mrs. Halprin's care. Both the second-year resident, Dr.

Barton, and the third-year medical student, Charles Covici, examined Mrs. Halprin on the day she was admitted to Boston Central Hospital. Dr. Barton presented her findings and analysis the next morning to Dr. Harold Williams, the attending physician. As we pointed out, the case presentation and the written history are both stylized summaries of the information obtained by the examiner. They differ slightly from each other, primarily because the case presentation is more abbreviated, but both contain the major elements—the chief complaint, history of present illnesses, and so on.

Both these formats are rational reconstructions of the events, rather than a verbatim transcript of the conversation. To reconstruct the information, the examiner needs hypotheses that suggest what information to include and what to discard as irrelevant. In general, certain findings are obligatory information in any general examination-for example, the age, gender, and name of the patient, as well as vital signs (temperature, blood pressure, pulse rate, and respiratory rate). In addition, a checklist of findings related to the major organ systems is usually included. More detailed descriptions are reserved for more important findings relevant to the patient's current problem. The absence of findings consistent with possible causes of the patient's disorder are noted as pertinent negatives.

The language used to describe the findings, in either the written or spoken format, is technical. "A red, itchy, bumpy rash" does not convey the same precise information as "an erythematous papular pruritic rash" does. Erythema is a distinctive kind of redness, caused by dilated blood vessels in the skin, and papules are discrete bumps between 1 mm and 5 mm in diameter. Using this vocabulary allows a more precise and condensed account of the problem .What is more, such terms are often implicit causal ascriptions. To call a rash erythematous is not merely to describe it as a certain shade of red, it is also to assert that the rash is one produced by certain underlying physiologic mechanisms.

Not all the vocabulary of medicine can be justified in this manner. Some words are simply holdovers and could be replaced with modem terms without a loss of information content. For example, pruritic and itchy are synonymous.

Some patients are annoyed by this vocabulary, the use of which they perceive as a deliberate attempt to cloak the field in a shroud of mystery. Although the vocabulary can be used in this manner, that is not its intended function.

Two interesting aspects of Dr. Barton's examination are worth elaborating. First, when Dr. Barton talked with her, Mrs. Halprin failed to recall having a urinary tract infection and unwittingly conveyed false information about her experience in taking a sulfa antibiotic. This kind of unreliability is common, although in the academic setting it is typically exposed by taking multiple histories. In general, the validity and reliability of clinical findings are hard to assess, particularly if they are nonspecific findings compatible with many diagnostic possibilities. The potential for incorrect diagnostic hypotheses is magnified by an incorrect history. Second, it is useful to note that what a patient considers most important medically is not necessarily the same as what the physician considers most important. Patients often focus on what can quite literally be seen to be wrong and tend to dismiss or question symptoms that cannot be visually displayed to the physician or to another observer. Thus it was Mrs. Halprin's alarm at her rash that prompted her return to Dr. Kline.

Dr. Barton, in presenting her clinical findings, noted a pertinent negative result-the absence of a pleural rub. She had noticed a dull sound when the chest was tapped, which is a sign of fluid in the lung or in the space between the lung and the chest wall, the pleural cavity. She specifically mentioned the absence of a grating sound that occurs during breathing, because the sound often accompanies "dullness to percussion," if that dullness is due to fluid in the pleural cavity (pleurisy) rather than in the lung. If both findings are present, it is strong evidence for inflammation of the membranes that cover the lung and line the pleural cavity (pleurisy) rather than of the lung itself.

While admitting that gonococcal arthritis-dermatitis syndrome was a diagnostic possibility, one might question Dr. Barton's decision to culture Mrs. Halprin's cervix, rectum, and pharynx for gonorrhea. It is clear from experience in venereal disease clinics that the sensitivity of testing for gonorrhea increases with the number of sites cultured, so Dr. Barton was technically correct in her decision to culture the three sites. However, the clinic information may not be directly applicable to Mrs. Halprin, for VD clinics generally see a different patient population from the one to which Mrs. Halprin is likely to belong. This issue of the generalizability of reported findings is always present when one extrapolates from the literature to particular patients.

After Mrs. Halprin's history was recited, Dr. Williams paused to try to organize the material Dr. Barton presented. When the clinical picture is ambiguous or complicated, it is often useful to summarize the findings. While he did identify the disorder as systemic, he did little to clarify the situation. It is likely that he would have been more successful if he had recited the major findings in an organized fashion.

The usual framework for such a recapitulation is to categorize the findings by organ system. For example, Dr. Williams could have described Mrs. Halprin in the following way:

> The patient is a previously healthy thirty-one-year-old mother of two young children with a four-week history of a systemic disorder characterized by constitutional symptoms including fever, an unproductive cough, and symptoms of an upper respiratory tract infection which was initially treated with Septra and an antihistamine. She briefly improved but relapsed with increased constitutional symptoms, a rash, abdominal pain, and arthralgias that did not improve after her medicine was discontinued.

If Dr. Williams had then attempted to generate a complete list of possible diagnoses, he would have been unsuccessful. A more cogent approach would have been to list broad categories of disorders and perhaps a few possibilities within them. Neoplastic, infectious, and immunologic disorders could result in a compatible clinical picture, whereas it would be difficult to imagine a hereditary or degenerative possibility. Alternatively, he would have tried to develop differential diagnoses around each of the outstanding abnormalities, such as proteinuria eosinophilia, and so forth. It is during the procedure of trying to establish a diagnosis that most theoretic reasoning in clinical medicine occurs. There is an attempt to categorize the findings into theoretic entities (diagnoses) and employ inferential reasoning to support the conclusion.

The third-year medical student appropriately named viral hepatitis as a possible cause, but he inappropriately stated that it was the probable cause of Mrs. Halprin's disorder. There was simply not enough information to establish even ballpark probabilities with any degree of certainty. In general, it is unwise to attempt to establish probabilities before enough information is acquired to determine a complete list of possibilities.

Probability assignments are made by comparing the item on a list of possibilities, and if that list is radically incomplete, no reliable comparisons can be made among the items. For example, a physician who is unclear about the diagnosis of a patient's disorder is not likely to list as possibilities two relatively rare diseases with explicit but low probabilities, while listing the other probabilities under the general heading of "others." Usually, physicians prefer to have a list of definite possibilities and an ordinal ranking of the likelihood of each before they make explicit probability assignments.

The ability to generate diagnostic hypotheses is limited by the knowledge base of the individual attempting to make the diagnosis. This is illustrated by the relatively long list of possibilities given by the second-year resident, compared to the suggestions of the medical student. The importance of a broad knowledge base, both in terms of symptoms that are associated with certain disorders and of diseases that can account for sets of symptoms, cannot be overestimated. As a medical aphorism puts the point, "What you don't know, you can't use."

Dr. Williams was correct in rebuking Charles Covici's intimation that an argument could be properly formulated to confirm or deny that Mrs. Halprin had viral hepatitis by employing the results of a small number of chemical tests on serum. The tests are designed to reveal the presence or absence of enzymes normally found in liver tissue that are released into the blood stream when the liver is damaged. The argument might be stated this way:

> Assumption: Mrs. Halprin has disease x.
> Assumption: Disease x is viral hepatitis, if, and only if, Mrs. Halprin has
> abnormal liver function tests.
> Test Result: Mrs. Halprin has abnormal liver function tests.
> Conclusion: Mrs. Halprin has viral hepatitis.

Dr. Williams properly disputed the second assumption of this tacit argument.

Dr. Williams next decided to question the patient, before hearing the results of her laboratory studies. His questions fell into several categories. First, there were questions of clarification. He wanted to hear for himself that the illness began about four weeks ago. This is especially important when the onset is somewhat insidious. Second, there were questions to test hypotheses. Shellfish-borne hepatitis would require eating uncooked shellfish, and drug reaction to a sulfa antibiotic is unlikely if the individual has taken the drug previously with no ill effects. Finally, Dr. Williams tested two other hypotheses—sub-acute bacterial endocarditis and systemic lupus erythematosus—with questions about any recent dental procedures and about the rash, which might be a dermal manifestation of SLE.

At the end of this first conversation with the patient, Dr. Williams was unable to offer a prognosis. His explanation was straightforward: without a sufficiently confirmed diagnostic hypothesis, one cannot generate a reasonable prognosis. Thus, he implicitly appealed to the symmetry of explanation and prediction that we discussed in connection with scientific hypotheses. Loosely speaking, the extent to which a diagnostic hypothesis is an adequate explanation for the patient's disorder is the degree to which the prognosis based on that hypothesis is justified. The stronger the evidence for a given diagnosis, the more accurate and reliable the prognosis based on that diagnosis.

The laboratory data were, for the most part, abnormal, but they were also nonspecific. That is, they did not single out any one diagnosis as being more likely than some other. In addition, the data did not raise any new diagnostic considerations. The initial laboratory screening examinations done at most academic medical centers have not been rigorously tested for their sensitivity and specificity or their predictive value in hospitalized populations.

In addition to these routine screening tests, Dr. Barton ordered some more specific laboratory studies. These included hepatitis antigen for viral hepatitis prodome, antinuclear antibodies and complement studies for lupus, and blood cultures for subacute bacterial endocarditis. Here at the beginning of the clinical encounter with Mrs. Halprin, Dr. Barton was already testing diagnostic hypotheses. She used the hypotheses to select appropriate laboratory studies. What she did not do was to order a variety of tests with no purpose in mind, hoping to acquire information that might prove diagnostically relevant. Such a "fishing expedition" is virtually always pointless and unproductive.

For better or worse, a clinician must make some choices and decisions at the termination of an examination. The choices made by Dr. Barton reflected a number of factors. First, the findings at that point suggested certain disorders. Second, the prevalence of those disorders in the population of individuals similar to Mrs. Halprin suggested how likely they were in that setting. Thus, viral hepatitis is a common disease, and even if the patient's findings were accounted for by lepromatous leprosy, the rarity of that disorder in individuals like Mrs. Halprin would make it an unlikely possibility. As we saw in chapters 4 and 9, these considerations may be formalized by the use of Bayes' theorem. While we approve of Dr. Barton's decision to forego a diagnostic evaluation for leprosy (assuming it occurred to her), we might chide her for ignoring another common viral disorder—infectious mononucleosis.

At this stage of the investigation Dr. Barton appropriately chose among possible tests for those that screen for disease, rather than those that confirm diagnoses. These tests are sensitive. That is, they are usually positive when the disease is present. How predictive they are depends on an estimate of the probability of the disorder before the test was ordered (prior probability). For example, Dr. Barton ordered an antinuclear antibody test for systemic lupus erythematosus. This test is quite sensitive, perhaps as high as 96 percent. This is a fine choice for a screening test. In addition, since lupus is relatively common (with a prevalence of 1 in a 1,000 women of this age-group) and is compatible with Dr. Barton's findings, the test is quite predictive, if positive. We earlier described lupus as an "uncommon" disorder in discussing Mrs. Halprin's evaluation by Dr. Kline, and now we have called it a "common" disorder in discussing her evaluation by Dr. Barton. These two descriptions are only apparently inconsistent. In the first instance, the patient was presenting as a previously healthy young woman with an upper respiratory tract infection. The incidence of SLE in the general population is about 5 to 7 per 100,000 per year. Thus, a case of SLE is a relatively rare occurrence. To focus on SLE as a possibility in the first set of circumstances would be absurd.

By contrast, by the time Mrs. Halprin was examined by Dr. Barton, she had an unknown multisystemic disease, a compatible rash possibly produced by a sulfa drug, and had become part of a hospitalized population. Under these conditions, the prior probabilities increased dramatically, justifying the characterization of the disease as relatively "common." Indeed, the prior probabilities for SLE became far higher than even the prevalence figures for black women of childbearing age, which are as high as 1 in 250 individuals. At the time Mrs. Halprin was seen by Dr. Barton, many clinicians would estimate the prior probability of SLE as 20 percent or more.

If a disorder is uncommon or unlikely but the test for it highly sensitive, the test might still be a good screening test. Whether it is considered good or not depends on the aim of screening. If the aim is to identify a group of individuals who have the disease, then such a test may be useful. However, this group will need further study to determine which among its members are truly diseased, since there will be a large number of false positives identified by the first test. By contrast, if the aim is to identify in a cost-effective, reliable fashion diseased individuals within a general population, then these are much more difficult criteria to satisfy. A test may be good judged by the first aim but not by the second, which requires high sensitivity, high specificity, and cost-effectiveness.

Consider another aspect of Dr. Barton's decision to order cultures of Mrs. Halprin's cervix, rectum and pharynx to test for disseminated gonococcal infection. While DGI is common, up to 50 percent of those who have the syndrome have negative cultures. Let us ignore the possibility that some of those 50 percent who are negative really do not have DGI and assume that all of them have it. If this is the case, then the test is quite insensitive. It is also very expensive and a poor screening test. Then why did Dr. Barton order this test? Simply because she had no choice; there is no screening test for DGI. However, if positive, this test is quite good at confirming the presence of DGI, for there are few false positives. That is, the test has high specificity.

The last aspect of Dr. Barton's management was her choice not to institute therapy. Most physicians would agree with this choice, but probably not all. Some might argue that Dr. Barton had an adequate number of blood cultures and that there would be little harm in starting broad spectrum antibiotics for subacute bacterial endocarditis. There is good evidence to support the claim that the earlier antibiotics are administered, the less damage to the heart valves will ensue and, consequently, the fewer the complications. On the harm side, there is a real risk, albeit small, in the use of these antibiotics. Also, there is the possibility that they will confuse the clinical picture over the few days during which the physicians are trying to sort things out. An intermediate position might be to obtain an echocardiogram to attempt to locate vegetations on the heart valves, but it is insensitive and quite expensive.

Other physicians might argue analogously for the institution of therapy for DGI. Theoretically, both these questions could be answered definitively by decision analysis. (Those interested may refer to chap. 9 and work out a decision tree.) For both SLE and DGI, toward the low end of the prior probability of each disease, there will be a "test-notest" threshold. Toward the other end of the spectrum of prior probabilities, there will be a "test-treat" threshold. Dr. Barton apparently thought that the prior probability of each of these disorders lay between these two thresholds and made the choice to test for them. Unfortunately, at the present time, clinical medicine is unable to employ decision analysis at appropriate junctures such as this. There is not enough time, expertise, or information to make its use a routine procedure in most medical centers. For the moment, we believe that formal decision analysis is relegated to a role in policy making. In that context, the time constraints are not so crucial. However, within the decade we may see computer-assisted decision analysis done on the wards of teaching hospitals. Software programs for several microcomputers are available now that construct a decision tree by obtaining the information from the user in an interactive mode.

The final portion of the first attending conference ended with a summing up by Dr. Williams. In a lengthy discussion, he weighed the pros and cons of the diagnostic possibilities mentioned earlier and several others that he introduced. He presented a pathogenic model of disease-the immune complex model that stimulated him to consider other diagnostic entities that are caused by immune complex deposition. When pathogenic models of disease are available, physicians often argue by analogy from the model to explain manifestations of the patient's presentation. The correctness of their conclusions depends on the strength of the relationship between the model and the disorder. At best, one can make only a semiquantitative estimation of the validity of the conclusion based on the strength of the analogy. A further use of analogical reasoning is to enlarge the diagnostic field by the process of association. The introduction of the idea of lupus as an immune complex disease led Dr. Williams to think of other immune complex diseases.

In the discussion of systemic lupus erythematosus, Dr. Williams introduced a new concept—the notion that diseases can be diagnosed by fulfilling certain criteria. He used the updated ARA criteria for SLE and suggested obtaining data relevant to all eleven criteria to establish whether the patient had SLE. This discussion opens a Pandora's Box of problems. For example, is SLE a syndrome or a disease? If it is a syndrome, are these the agreed-upon criteria for the disorder? If so, then it makes no sense to say that fulfilling them is 96 percent sensitive for the disorder. To say this implies *another* set of criteria. Assuming that the framers of the criteria and Dr. Williams both view SLE as a disease, we really do not know which criteria were used to decide whether someone was a case of SLE or a comparison case of a related but different disorder. It is important to realize that, in the absence of a pathognomonic finding, the "gold standard" is always the judgment of experts. Employing such criteria standardizes clinical studies, but the criteria have little bearing on the individual patient. Often, the individual who is difficult to categorize is at an early stage in the course of a chronic disorder and may not have had time to express all the manifestations of the disease. By contrast, those individuals considered in formulating the criteria have stable, fully developed manifestations. Parenthetically, the diagnostic artificial intelligence program for rheumatology (AI/RHEUM) uses criteria mapping (of the patient's manifestation onto criteria) as its primary inferential tool.

Later, Dr. Williams attempted to amalgamate the clinical findings suggestive of a vasculitic disorder with Mrs. Halprin's eosinophilia. However, he rejected the specific diagnoses in the intersection of those two sets— Churg-Strauss disease, polyarteritis nodosa, and hypersensitivity angiitis- because of the absence of other compatible findings.

The cyclical diagnostic model appropriately represents these deliberations. Dr. Barton initiated the diagnostic cycle by ordering tests for viral hepatitis, subacute bacterial endocarditis, disseminated gonoccal infection, and SLE, in addition to the normal screening tests. The screening tests reveal an additional significant datum-eosinophilia-which caused Dr. Williams to enlarge the field of diagnostic possibilities. In effect, he cycled back through the diagnosis-generation phase of the model.

In seeking a single explanation for the eosinophilia and the other disease manifestations, Dr. Williams introduced the one-disease assumption as a thought plan. When this plan failed, he treated the eosinophilia as diagnostically irrelevant. However, the findings suggested a systemic immunecomplex disease, and Dr. Williams utilized this as a disease class in his diagnostic evaluation. This thought plan led to management plans that included additional laboratory studies and seeking the opinion of colleagues (the dermatologists).

Although we do not have an account of the dermatologists' conversation about Mrs. Halprin, it is safe to assume that they focused on different aspects of the findings. While they might have approached the patient from the standpoint of certain disease categories (such as neoplastic, infectious, vasculitic, etc.), they also might have approached her from the character of the rash. In this case they might have run down a list of papular pruritic rashes, such as contact dermatitis, urticaria, certain types of eczema, or types of porphyria. Consultants may be useful both for a different knowledge base and also for a different approach, one that reflects a different way of systematizing their knowledge. Although the high-titer ANA, low-serum complement, and low-titer VDRL strongly suggested SLE, it was not until the anti-DNA antibody test was reported as positive that Dr. Williams ended the diagnostic cycle and concluded that Mrs. Halprin had SLE.

Had Dr. Williams been called upon to justify this diagnostic conclusion, he could have offered the following inductive-probabilistic argument:

> Mrs. Halprin's prior probability for SLE at the time of her hospitalization was 20 percent. The sensitivity of the ANA test for SLE is 95 percent, and the specificity is 80 percent. Thus, after the positive ANA results, the prior probability for SLE became 54 percent. After the anti-DNA antibody test, which has a specificity of 99 percent and a sensitivity of 60 percent, was reported positive, assuming independence, the posterior probability of Mrs. Halprin's having SLE was 99 percent. This is probably sufficient for diagnostic confirmation.

The information contained in such a justification would also have allowed Dr. Williams to arrive at the same conclusion in a way that can be represented by a simple deductive argument:

> Satisfying at least four out of the eleven American Rheumatism Association criteria establishes the diagnosis of lupus.
> Mrs. Halprin satisfies at least four out of the eleven ARA criteria.
> The diagnosis of lupus is established for Mrs. Halprin.

Dr. Williams outlined a decision analysis when considering whether to perform a renal biopsy, although he did not perform the analysis in a formal fashion. The decision to perform the biopsy was embedded in considerations of more general strategies concerning stopping certain medications and starting others. Dr. Williams used some general heuristic rules to help sort out the available options. For example, Dr. Williams mentioned that it is generally unwise to perform two therapeutic maneuvers (stopping indomethacin and starting corticosteroids) at the same time. This led him to suggest stopping the indomethacin, then observing her. This was done, but later Mrs. Halprin elected to have the renal biopsy, over Dr. Williams's objections, because of the potential for acquiring prognostic information. It could be that Mrs.

Halprin was concerned with avoiding high-dose steroids and immunosuppressives and hoped that the biopsy would provide her with another option. Apparently, she put more weight on the biopsy findings than her physicians did. While this is unusual (typically, the situation is the reverse), it is not unique. This is one aspect of clinical reasoning and decision making that runs straight into ethical considerations. Sometimes this "need to know" can actually be detrimental to decision making since the accuracy of the information can plateau or even decline with additional testing.

It is clear from our analysis in chapter 9 that a biopsy can provide useful information, but whether the biopsy will affect a therapeutic decision depends on the precise clinical situation. For example, the decision to administer high-dose corticosteroids or immunosuppressives for reasons other than renal disease will not be affected by a biopsy. The difficulty is that while the biopsy may not contribute any decision-making information useful at the moment, it may provide information that will be useful in the future in a way unforseen at the moment. For example, suppose the apparent need for immunosuppressives disappeared after a few months, but the biopsy revealed a need for longer-term therapy. In this unforseen fashion, the biopsy would have turned out to be useful. Unfortunately, we cannot perform every test merely because it may tum out to be useful in the future.

The renal biopsy is a classic example of a test that has gone in and out of fashion as a prognostic indicator. In the early days of biopsy, the information was interpreted as "mild," "moderate," and "severe." Later, more sophisticated classification schemes came into general use. These appeared to have pragmatic and therapeutic value, but later still it became clear that patients often switched classes if they were rebiopsied. Furthermore, those thought to have the most severe disease (diffuse proliferative lupus glomerulonephritis) did better than expected and, according to some studies, survived as long as those with mild disease (focal proliferative). This finding led to the biopsy's going out of favor. Later still, additional microscopic characteristics of the biopsy material were examined (basically, degree of scarring) and were found to be prognostically important. Thus the biopsy has now returned to favor as a tool for prognostication and therapeutic intervention in SLE.

When Mrs. Halprin became an outpatient, Dr. Barton was faced with the challenge of tailoring Mrs. Halprin's therapy to her varying levels of disease activity. This problem faces all physicians caring for patients with chronic diseases (the majority of outpatient internal medicine) and is given virtually no consideration in studies of disease. We know a great deal about features that form diagnostic criteria, somewhat less about prognostic characteristics, and very little about features that correlate with disease activity and allow us to monitor significant changes and plan appropriate therapeutic programs.

The last hospital admission of Mrs. Halprin was a tangled web of confusion. Procedures were performed against her wishes and were to no avail. (The issue of informed consent arises here. Accompanying this is the issue of competence, for legitimate consent requires that a person be able to make an autonomous decision.) She apparently was treated overaggressively for her SLE but not at all for a second disease that was masquerading as a manifestation of SLE. Both the diseases contributed to her acquiring the pneumonia that resulted in her death. Though luck had some role to play in Mrs. Halprin's fatal course, there were clearly errors of omission, errors of commission, and errors of reasoning.

What were those errors? Mrs. Halprin's physicians worried about the possibility that her comatose state was due to something in addition to lupus. They worried about an infection and treated her for that possibility. So what went wrong? From the medicolegal standpoint of adequate care or the "standard of care in the community," they clearly did no wrong. However, just as clearly, the patient died of an undiagnosed treatable disease. The clinical team continued to adhere to the one-disease assumption that had served successfully in the diagnostic cycle. The diagnosis of lupus served as a basis for therapeutic intervention, but the therapy itself caused changes that modified the clinical picture. It was reasonable to rely on the one-disease assumption (and the diagnosis of lupus in particular) to account for coma of unknown etiology, but there were some worrisome aspects that the team failed to consider. It is uncommon (although not impossible) for central-nervous-system lupus to cause coma with simultaneous renal failure. Further, Mrs. Halprin had an abnormal number of lymphocytes in her spinal fluid, something also uncommon with CNS lupus. The clearest explanation of what happened is that the class of diagnostic entities known as infectious diseases were thought to be of low probability and were believed to be effectively excluded by a negative spinal fluid culture. Ironically, if the physicians had pursued diagnostically what was considered the most likely possibility, lupus cerebritis, with newer modalities, such as nuclear magnetic reasonance or a leptomenigeal biopsy (for CNS vasculitis), they might have stumbled on the correct diagnosis. In any case, it was a clear error of omission not to test the spinal fluid for cryptococcal antigen. The error of commission was the aggressive treatment for lupus cerebritis by using high-dose corticosteroids and immunosuppressive agents-treatments that could only worsen the body's defense against cryptococcal meningitis. This is not an unusual situation. Up to 10 percent of autopsies reveal a disorder unexpected by the clinicians caring for the patient.

Could decision analysis have helped them? Perhaps it could have helped in enumerating the evidence for and against lupus cerebritis. In evaluating further diagnostic tests, it might have pointed out the lack of findings supporting CNS lupus. However, decision analysis is most effective in comparing one strategy with another, and it presumes that the options available are exclusive ones. In Mrs. Halprin's case, the relevant diagnostic option of cryptococcal meningitis (with its therapeutic implications) was not even entertained by her physicians. Thus, it was not susceptible to scrutiny by decision analysis. If her physicians had considered the infection as a possibility, they certainly would have tested for it, since the test itself is simple, sensitive, and specific. A decision analysis would not be necessary for this manuever. If, however, the team wanted to "cover all possible bases" without thinking of cryptococcal meningitis in particular and start appropriate therapy for systemic fungal disease, this move could have been evaluated by decision analysis. In every case, much depends on who formulates the decision analysis, what options are considered, and what probabilities are used. Decision analysis is not a panacea, but it can force a clinician to face the information available squarely and openly. The very act of doing this may suggest alternative viewpoints.

"At least do not harm" is perhaps the greatest of all the Hippocratic dicta. But any clinician who cares for patients runs the very real risk of doing harm. Risk cannot be eliminated. However, it can be minimized, and the most important factor in minimizing risk is knowledge. Knowledge of pathophysiological processes, pharmacological actions, diagnostic categories, and management procedures is undeniably essential. But the knowledge necessary for the best possible patient care cannot stop here. It must include the skills of reasoning, acquiring and evaluating data, and making decisions.

The good clinician must be well informed, but more than that, the good clinician must be intellectually sophisticated. This means being able to employ the logical, conceptual, and mathematical tools that have been developed to deal with the problems presented by human illness. It also means knowing enough about the tools to judge their strengths and weaknesses, to know their limits as well as their uses.

CPSIA information can be obtained
at www.ICGtesting.com
Printed in the USA
FSHW020622180119
55111FS